Prevention of Stroke

John W. Norris   Vladimir C. Hachinski
Editors

Prevention of Stroke

With 106 Illustrations, 3 in Full Color

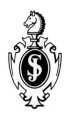

Springer-Verlag

New York Berlin Heidelberg London Paris
Tokyo Hong Kong Barcelona Budapest

John W. Norris, M.D.
Department of Neurology
University of Toronto
Sunnybrook Health Science Centre
Toronto, Ontario M4N 3M5
Canada

Vladimir C. Hachinski, M.D.
Department of Clinical Neurological Sciences
University of Western Ontario
London, Ontario N6A 5A5
Canada

Library of Congress Cataloging-in-Publication Data
Prevention of stroke / J.W. Norris, V.C. Hachinski, editors.
        p.   cm.
        Includes bibliographical references and index.
    ISBN 0-387-97442-3 (alk. paper). — ISBN 3-540-97442-3 (alk.
paper)
    1. Cerebrovascular disease — Prevention.   I. Norris, John W.
II. Hachinski, Vladimir.
    [DNLM: 1. Cerebrovascular Disorders — drug therapy.
2. Cerebrovascular Disorders — prevention & control.
3. Cerebrovascular Disorder — surgery.   WL 355 P9445]
RC388.5.P66   1991
616.8'1 — dc20
DNLM/DLC
for Library of Congress   90-10390
                                                 CIP

Printed on acid-free paper.

Typeset by Publishers Service of Montana, Bozeman, Montana, USA.
Printed and bound by Edwards Brothers, Inc., Ann Arbor, Michigan, USA.
Printed in the United States of America.

9 8 7 6 5 4 3 2

ISBN 0-387-97442-3 Springer-Verlag New York Berlin Heidelberg
ISBN 3-540-97442-3 Springer-Verlag Berlin Heidelberg New York

Read not to contradict and confute nor to believe and take for granted, but to weigh and consider.

Francis Bacon, 1620
Novum Organum

Preface

Prevention of stroke is infinitely more effective than its treatment and rehabilitation of patients; it is also infinitely less costly. In spite of rapid progress in knowledge of the etiology and pathogenesis of stroke, the physician faced with the hemiplegic patient is almost as helpless today as in the past. The decrease in mortality, and in the incidence of stroke, is due largely to the control of risk factors, not treatment. Investment in stroke prevention is the best avenue for today's shrinking economic resources.

Our knowledge of the major causes of stroke is still pathetically inadequate. Much of ischemic stroke is due to carotid artery atherosclerosis, but most cases remain unexplained. Debate continues concerning the role of artery-to-artery embolism versus hemodynamic effects. Even today, with all our potential for imaging the heart and extracranial and intracranial blood vessels, we cannot with certainty identify strokes of cardiac origin. We know that asymptomatic carotid disease causes stroke, but we do not know which patients need surgery. Despite the dramatic effect of the treatment of hypertension on stroke prevention, all known risk factors account for less than half the risk of stroke. Details of the genetic risk of stroke and other forms of vascular disease are unknown, yet genetic engineering could prove a valuable tool in future prophylaxis. Identification and control of risk factors offer the best current and potential avenue for modifying the occurrence and nature of stroke.

Information about stroke prevention is available in journals, proceedings, and book chapters, but this book is an attempt to sum up and critically analyze our present knowledge and understanding of the subject. It brings together experts to cover all major aspects of stroke prophylaxis. We hope that it will appeal not only to neurologists and neurosurgeons directly involved with stroke patients, but also to experts from many other disciplines, including vascular surgeons, psychiatrists, internists, family physicians, health planners, and others. This text will help stimulate further interest in this relatively new concept of stroke care and so help diminish the terrible toll in death and chronic disability that stroke claims every year.

John W. Norris, M.D.
Vladimir C. Hachinski, M.D.

Acknowledgment

This book would not be the same without the invaluable help of Mrs. Jean Twiner. Not only did she devote many hours (often of her own) to ensuring the manuscripts were word perfect, she also helped edit prose and reviewed layout; her comments and criticisms were invaluable.

Contents

Preface vii
Contributors xiii

Chapter 1   Stroke Prevention: Past, Present, and Future   1
             John W. Norris and Vladimir C. Hachinski

PART I   Medical Prevention of Stroke

Chapter 2   Cellular Basis of Atherosclerosis   19
             Marc Fisher

Chapter 3   Prevention of Atherothrombotic Brain Infarction:
             Role of Lipids   37
             Frank M. Yatsu and Thomas J. DeGraba

Chapter 4   Regression of Atherosclerosis   49
             Michael G. Hennerici

Chapter 5   Drug Inhibition of Experimental
             Carotid Atherogenesis   65
             Eberhard L. Betz

Chapter 6   Stroke Risk Factors   83
             Mark L. Dyken

Chapter 7   Head and Neck Bruits in Stroke Prevention   103
             John W. Norris

Chapter 8   Hypertension and Stroke Prevention   113
             J.D. Spence

Chapter 9   Aspirin in Stroke Prevention   121
             James C. Grotta

Chapter 10   Ticlopidine: A New Drug to Prevent Stroke   127
             William K. Hass

Chapter 11   Present Status of Anticoagulant Prophylaxis   139
              J. Donald Easton

Chapter 12   Prevention of Cardioembolic Stroke   149
              David G. Sherman

Chapter 13   Clinical Trials in Stroke: A New Approach   161
              John A. Blakely

PART II   Surgical Prevention of Stroke

Chapter 14   Carotid Endarterectomy: A Challenge for
              Scientific Medicine   171
              H.J.M. Barnett

Chapter 15   Carotid Endarterectomy in Patients with
              Asymptomatic Carotid Stenosis   177
              J.J. Ricotta

Chapter 16   Does Carotid Endarterectomy Prevent Stroke?   195
              Saran Jonas

Chapter 17   Balloon Transluminal Angioplasty of the Carotid
              Artery in the Head and Neck   205
              Fong Y. Tsai and Randall Higashida

Chapter 18   Preventing Cerebral Complications
              of Cardiac Surgery   219
              Marc I. Chimowitz and Anthony J. Furlan

Chapter 19   Prevention of Stroke from Cerebral Vascular
              Malformations   229
              *Ricardo Garcia-Monaco, Pierre Lasjaunias,
              and Alex Berenstein*

Chapter 20   Prevention of Aneurysmal Subarachnoid
              Hemorrhage   247
              J.M. Findlay and B.K.A. Weir

Chapter 21   Prevention of Recurrent Stroke   261
              N.M. Bornstein and A.D. Korczyn

Index   269

Contributors

H.J.M. Barnett, O.C., M.D., F.R.C.P.C. President and Scientific Director, The John P. Robarts Research Institute, London, Ontario, N6A 5K8, Canada

Alex Berenstein, M.D. Professor of Radiology and Neurosurgery, New York University School of Medicine, New York, New York 10016, USA

Eberhard L. Betz, M.D. Professor, Institute of Physiology, University of Tübingen, D07400 Tübingen, Germany

John A. Blakely, M.D., F.R.C.P.C. Assistant Professor of Medicine, University of Toronto, Toronto, Ontario M5S 1A1, Canada

N.M. Bornstein, M.D. Department of Neurology, Sackler Faculty of Medicine, Tel Aviv University, Tel Aviv, Israel 64239

Marc I. Chimowitz, M.D. Assistant Professor of Neurology, University of Michigan, Ann Arbor, Michigan 48109, USA

Thomas J. DeGraba, M.D. Department of Neurology, University of Texas Health Science Center, Houston, Texas 77030, USA

Mark L. Dyken, M.D. Professor and Chairman, Department of Neurology, Indiana University School of Medicine, Indianapolis, Indiana 46202, USA

J. Donald Easton, M.D. Professor and Chairman, Department of Clinical Neurosciences, Brown University, Rhode Island Hospital, Providence, Rhode Island 02903, USA

J.M. Findlay, M.D., Ph.D., F.R.C.S.C. Assistant Professor of Neurosurgery, University of Alberta, Edmonton T6G 2M7, Canada

Marc Fisher, M.D. Professor and Chief, Department of Neurology, Medical Center of Central Massachusetts – Memorial, Worcester, Massachusetts 01605, USA

Anthony J. Furlan, M.D.   Director, Stroke Program, The Cleveland Clinic Foundation, Cleveland, Ohio 44106, USA

James C. Grotta, M.D.   Professor of Neurology, Department of Neurology, University of Texas Health Science Center, Houston, Texas 77225, USA

Vladimir C. Hachinski, M.D., F.R.C.P.C., D.Sc. (Med.)   Richard and Beryl Ivey Professor and Chairman, Department of Clinical Neurological Sciences, University of Western Ontario, London, Ontario N6A 5A5, Canada

William K. Hass, M.D.   Professor of Neurology, New York University School of Medicine, New York, New York 10016, USA

Michael G. Hennerici, M.D.   Professor and Chairman, Department of Neurology, University of Heidelberg, Klinikum Mannheim, 6900 Heidelberg, Germany

Randall Higashida, M.D.   Associate Professor of Radiology and Neurological Surgery, University of California, San Francisco, California 94122, USA

Saran Jonas, M.D.   Professor of Clinical Neurology, New York University School of Medicine, New York, New York 10016, USA

A.D. Korczyn, M.D.   Professor of Neurology, Sackler Faculty of Medicine, Tel Aviv University, Tel Aviv, Israel 64239

Pierre Lasjaunias, M.D., Ph.D.   Professor of Radiology, Neuroradiologie Vasculaire Centre, Hospitalier De Bicetre, 94275 Le Kremlin-Bicêtre, France

Ricardo Garcia-Monaco, M.D.   Neuroradiologist, Neuroradiologie Vasculaire Centre, Hospitalier De Bicetre, 94275 Le Kremlin-Bicêtre, France

John W. Norris, M.D., F.R.C.P., F.R.C.P.C.   Professor of Neurology, University of Toronto, Stroke Research Unit E-428, Sunnybrook Health Science Centre, Toronto, Ontario M4N 3M5, Canada

J.J. Ricotta, M.D.   Professor of Surgery, Division of Vascular Surgery, State University of New York, Buffalo, New York 14209, USA

David G. Sherman, M.D.   Professor and Chief, Division of Neurology, University of Texas, San Antonio, Texas 78284, USA

J.D. Spence, M.D., F.R.C.P.C., F.A.C.P.   Professor, Clinical Pharmacology and Neurology, Victoria Hospital and University of Western Ontario, London, Ontario, N6A 4G5, Canada

Fong Y. Tsai, M.D. Professor and Chairman, Department of Radiology, University of Missouri, Kansas City, Missouri 64110, USA

B.K.A. Weir, M.D.C.M., M.Sc., F.R.C.S.C., F.A.C.S. Walter Stirling Anderson Professor and Chair, Department of Surgery, University of Alberta, Edmonton, T6G 2B7, Canada

Frank M. Yatsu, M.D. Professor and Chairman, Department of Neurology, University of Texas Health Science Center, Houston, Texas 77030, USA

1
Stroke Prevention: Past, Present, and Future

John W. Norris and Vladimir C. Hachinski

He that will not apply new remedies must expect new evils; for time is the greatest innovator.

Francis Bacon 1561–1626

A Caveat

Strokes of all types have yet to yield to any past or current medical intervention. Preventing stroke is much easier than treating it, as in other forms of vascular disorders, such as ischemic heart disease. In spite of dramatic claims for the prevention of coronary heart disease in both lay and medical media, a review of scientific evidence suggests that they are premature.

For instance, in the Multiple Risk Factor Intervention Trial (MRFIT), in over 10 000 individuals, there was little difference in cardiac mortality between those "treated" with aggressive risk factor intervention and those treated with benign neglect.[1] In a critical review by McCormick and Skrabanek[2] of all published major intervention studies as of 1988, the authors concluded that "present experimental evidence that we can prevent much coronary heart disease provides no data to justify the time, energy and money which are being devoted to this crusade." Although correct diet and exercise can do no harm, what of the cost and potential harm of hypertensive drugs in the elderly, or the increase in stroke and association of colonic cancer in patients with cholesterol levels artificially lowered by drugs?[3,4]

More positive thinking implies that we are only on the threshold of knowledge of prevention in any area and that effective prevention can only begin with the correct lifestyle in infancy or childhood; to await definitive evidence is to allow many individuals to develop preventable disease.[2]

Clearly, a healthy scepticism must be maintained by a rigorous scientific approach to the alleged benefits of life-style changes as well as to attempts at stroke prophylaxis.

Historical Perspective

Prevention of disease is most effective when based on knowledge of its causes. Although the pathogenesis of stroke has become clearer in the last few decades, it remains poorly understood. The concept of systemic emboli lodging in the brain to cause stroke was described by Virchow in 1847,[5] but the therapeutic potential was not realized for a further century.[6] Chiari described "cerebral softening" secondary to carotid artery stenosis in 1905,[7] but its major role in causing ischemic stroke only emerged with Fisher's 1951 classic paper.[8]

Many of the concepts now taken for granted, such as transient ischemic attacks (TIAs) as harbingers of stroke, were only recognized in the 1950s,[9] and their outcome evaluated in the 1960s.[10,11] The characteristic clinical picture and the clinicopathological correlation of lacunar strokes were reaffirmed and refined in the late 1960s mainly by C.M. Fisher, and later corroborated by pathology and computerized tomography (CT).[12] Although asymptomatic carotid stenosis was long believed to be a risk factor for stroke, outcome data were only documented in the past 10 years[13,14]; their role in medical or surgical intervention remains controversial.[15]

It was as recent as 1973 that Brown and Glassenberg published autopsy data that first showed that death in acute stroke was mainly due to cerebral edema and recurrent cerebral hemorrhage, while mortality after this immediate period was due to pulmonary, cardiac, and other systemic complications.[16] About the same time it became clear that the greatest threat in patients with TIAs, carotid surgery, and asymptomatic carotid stenosis was cardiac, not cerebral, ischemia.[17,18]

Charcot and Bouchard described miliary aneurysms responsible for cerebral hemorrhage in the brains of hypertensives in 1868.[19] It took another 100 years before Cole and Yates, after painstakingly mapping these lesions in autopsy specimens, concluded that preventing hypertension might prevent the strokes.[20] The decline of stroke in recent decades has focused attention on its pathogenesis and is generally attributed to the control of hypertension,[21] although there is good epidemiological evidence that this is only a partial explanation.[22] Factors previously deemed insignificant, such as smoking[23] and mitral valve prolapse,[24] have become important because of the increasing sophistication of epidemiological methods.

Anticoagulants came into general clinical use in the 1950s, but their early promise as the first drug for stroke prophylaxis remains unfulfilled. By the late 1960s, following a series of negative trials of anticoagulants in patients with TIAs,[25,26] their popularity rapidly waned. Their role in stroke prevention remains undecided.[27] Antiplatelet drugs appeared later, with the advantage of superior methodology and statistics; both aspirin and ticlopidine have an established role in stroke prevention.[28-30]

Technical advances in vascular and brain imaging have also shed new light on stroke pathogenesis. Initially, angiography was introduced to study peripheral blood vessels, but Moniz's first successful cerebral angiographic techniques[31] had to wait nearly 30 years before their potential in stroke prevention was realized. In 1954 Eastcott and colleagues published the first case of prophylactic carotid surgery.[32] Unfortunately, as vascular imaging methods became less hazardous, carotid surgery became fashionable for increasingly flimsy indications. In 1984 a plea for reappraisal was made,[33] and at present several large, multicenter studies in progress throughout the world are evaluating the procedure scientifically. Surgical prevention of stroke in patients with TIAs using extracranial-intracranial bypass techniques was demonstrated to be ineffective in a definitive multicenter trial and is now largely abandoned.[34]

Advances in methodology and biostatistics have been at least as important as progress in clinical knowledge and diagnostic and therapeutic techniques. For instance, anticoagulant trials employing a total of < 40 patients with follow-up < 1 year were considered adequate in the 1960s,[35] but in today's terms are only of historic interest. Another 10 years later, stroke prophylaxis trials with < 500 patients and < 2 years' follow-up were considered inadequate.[36] By the 1980s, similar trials demanded 1000 to 2000 patients.[29,30] With the newly evolved strategy of meta-analysis, where results are pooled retrospectively from many trials, populations of nearly 30,000 patients can be analyzed.[37] Today the only feasible way to conduct clinical trials in stroke prophylaxis is by large, multicenter studies. There is no longer any excuse for the proliferation of small, individual trials, often incomparable in methods and contradictory in results.[38] This major step in progress reflects not only growing sophistication in statistical techniques, facilitating data processing, but also the electronic and computer revolution, accelerating communication in hitherto unimagined ways.

Stroke Prevention in the 1990s

The prevention of stroke can be implemented at all stages of cerebrovascular disease (Table 1.1), although its impact diminishes with each advancing stage.

Stroke Prevention in the Asymptomatic Stage

Age, Sex, and Race

Age is a powerful risk factor for stroke (Table 1.2).[39] Men are more prone than women in almost all age categories. Moreover, an analysis of a cohort of 789 born in 1913 showed that men whose mothers had died of stroke had a threefold increase in the incidence of stroke compared to men without such a maternal history.[40] A doubt lingers. Since

TABLE 1.1. Therapeutic opportunities in stroke prevention.

Asymptomatic stage
Treatment of risk factors
Management of asymptomatic carotid artery bruits and stenoses
Warning stage
Management of TIAs and minor stroke
Recognition and management of the "warning leak" of subarachnoid hemorrhage
Recurrent stage
Prevention of recurrent stroke and myocardial infarction

TABLE 1.2. Risk factors for stroke.

Hypertension (diastolic and systolic)
Cardiac
ischemic/hypertensive
valvular
arrhythmias
Smoking
Fibrinogen
Diabetes
Erythrocytosis
Other
Physical inactivity
Hyperlipidemia
K+ dietary deficit
Age
Race
Maleness
Unknown

men's life expectancy is shorter, the fathers of the men in the study may have died from something else before they would have died from a stroke. Whites tend to have predominantly extracranial disease; Orientals, intracranial disease; and blacks, both. Moreover, known vascular risk factors cannot explain the differences, implying a role for genetic factors.[41]

Hypertension

Hypertension represents the most important treatable risk factor for stroke. The risk rises with increasing levels of systolic and diastolic blood pressure, beginning in the normal range.[42] Hypertension represents a risk for atherothrombotic, lacunar, and hemorrhagic stroke and for subarachnoid hemorrhage in both sexes and all ages. Treatment of hypertension decreases the hazard of stroke substantially and promptly.[43-45]

Cardiac Disease

Ischemic, hypertensive and valvular heart disease, and arrhythmias pose significant and largely treatable risks for stroke.[46]

Smoking

Smoking has long been recognized as a strong risk factor for myocardial infarction and sudden death. A meta-analysis of 32 separate studies leaves little doubt that smoking also represents an independent risk factor for stroke.[47] The overall risk of stroke associated with cigarette smoking is 1.5 (95% confidence interval 1.4–1.6). The risk of smoking for cerebral infarction is 1.9, for cerebral hemorrhage 0.7, and for subarachnoid hemorrhage 2.9. There

is a dose response relationship between the number of cigarettes smoked and the relative risk for stroke.

Fibrinogen

Raised fibrinogen levels (126-696 mg/dl) correlate with the risk for coronary artery disease and stroke in both men and women. The risk of stroke increases progressively in men but not women, although next to hypertension it is the most powerful predictor of stroke.[48]

Fibrinogen levels correlate with smoking,[49] and smoking cessation reduces fibrinogen levels.[48] Fibrinogen increases blood viscosity, affects the "distortability" of red blood cells, and may promote platelet aggregation. High-cholesterol diets raise fibrinogen levels in rats,[50] and high fibrinogen levels have been noted in human type 2 hyperlipoproteinemia.[51]

Diabetes Mellitus

Glucose intolerance increases the risk for stroke two- to threefold,[42] and hyperglycemics tend to suffer larger cerebral infarcts than normoglycemic patients.[52] Unfortunately, controlling blood glucose levels does not halt the progression of the vascular complications.

Erythrocytosis

A raised hematocrit value carries a risk for stroke, beginning in the normal range, in part from associated hypertension,[53] and in part from increased

TABLE 1.3. Risk factors for stroke in the young.

Cardiac disease	Trauma
Valvular	Infections
Cardiomyopathy	Neurosyphilis
Atrial myxoma	AIDS
Anticardiolipin antibodies	Drugs
Hypertension	Alcohol
Juvenile diabetes	Amphetamines
Migraine	Cocaine
Oral contraceptives	Crack
Hyperlipidemias	Smoking
Homocysteinuria	

viscosity and perhaps other factors. Although decreasing the hematocrit ameliorates symptoms in polycythemics, it remains unproven whether lowering the hematocrit diminishes the risk for stroke.

Physical Inactivity

Physical inactivity may be a risk for stroke,[54] but it is not a well-established one.

Hyperlipidemia

Elevated blood cholesterol poses only a small risk for stroke, an effect that dissipates after the age of 55 years. According to the Framingham data, there is an inverse relationship between blood levels of low-density lipoprotein (LDL) and the risk of stroke, especially in women.[42] On the other hand, other studies have documented low high-density lipoprotein (HDL) levels[55] in stroke patients, and it has recently been shown that stroke itself affects serum lipid levels.[56]

Dietary Potassium

A prospective study of 859 men and women (aged 50 to 79 years) followed for 12 years showed a 40% reduction in stroke mortality with an increase in dietary potassium of 10 mmol per day.[57] The number of stroke-related deaths was small[42] and the diagnosis largely derived from death certificates, which are notoriously unreliable. On the other hand, the increased intake of one or two servings of fresh fruits or vegetables is unlikely to be harmful, not to say enjoyable.

Unknown

Known risk factors for stroke account for only a fraction of the risk.[58] This suggests the existence of other risk factors potentially amenable to modification.

Cerebrovascular Risk Factors in the Young

The etiology of stroke in the age range 18 to 45 years is broader, with different entities predominating than at a later age.[59] The risk factors also differ (Table 1.3).

Cardiac Disease

Valvular heart disease is an important cause of stroke in the young. Rheumatic heart disease has dropped dramatically in North America in the past 25 years[60] but remains a menace in the developing world. Mitral stenosis, especially with associated atrial fibrillation, is the most common lesion leading to neurological sequelae.[46] Mitral valve prolapse, although innocent and symptomless in the vast majority of subjects, has become a leading cause of stroke and transient ischemic attacks in the young.[46] Bicuspid aortic valves, idiopathic hypertrophic subaortic stenosis, infective and idiopathic cardiomyopathies, and atrial myxoma represent uncommon, but important causes of stroke in the young. Paradoxical emboli may occur when increased pressure in the right heart forces an embolus into the left heart through a patent foramen ovale.[61] Increased blood pressure is an important risk factor for hemorrhage and ischemic stroke, especially if untreated or combined with other risk factors such as diabetes or a hyperlipidemia.

Anticardiolipin Antibodies

Two circulating immunoglobulins have proved important (though rare) causes of ischemic stroke: lupus anticoagulant and anticardiolipin antibodies. They produce systemic and cerebral thromboembolism, both venous and arterial.

Despite continuing confusion regarding their role in cerebrovascular disease, a few conclusions emerge: (1) The neurological complications of systemic lupus erythematosus (SLE) are not usually caused by vasculitis; (2) the misnamed lupus anticoagulant (which is an *in vivo* coagulant) occurs most commonly with conditions other than SLE; (3) cardiolipin antibodies are commonly associated with neurological complications.

In a series of 50 patients with SLE, 37 manifested neuropsychiatric disorders: 5 psychiatric, 15 neurological, and 17 both. Fourteen developed thrombotic thrombocytopenic purpura during their terminal illness, 10 had evidence of embolic brain infarctions, and remarkably *none* had evidence of cerebral vasculitis at autopsy.[62]

In 80 patients with raised anticardiolipin antibodies, 25 suffered from cerebral infarction, acute ischemic encephalopathy with evidence of fibrin thrombi in the cerebral vessels, headache, or ophthalmologic complications.[63] The name "CLEAT" syndrome has been suggested for the clinical manifestations associated with anticardiolipin antibodies (Table 1.4).[64]

Among 51 patients admitted to the neurology service at University Hospital, London, Ontario, with TIAs or strokes, 3 had definite raised anticardiolipin antibodies, and a further 5 had clinical features suggestive of the CLEAT syndrome but had no increases in the levels of cardiolipin antibody, primarily because they were on steroids.[65]

Migraine

Migraine is common and often occurs coincidentally in patients with strokes because of other causes. It should be a diagnosis of exclusion unless the deficit follows a previous series of transient deficits of the same nature. Controversial evidence hints that migraine compounds the risk of stroke in women taking oral contraceptives.[66]

Oral Contraceptives

Evidence for an association between oral contraceptives and risk for stroke was suggested by the large prospective study by the Royal College of General Practitioners,[67] showing that the risk of cerebral thrombosis and cerebral embolism among users is 19 times that of nonusers, although the absolute risk remains small. It was suggested that the risk for stroke rises sharply with increases in the level of blood pressure and also with increasing age, heavy smoking, and migraine.[66] However, the same group of investigators found no increased risk for cardiovascular disease, including stroke, if low-dose contraceptives are used.[68]

The relationship between the contraceptive pill and stroke remains controversial. When an expert committee met in 1984 under the auspices

TABLE 1.4. The "CLEAT" syndrome.

Cerebral ischemia (infarcts, TIA, "migraine")
Livedo reticularis
Endocardial lesions
Amaurosis fugax
Thrombosis

of the American Heart Association to assess risk factors in stroke, they concluded that there was no substantial evidence to incriminate the contraceptive pill.[69]

Sickle Cell Disease

Sickle cell disease carries a recognized risk for the development of stroke, especially in childhood.[70]

Hyperlipidemia

A direct correlation between serum cholesterol levels and risk of stroke exists up to the age of 55 years, although the association is not powerful.[40]

Homocysteinuria

Homozygote homocysteinuria has long been recognized as leading to premature arteriosclerosis and thromboembolic complications. Boers et al.[71] studied 75 patients under the age of 50 years with occlusive peripheral arterial disease, occlusive cerebrovascular disease, and myocardial infarction. Each category comprised 25 patients. After methionine loading and tests for cystathionine synthase deficiency, heterozygosity for homocysteinuria was established for 7 patients in each of the peripheral and cerebrovascular arterial disease categories but none in the myocardial infarction group. Since heterozygosity for homocysteinuria occurs in no more than 1 in 70 of the normal population, the authors conclude that this condition predisposes to the development of premature occlusive peripheral arterial disease, renovascular hypertension, and ischemic cerebrovascular disease.

Trauma

Direct trauma to the cervical arteries or damage from chiropractic manipulation may lead to dissection or occlusion and stroke.[72]

Infections

Neurosyphilis

Although neurosyphilis has declined considerably since the advent of penicillin, meningosyphilis accounts in a small, but significant proportion of strokes, especially among the young.[73]

AIDS

Stroke is more likely to occur in individuals under the age of 45 years infected with the human immunodeficiency virus than those free from the infection.[74] One to 12% of patients with acquired immunodeficiency syndrome (AIDS) may suffer a stroke,[75] usually infarction, although the mechanisms remain obscure. They may include an altered coagulant state, alterations in the lining of blood vessels, and associated infections.[76]

Drugs

Alcohol

Alcoholic intoxication has been suggested as a prelude to stroke.[77] Possible mechanisms include contraction of cerebral and systemic vessels, platelet activation, and unreported or forgotten trauma.

Amphetamines

Oral or intravenous amphetamines and intravenous heroin can lead to arteritis and cerebral infarction or hemorrhages.[78]

Cocaine

Cocaine abuse represents a risk both for ischemic and hemorrhagic stroke.[79,80]

Smoking

Cigarette smoking imposes a risk for stroke in inverse relationship to age. The relative risk for stroke below 55 years of age is 2.9; 55 to 74 years, 1.8; and ≥75 years, 1.1.[47]

Aggregation and Interaction of Risk Factors

The Framingham data show that the presence of one risk factor may potentiate that of another.[42] Moreover, there is some evidence that siblings of stroke patients are more likely to have multiple risk factors than the relatives of their spouses.[81] An example of potentiation among the young is the augmentation of risk for stroke by oral contraceptives in the presence of hypertension and smoking.[66]

The Need to Search for New Risk Factors

All the known risk factors account for only a fraction of the risk for stroke.[42] The search for genetic markers to identify patients at high risk may prove rewarding. New risk factors, such as raised fibrinogen levels,[49] and studies comparing the differing incidence of stroke and coronary heart disease among ethnically similar populations in Japan and Hawaii strongly suggest that lifestyle, diet, and environment play major roles.[82,83] The search for new risk factors is likely to be fruitful.

Management of Patients with Asymptomatic Bruits and Stenosis

Asymptomatic bruits signal an increased risk for stroke.[84,85] However, an infarct is as likely to occur in a silent carotid artery as it is in the territory of a noisy one. The incidence of ischemic stroke ipsilateral to the carotid bruit is between 0.1 and 0.4% per year,[86] compared with the average mortality rate of carotid endarterectomy of 2.8% and morbidity of one to five times greater.[87] Moreover, most patients with asymptomatic bruits and carotid lesions are likely to manifest first as TIA rather than stroke.[88,89] On balance, surgery appears unjustified.[90] Nevertheless, there may be individual cases in whom the indications are felt to be compelling, and referral to one of the multicenter trials is appropriate.[91,92]

Stroke Prevention in the Warning Stage

A general approach to the management of patients with transient ischemic attacks and minor strokes is outlined in Table 1.5

TABLE 1.5. Approach to the management of patients with TIA and minor strokes.

Modification of risk factors
Hypertension
Smoking
Surgical treatment
Carotid endarterectomy
Drug therapy
Anticoagulants (in cases of cardiac embolism)
Heparin
Coumadin
Platelet inhibitors
Aspirin 325 mg four times a day (dose may be reduced if side effects occur)
Ticlopidine 250 mg twice a day (not yet available)

Modification of Risk Factors

Although a number of risk factors affects the likelihood of stroke,[42] two stand out as important and modifiable, namely, hypertension[43-45] and cessation of smoking.[93] The cessation of smoking not only decreases the risk of cerebral infarction but effectively reduces the risk of myocardial infarction and sudden death.[94,95] Myocardial infarction and cardiac death is common among patients with transient ischemic attacks.[42] Cessation of smoking appears to be a particularly worthwhile endeavor in these patients.

Carotid Endarterectomy

Until recently, carotid endarterectomy was one of the most commonly performed vascular operations in the United States and Canada. Its recent decline[96] may be no more justified than its spectacular rise. Nevertheless, better knowledge of the natural history of cerebrovascular diseases, improved medical therapy, and awareness of the wide range of results of this operation call for a cautious approach.[97] The price of progress is constant reevaluation. Both patients and society at large are most likely to benefit if appropriate candidates are referred to one of the multicenter trials on symptomatic[98] or asymptomatic[91,92] patients with appropriate carotid lesions.

Anticoagulants

Although the evidence suggests that patients with TIAs of cardiac origin may benefit from anticoag-

ulation,[99,100] no appropriate studies have been done to address this question since the advent of CT scanning, which allows the differentiation of hemorrhagic infarction from primary intracerebral hemorrhage.

Antiplatelet agents

A Canadian[101] and a French[102] multicenter study established the effectiveness of aspirin 325 mg four times a day in the prevention of stroke and death in patients with TIA and minor stroke. Two issues have remained: that of dose and that of sex. The UK-TIA Aspirin Trial[103] found no difference in risk reduction between the group taking one (325 mg) and the group taking four aspirins a day. However, absence of proof is no proof of absence. Since the patients entered in the British trial seemed to be at a lower risk of stroke than in other series, and since the most dramatic finding was a reduction in the mortality from cancer, it may be prudent to await the results of other comparative studies of aspirin dose before reducing the dose from four tablets to one a day. Nevertheless, since there is a direct relationship between dose and side effects, a reduction may well be dictated by patient intolerance.

Although both sulfinpyrazone and dipyridamole have proven antiplatelet effects, randomized clinical trials do not justify a therapeutic role for either. The Canadian study[101] found sulfinpyrazone to be ineffective. Despite the theoretical possibility of a synergistic action of sulfinpyrazone with aspirin[104] such an interaction is unlikely.[105,106]

The sex question in the effect of aspirin remains controversial. Aspirin benefited French[102] but not Canadian,[101] women. The obvious conclusion is that French women are different from Canadian women. However, the more likely explanation for the differential effect is that not enough women entered either study and that the risk of stroke for women with TIA may be lower than in men.[107] In a recently completed European study[108] where females represented 45% of the study population, an aspirin-dipyridamole combination proved effective both in men and in women.

Dipyridamole appears to have no independent ability to prevent stroke, and when used in combination with aspirin, the combination performs no better than aspirin alone.[102,108,109] There is little

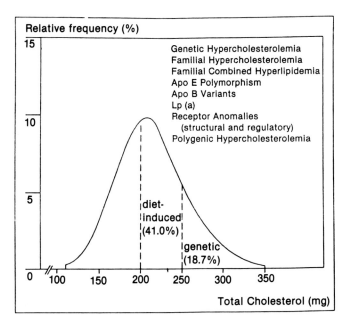

FIGURE 1.1. Distribution of cholesterol levels in 11,091 men aged 20–50 years. (From Bertelsmann Foundation, Gutersloh, West Germany. In: Assman G: Lipoproteins, myocardial infarction and stroke. In: Hennerici M, Sitzer G, Weger L-H, eds. *Carotid Artery Plaques*. Basel: Karger. 1987:31. Reprinted by permission.)

that justifies the use of dipyridamole in patients with TIA and stroke.

Ticlopidine hydrochloride 250 mg twice daily reduced the risk of stroke and vascular death by 21% compared to an aspirin-treated group of patients with TIAs and minor stroke.[29] Since the drug is as yet unavailable and both its advantages and disadvantages compared to aspirin have not been fully assessed, it will be at least a year before the drug and its indications become part of daily decision making for patients with TIA and minor stroke.

Stroke Prevention in the Recurrent Stage

Management of Patients with Recurrent Stroke

A Swedish study[110] compared the efficacy of aspirin (1500 mg/d) with that of placebo in preventing recurrent stroke in 505 patients with minor and major stroke. Aspirin did not affect the mortality, the incidence of recurrent stroke, or that of myocardial infarction. The study may have been too small to rule out benefits from aspirin, but it may be that the mechanism of recurrent stroke differs from that of stroke after transient ischemic attacks or minor strokes.

The Canadian American Ticlopidine Study (CATS) was a randomized double-blind placebo-controlled clinical trial to assess the benefit of ticlopidine 250 mg twice daily in reducing the rate of recurrent stroke, myocardial infarction, and vascular death in 1072 patients who had suffered a thromboembolic stroke no less than one week and no more than four months after a thromboembolic stroke.[111,30] The ticlopidine group experienced a relative risk reduction of 31% compared to the placebo group in both males and females. Adverse effects included transient severe neutropenia in 1% of cases and severe transient rashes and diarrhea in 2% of individuals on ticlopidine.

The study merits further discussion, peer review, and the clarification of a number of issues, including its precise role in stroke and vascular death prevention in males and females, and its limitations, including cost and serious side effects in a minority of patients. Nevertheless, this is a welcome development in an area where hitherto there had been no proven therapy to reduce the risk of recurrent stroke, and it appears to be equally effective in females.

Future Possibilities

The cause of most ischemic strokes at present remains largely unknown. In stroke data banks, investigating prospectively large numbers of stroke patients, about 40% of cases remain unexplained even after exhaustive diagnostic procedures.[112] The remaining 60% are attributed to carotid artery disease, cardioembolic stroke, lacunar infarction, and others. Even so, this represents a major advance from the classification only a few decades ago of "thrombosis, embolism and hemorrhage." At least now we know how much we do not know.

The Nature of Atherosclerosis

Extracranial carotid atherosclerosis remains one of the commonest causes of ischemic stroke. Damage to the vascular endothelium, mainly at bifurcations, by a variety of noxious stimuli, is probably the initiating factor.[113] Macrophages are critical for cholesterol metabolism at the vascular endothelial surfaces, and if they become overloaded with cholesteryl esters, they become "foamy" and are deposited under the endothelium.[114] It is now widely accepted that serum cholesterol levels should not exceed 200 mg/dl, and there is a linear risk of coronary artery disease (if not diffuse atherosclerosis) above this level.[1] At 200–250 mg/dl, hypercholesterolemia can be corrected by diet, but >250 mg/dl it is probably genetically determined and needs pharmacological intervention (Fig. 1.1).

The predilection for early atherosclerotic lesions to appear at arterial bifurcations, irrespective of the noxious agent (hypertension, hypercholesterolemia, etc.) is probably determined by flow patterns. For instance, the carotid bulb has a distinctive velocity pattern of blood flow producing an inappropriate "wear and tear" on the arterial wall (Fig. 1.2).

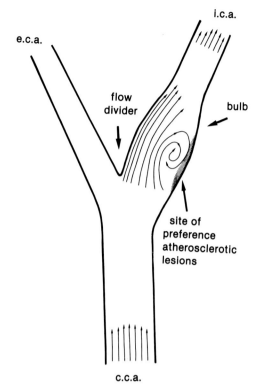

FIGURE 1.2. Schematic representation of axial velocity patterns in the carotid artery bifurcation. (From Bertelsmann Foundation, Gutersloh, West Germany. In: Reneman RS, van Merode T, Smeets FAM, Hoeks APG: Velocity patterns and vessel wall properties in the carotid artery bulb in man – their relation to atherogenesis. In: Hennerici M, Sitzer G, Weger L-H, eds. *Carotid Artery Plaques.* Basel: Karger; 1987:159. Reprinted by permission.)

Atherosclerotic Regression

The rate of progression of atherosclerosis, determined by a variety of noninvasive means of vessel imaging, is now well documented.[115-117] Unfortunately, the factors responsible for progression, such as smoking and hypertension, which are potentially amenable to prevention, remain controversial. Different rates of progression of carotid stenosis in each artery in the same individual point to a superadded mechanical factor influencing flow patterns that are different for each artery. Malinow has shown that a variety of therapeutic interventions, such as drugs or a cholesterol-free diet, regresses atherosclerosis in experimental

animals.[118] Most plaques are in constant flux, and progress and regress with a number of factors, both systemic and mechanic. This is observed on B-mode real-time imaging of the carotid arteries,[116] and plaque volume may change dramatically because of major changes in morphology, such as plaque hemorrhage.[119]

The discovery that Inuit have a disproportionately low incidence of cardiovascular disorders and eat disproportionately high amounts of fish oils has stimulated attempts to reduce atherosclerosis by the essential fish-oil ingredient, Omega-3 fatty acids.[120] Coronary atherosclerosis is reduced in hyperlipidemic pigs fed a diet rich in Omega-3 fatty acids.[121] This is unassociated

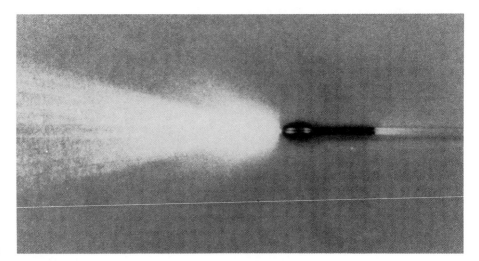

a

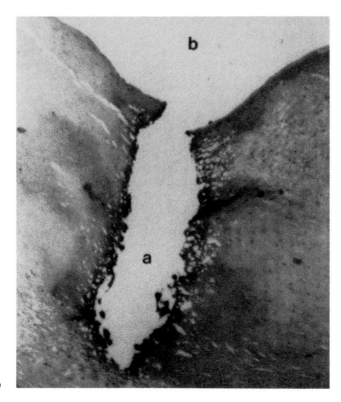

b

FIGURE 1.3. (a) Tip of laser angioplasty probe. (b) Lesion in plaque produced by laser angioplasty. (From *J Vasc Surg* 1987; 6:60–65. Reprinted by permission.)

with any lipid lowering effect, but it reduces platelet aggregation.

Homocysteinemia is a rare, autosomal-recessive, inborn error of metabolism producing early death by premature atherosclerosis. The arterial lesions are indistinguishable from those seen in normal aging, and it is postulated that a major factor in "normal" atherosclerosis is a defect in homocysteine metabolism. In a pilot study, 19 patients with ischemic cerebral symptoms were matched with 17 asymptomatic controls and had significantly higher levels of plasma homocysteine.[122] If such metabolic deficits were found to play a significant role in the genesis of atherosclerosis, possibly they could be prevented by genetic engineering.

Decline of Stroke

The decline of stroke in recent years might be partly attributable to antiplatelet agents, now widely prescribed and often self-administered by our aging population. The Physicians Health Study in the United States involving 22 000 male physicians demonstrated conclusively that aspirin reduces the rate of myocardial infarction.[123] There is similar evidence from meta-analysis that the rate of ischemic stroke is also reduced.[37] The synthesis of even more effective antiplatelet drugs may have a major impact on prevention of all types of atherosclerotic outcomes, including stroke.[29,30]

The effect of surgical prevention by carotid endarterectomy is at present under scrutiny[124] but in any case could be superseded by much less invasive, radiological techniques.

Recent trends in plaque destruction by the transluminal approach are more promising. Balloon angioplasty, either percutaneous or by operative exposure of the artery, allows inflation of a distal balloon inside the artery to compress and destroy the plaque.[125] Laser angioplasty represents a further refinement, vaporizing the plaque using a laser beam at the tip of the arterial catheter (Fig. 1.3).[126] With the use of special techniques, the plaque can be sensitized to laser beams that do not damage normal artery, since a serious, though unusual, complication is perforation of the vessel.[127]

The general decline in vascular disease must be due partly to the increasing awareness of demonstrated risk factors such as hypertension and smoking. A recent apparent reversal of this decline may be associated with improved survival of patients with ischemic heart disease, thus increasing the pool of potential stroke candidates.[128] Screening of the population to identify stroke-prone persons has not yet been successfully achieved. Self-administered TIA questionnaires produce a large number of nonspecific symptoms and would need costly and skilled clinical and laboratory follow-up as a next phase.[129]

Duplex-screening of people attending community gatherings such as health fairs have also shown low cost effectiveness. About 4% of "normal" adults have detectable carotid stenosis, but only about 1% have stenosis >75%.[130]

Cerebral Aneurysm

The increasing awareness of the "sentinel" headache in predicting the presence of unruptured cerebral aneurysm may allow prophylactic clipping of aneurysms that might otherwise produce mortality and morbidity (Chapter 16). Prophylactic aneurysm clipping is also possible in patients presenting with otherwise uncomplicated cranial nerve signs, such as third nerve palsies, and when asymptomatic aneurysms are found during angiography for other reasons or following rupture of another cerebral aneurysm.

At present, angiographic screening for vulnerable subgroups (eg polycystic kidneys or Marfan's syndrome) is probably not justified, but may be in those with close relatives undergoing aneurysmal rupture. Future development of noninvasive technologies such as magnetic resonance imaging (MRI) may make this feasible, however, and justify prophylactic aneurysmal surgery.

Conclusion

Although stroke has been recognized since antiquity, only since the middle of our century have the scientific bases for its prevention been established. While much can be done to prevent stroke through the recognition and treatment of risk factors and the management of stroke-prone individuals, much more remains to be discovered. Growing awareness of the heterogeneity of stroke, the complex interplay of genetic and environmental factors, and the expanding possibilities provided by technology, epidemiology, and clinical methodology offer to make the 1990s not only the decade of the brain but a decade of great advances in preventing its damage by stroke.

References

1. Multiple Risk Factor Intervention Trial Research Group: Multiple Risk Factor Intervention Trial.

Risk factor changes and mortality results. *JAMA*. 1982;248:1465–1477.

2. McCormick J, Skrabanek P: Coronary heart disease is not preventable by population intervention. *Lancet*. 1988;2:839–841.

3. Iso H, Jacobs DR, Wentworth D, et al. Serum cholesterol levels and six-year mortality from stroke in 350,977 men screened for the Multiple Risk Factor Intervention Trial. *N Engl J Med*. 1989;320:904–910.

4. Sherwin RW, Wentworth DN, Cutler JA, et al. Serum cholesterol levels and cancer mortality in 361,622 men screened for the Multiple Risk Factor Intervention Trial. *JAMA*. 1987;257:943–948.

5. Virchow R: Über die akut Entzundung der Arterien. *Virchow's Arch A*. 1847;1:272–378.

6. Fisher CM, Adams RD: Observations on brain embolism with special reference to hemorrhagic infarction. In: Furlan Anthony J, ed. *The Heart and Stroke*. New York, NY: Springer-Verlag; 1987:1 pp 17–36.

7. Chiari H: Uber das Verhalten des Tielungswinkels der Carotis communis bei der Endarteritis chronica deformans. *Verhandl d deutsch path Gesellsch*. 1905;9:326–330.

8. Fisher CM: Occlusion of the internal carotid artery. *Arch Neurol Psychiat*. 1951;65:346–377.

9. Fisher CM, Cameron DG: Concerning cerebral vasospasm. *Neurology*. 1953;3:468–473.

10. Marshall J: The natural history of transient ischaemic cerebro-vascular attacks. *Q J Med*. 1964;33:309–324.

11. Whisnant JP, Matsumoto N, Elveback LR: Transient cerebral ischemic attacks in a community: Rochester, Minnesota, 1955 through 1969. *Mayo Clin Proc*. 1973;48:194–198.

12. Miller VT: Lacunar stroke: a reassessment. *Arch Neurol*. 1983;40:129–134.

13. Thompson JE, Patman RD, Talkington CM: Asymptomatic carotid bruit. *Ann Surg*. 1978;3:308–316.

14. Heyman A, Wilkinson W, Heyden S, et al. Risk of stroke in asymptomatic persons with cervical arterial bruits. *N Engl J Med*. 1980;302:838–841.

15. Dyken ML: Carotid endarterectomy studies: a glimmering of science. *Stroke*. 1986;17:355–358.

16. Brown M, Glassenberg M. Mortality factors in patients with acute stroke. *JAMA*. 1973;224:1493–1495.

17. Whisnant JP, Matsumoto N, Elveback LR. The effect of anticoagulant therapy in the prognosis of patients with transient cerebral ischemic attacks in a community: Rochester, Minnesota, 1955 through 1969. *Mayo Clin Proc*. 1973;48:844–848.

18. Norris JW, D'Alton JG. Outcome of patients with asymptomatic carotid bruits. In: Reivich M, Hurtig HI, eds. *Cerebrovascular Diseases*. New York, NY: Raven Press;1983:1 pp 63–71.

19. Charcot JM, Bouchard C. Nouvelles recherches sur la pathogenie de l'hemorrhagie cerebrale. *Arch Physiol Norm Path*. 1868;1:110–127;643–645; 725–734.

20. Cole FM, Yates PO. The occurrence and significance of intracerebral microaneurysms. *J Path Bact*. 1967;93:393–411.

21. Whisnant, JP. The role of the neurologist in the decline of stroke. *Ann Neurol*. 1983;14:1–7.

22. Bonita R, Beaglehole R. Increased treatment of hypertension does not explain the decline in stroke mortality in the United States 1970–1980. *Hypertension*. 1989;13 (suppl 1):I-69–I-73.

23. Wolf PA, d'Agostino RB, Kannel WB, et al. Cigarette smoking as a risk factor for stroke. *JAMA*. 1988;259:1025–1029.

24. Barnett HJM, Boughner DR, Taylor DW, et al. Further evidence relating mitral-valve prolapse to cerebral ischemic events. *N Engl J Med*. 1980;302:139–144.

25. Baker RN, Broward JA, Fang HC, et al. Angicoagulant therapy of cerebral infarction: report of a national cooperative study. In: Millikan CH, ed. *Cerebrovascular Disease, Proceedings of Association for Research in Nervous and Mental Disease*. Baltimore, MD: William and Wilkins; 1966:1 pp 287–302.

26. Whisnant JP, Cartlidge NEF, Elveback LR. Carotid and vertebral-basilar transient ischemic attacks: effect of anticoagulants, hypertension, and cardiac disorders on survival and stroke occurrence – a population study. *Ann Neurol* 1978; 3:107–115.

27. Jonas S. Anticoagulant therapy in cerebrovascular disease: review and meta-analysis. *Stroke*. 1988; 19:1043–1048.

28. Peto R, Gray R, Collins R, et al. Randomised trial of prophylactic daily aspirin in British male doctors. *Br Med J*. 1988;296:313–316.

29. Hass W, Easton JD, Adams HP Jr, Pryse-Phillips W, et al. A randomized trial comparing ticlopidine hydrochloride with aspirin for the prevention of stroke in high-risk patients. *N Engl J Med*. 1989; 321:501–507.

30. Gent M, Easton JD, Hachinski VC, et al. The Canadian–American Ticlopidine Study (CATS) in thromboembolic stroke. *Lancet*. 1989;1:1215–1220.

31. Moniz E. L'encephalographie arterielle, son importance dans la localisation des tumeurs cerebrales. *Rev Neurol* 1927;2:72–90.

32. Eastcott HHG, Pickering GW, Rob CG. Reconstruction of internal carotid artery in a patient with intermittent attacks of hemiplegia. *Lancet*. 1954; 2:994–996.

33. Barnett HJM, Plum F, Walton JN. Carotid endarterectomy—an expression of concern. *Stroke*. 1984;15: 941–943.

34. The EC/IC Bypass Study Group. Failure of extracranial-intracranial arterial bypass to reduce the risk of ischemic stroke. Results of an international randomised trial. *N Engl J Med*. 1985;313:1191–1200.

35. Pearce JMS, Gubbay SS, Walton JN. Long-term anticoagulant therapy in transient cerebral ischemic attacks. *Lancet*. 1965;1:6–9.

36. The Canadian Cooperative Study Group. A randomized trial of aspirin and sulfinpyrazone in threatened stroke. *N Engl Med*. 1978;299:53–59.

37. Antiplatelet Trialists' Collaboration. Secondary prevention of vascular disease by prolonged antiplatelet treatment. *Brit Med J*. 1988;296:320–331.

38. Taylor DW, Sackett DL, Haynes RB. Sample size for randomized trials in stroke prevention. How many patients do we need? *Stroke*. 1984;15:968–971.

39. Robins M, Baum HM. National survey of stroke. Incidence. *Stroke*. 1981;12(suppl 2):1–45, 1–57.

40. Welin L, Svardsudd K, Wilhelmsen L, et al. Analysis of risk factors for stroke in a cohort of men born in 1913. *N Engl J Med*. 1987;317:521–526.

41. Inzitari D, Hachinski VC, Taylor DW, et al. Racial differences in the anterior circulation of cerebrovascular disease: how much can be explained by risk factors? *Arch Neurol*. 1990;47:1080–1084.

42. Wolf PA, Kannel WB, Verter J. Current status of risk factors for stroke. *Neurol Clin North Am*. 1983;1:317.

43. Veterans Administration Cooperative Study in Antihypertensive Agents. Effects of treatment on morbidity in hypertension: results in patients with diastolic blood pressures averaging 115 through 129 mm Hg. *JAMA*. 1967;202:1928–1034.

44. Veterans Administration Cooperative Study in Antihypertensive Agents. Effects of treatment on morbidity in hypertension: results in patients with diastolic blood pressures averaging 90–144 mm Hg. *JAMA*. 1970;213:1143–1152.

45. Veterans Administration Cooperative Study in Antihypertensive Agents. Effects of treatment on morbidity in hypertension. III. Influence of age, diastolic pressure and prior cardiovascular disease; further analysis of side effects. *Circulation*. 1972; 45:991–1004.

46. Barnett HJM. Heart in ischemic stroke—a changing emphasis. *Neurol Clin North Am*. 1983;1:291–315.

47. Shinton R, Beevers G. Meta-analysis of relation between cigarette smoking and stroke. *Br Med J*. 1989;298:789–794.

48. Kannel WB, Wolfe PA, Castelli WP, et al. Fibrinogen and risk of cardiovascular disease. *JAMA*. 1987;258:1183–1186.

49. Wilhelmsen L, Svardsudd K, Korsan-Bengtsen K, et al. Fibrinogen as a risk factor for stroke and myocardial infarction. *N Engl J Med*. 1984;311: 501–511.

50. Mershey C, Wohl H. Changes in blood coagulation and fibrinolysis in rats fed atherogenic diets. *Thromb Diathes Haemorrh*. 1964;10:295.

51. Lowe GDO, Drummond MM, Third JLH, et al. Increased plasma fibrinogen and platelet aggregates in type II hyperlipoproteinemia. *Thromb Haemost*. 1979;42:1503–1507.

52. Plum F. What causes infarction in ischemic brain? The Robert Wartenberg Lecture. *Neurology*. 1983; 33:222–233.

53. Kannel WB, Gordon T, Wolf PA. Hemoglobin and the risk of cerebral infarction: the Framingham Study. *Stroke*. 1972;3:409.

54. Herman B, Leyten ACM, van Lujik CWGM. An evaluation of risk factors for stroke in a Dutch community. *Stroke*. 1982;13:334–339.

55. Murai A, Tanaka T, Miyahara T, et al. Lipoprotein abnormalities in the pathogenesis of cerebral infarction and transient ischemic attack. *Stroke*. 1981;12:167–172.

56. Mendez I, Hachinski VC, Wolfe BM. Serum lipids after stroke. *Neurology*. 1987;37:501–511.

57. Khaw K, Barrett-Connor E. Dietary potassium and stroke-associated mortality: a 12-year prospective population study. *N Engl J Med*. 1987;316:235–240.

58. Wolf PA, et al. Epidemiologic assessment of chronic atrial fibrillation of risk of stroke: the Framingham Study. *Neurology*. 1978;28:973–977.

59. Hachinski VC, Norris JW. The acute stroke. In: Plum F, ed. *Contemporary Neurology Series*. vol 27. Philadelphia, PA: FA Davis; 1985. pp. 141–163.

60. Statistics Canada. *Statistics Canada: Causes of Death 1978*. Ottawa: Queen's Printer; 1980.

61. Jones HR, Jr, et al. Cerebral emboli of paradoxical origin. *Ann Neurol*. 1983;13:314.

62. Devinsky O, Petito CK, Alonso DR. Clinical and neuropathological findings in systemic lupus erythematosus: the role of vasculitis, heart emboli, and thrombotic thrombocytopenic purpura. *Ann Neurol*. 1988;23:380–384.

63. Briley DP, Coull BM, Goodnight SH Jr. Neurological disease associated with antiphospholipid antibodies. *Ann Neurol*. 1989;25:221–227.

64. Bell DA (personal communication).

65. Trimble M, Bell D, Brien W, et al. The antiphospholipid syndrome: prevalence among patients with stroke and transient ischemic attacks. *Am J Med*. 1990;88:593–597.

66. Collaborative Group for the Study of Stroke in Young Women. Oral contraceptives and stroke in young women; associated risk factors. *JAMA*. 1975;231:718–722.

67. Royal College of General Practitioners. Incidence of arterial disease among oral contraceptive users. *J Roy Coll Gen Pract*. 1983;33:75–82.

68. Vessey MP, Villard-Mackintosh L, McPherson K, et al. Mortality among oral contraceptive users: 20-year follow up of women in a cohort study. *Br Med J*. 1989;299:1487–1491.

69. Dyken ML, Wolf PA, Barnett HJM, et al. Risk factors in stroke. *Stroke*. 1984;15:1105–1111.

70. Powars D, Wilson B, Imbus C, et al. The natural history of stroke in sickle cell disease. *Am J Med*. 1978;64:461–471.

71. Boers GHJ, Smals AGH, Trijbels FJM, et al. Heterozygosity for homocystinuria in premature peripheral and cerebral occlusive arterial disease. *N Engl J Med*. 1985;313:709–715.

72. Easton JD, Sherman JD, Sherman DG. Cervical manipulation and stroke. *Stroke*. 1977;8:594–597.

73. Simon RP. Neurosyphilis. *Arch Neurol*. 1985;42:606–613.

74. Engstrom J. Reported by Goldsmith MF. Neurologists study abnormal CSF, stroke associated with AIDS. *JAMA*. 1988;259:2957.

75. Snider WD, Simpson DM, Nielsen S, et al. Neurological complications of acquired immune deficiency syndrome: analysis of 50 patients. *Ann Neurol*. 1983;14:403–418.

76. Levy RM. Central nervous system disorders in AIDS. In: Levy JA, ed. *AIDS: Pathogenesis and Treatment*. New York, NY: Marcel Dekker Inc., 1988; pp 371–401.

77. Hillbom M, Kaste M, Rasi V. Can ethanol intoxication affect hemocoagulation with increased risk of infarction in young adults? *Neurology*. 1983;33:381–384.

78. Caplan LR, Hier DB, Banks G. Stroke and drug abuse. *Stroke*. 1982;13:869–872.

79. Klonoff DC, Andrews BT, Obana WG. Stroke associated with cocaine use. *Arch Neurol*. 1989;46:989–993.

80. Mangiardi JR, Daras M, Geller ME, et al. Cocaine-related intracranial hemorrhage. Report of nine cases and review. *Acta Neurol Scan*. 1988;77:177–180.

81. Diaz JF, Hachinski VC, Pederson L, et al. Aggregation of multiple risk factors for stroke in siblings of patients with brain infarction and transient ischemic attacks. *Stroke*. 1986;17:1240–1242.

82. Kagan A, Harris BR, Winkelstein W Jr, et al. Epidemiologic studies of coronary heart disease and stroke in Japanese men living in Japan, Hawaii and California: demographic, physical, dietary and biochemical characteristics. *J Chronic Dis*. 1974; 27:345–364.

83. Kagan A, Popper JS, Rhoads GG. Factors related to stroke incidence in Hawaiian Japanese men: the Honolulu heart study. *Stroke*. 1980;11:14–21.

84. Hennerici M, Hulsbomer HB, Hefter H, Lammerts D, Rautenberg W. Natural history of asymptomatic extracranial arterial disease. *Brain*. 1987;110:777–791.

85. Wolf PA, Kannel WB, Sorlie P, et al. Asymptomatic carotid bruit and risk of stroke: the Framingham study. *JAMA*. 1981;245:1442–1445.

86. Yatsu FM, Fields WS. Asymptomatic carotid bruit: stenosis or ulceration, a conservative approach. *Arch Neurol*. 1985;42:383–385.

87. Dyken ML, Pokras R. The performance of endarterectomy for disease of the extracranial arteries of the head. *Stroke*. 1984;15:948–950.

88. Hennerici M, Rautenberg W, Mohr S. Stroke risk from symptomless extracranial arterial disease. *Lancet*. 1982;2:1180–1183.

89. Chambers BR, Norris JW. Outcome in patients with asymptomatic neck bruits. *N Engl J Med*. 1986;315:860–865.

90. Chambers BR, Norris JW. The case against surgery for asymptomatic carotid stenosis. *Stroke*. 1984; 15:964–967.

91. Ford CS, Frye JL, Toole JF, et al. Asymptomatic carotid bruit and stenosis. A prospective follow-up study. *Arch Neurol*. 1986;43:219–222.

92. Veterans Administration Cooperative Study. Role of carotid endarterectomy in asymptomatic carotid stenosis. *Stroke*. 1986;17:534–539.

93. Wolf PA, D'Agostino RB, Kannel WB, et al. Cigarette smoking as a risk factor for stroke: the Framingham Study. *JAMA*. 1988;259:1025–1035.

94. Abbott RD, Yin Y, Reed DM, et al. Risk of stroke in male cigarette smokers. *N Engl J Med*. 1986; 315:717–720.

95. Colditz GA, Bonita R, Stampfer MJ, et al. Cigarette smoking and risk of stroke in middle-aged women. *N Engl J Med*. 1988;318:937–941.

96. Pokras R, Dyken ML. Dramatic changes in the performance of endarterectomy for disease of the extracranial arteries of the head. *Stroke*. 1988;19: 1289–1290.

97. Warlow CP. Carotid endarterectomy: does it work? *Stroke*. 1984;15:1068–1076.

98. North American Symptomatic Carotid Endarterectomy Study Group. Carotid endarterectomy:

three critical evaluations (editorial). *Stroke.* 1987; 18:987–989.

99. Genton E, Barnett HJM, Fields WS, et al. Report of the Joint Committee for Stroke Resources: 14. Cerebral ischemia: the role of thrombosis and of antithrombotic therapy. Study group on antithrombotic therapy. *Stroke.* 1977;8:150–175.

100. Weksler BB, Lewin M. Anticoagulation in cerebral ischemia. *Stroke.* 1983;14:658–663.

101. Canadian Cooperative Study Group. A randomized trial of aspirin and sulfinpyrazone in threatened stroke. *N Engl J Med.* 1978;299:53–59.

102. Bousser MG, Eschwege E, Haguenau M, et al. "AICLA" controlled trial of aspirin and dipyridamole in the secondary prevention of athero-thrombotic cerebral ischemia. *Stroke.* 1983;14:5–14.

103. UK-TIA Study Group. The United Kingdom transient ischaemic attack (UK-TIA) aspirin trial: interim results. *Brit Med J.* 1988;296:316–320.

104. Kurtzke JF. Controversy in neurology: the Canadian study on TIA and aspirin. A critique of the Canadian TIA study. *Ann Neurol.* 1979;5:597–599.

105. Armitage P. Controversy in the interpretation of clinical trials. *Ann Neurol.* 1979;5:601–602.

106. Candelise L, Landi G, Perrone P, et al. A randomized trial of aspirin and sulfinpyrazone in patients with TIA. *Stroke.* 1982;13:175–179.

107. Dyken ML. Transient ischemic attacks and aspirin, stroke and death; negativities and Type II error (editorial). *Stroke.* 1983;14:2–4

108. The European Stroke Prevention Study Group. The European stroke prevention study (ESPS): principal end-points. *Lancet.* 1987;2:1351–1354.

109. The American–Canadian Cooperative Study Group. Persantine-Aspirin trial in cerebral ischemia: 2. Endpoint results. *Stroke.* 1985;16:406–415.

110. Swedish Cooperative Study Group. High-dose acetylsalicylic acid after cerebral infarction. *Stroke.* 1987;18:325–334.

111. Gent M, Blakely JA, Easton JD, et al. The Canadian–American Ticlopidine Study (CATS) in thromboembolic stroke: design, organization and baseline results. *Stroke.* 1988;19:1203–1210.

112. Sacco RL, Ellenberg JH, Mohr JP, et al. Infarcts of undetermined cause: the NINCDS Stroke Data Bank. *Ann Neurol.* 1989;25:382–390.

113. Ross R, Glomset JA. The pathogenesis of atherosclerosis. *N Engl J Med.* 1976;295:369–425.

114. Brown MS, Goldstein JL. A receptor-mediated pathway for cholesterol homeostasis. *Science.* 1986;232:34–47.

115. Javid H, Ostermiller WE, Hengesh JW, et al. Natural history of carotid bifurcation atheroma. *Surgery.* 1970;67:80–86.

116. Hennerici M, Rautenberg W, Trockel U, et al.

Spontaneous progression and regression of small carotid atheroma. *Lancet.* 1985;1:1415–1419.

117. Roederer GO, Langlois YE, Jager KA, et al. The natural history of carotid arterial disease in asymptomatic patients with cervical bruits. *Stroke.* 1984; 15:605–613.

118. Malinow MR. Experimental models of atherosclerosis regression. *Atherosclerosis.* 1983;48:105–118.

119. Imparato AM, Riles TS, Mintzer R, et al. The importance of hemorrhage in the relationship between gross morphologic characteristics and cerebral symptoms in 376 carotid artery plaques. *Ann Surg.* 1983;197:195–203.

120. Fisher M, Levine PH, Weiner BH. The potential clinical benefits of fish oil consumption. *Arch Intern Med.* 1986;146:2322–2323.

121. Weiner BH, Ockene IS, Levine PH, et al. Inhibition of atherosclerosis by cod liver oil in a hyperlipidemic swine model. *N Engl J Med.* 1986;315:841–846.

122. Brattstrom LE, Herdebo JE, Hultberg BL. Moderate homocysteiremia—a possible risk factor for arteriosclerotic cerebrovascular disease. *Stroke.* 1984;15:1012–1016.

123. Steering Committee of the Physicians' Health Study Research Group. Preliminary report: findings from the aspirin component of the ongoing Physicians' Health Study. *N Engl J Med.* 1988;318: 262–264.

124. Hobson RW, Towne J. Carotid endarterectomy for asymptomatic carotid stenosis. *Stroke.* 1989; 20:575–576.

125. Hasso AN, Bird CR. Percutaneous transluminal angioplasty of carotid and vertebral arteries. In: Jang GC, ed. *Angioplasty.* New York, NY: McGraw-Hill Book Co., 1986: pp 104–115.

126. Yeng Y, Hashizume M, Arbutina D, et al. Argon laser angioplasty with a laser probe. *J Vasc Surg.* 1987;6:60–65.

127. La Muraglia GM, Mathews-Roth MM, Parrish JA, et al. Enhancing the carotenoid content of atherosclerotic plaque: implications for laser therapy. *J Vasc Surg.* 1989;9:563–567.

128. Kuller LH. Incidence rates of stroke in the eighties: the end of the decline in stroke (editorial). *Stroke.* 1989;20:841–843.

129. Wilkinson WE, Heyman A, Pfeffer RI, et al. A questionnaire for TIA symptoms: a predictor of subsequent stroke. In: Reivich M, Hurtig HI, eds. *Cerebrovascular Diseases.* New York, NY: Raven Press; 1983.

130. Colgan MP, Strode GR, Sommer JD, et al. Prevalence of asymptomatic carotid disease: Results of duplex scanning in 348 unselected volunteers. *J Vasc Surg.* 1988;8:674–678.

Part I
Medical Prevention of Stroke

2
Cellular Basis of Atherosclerosis

Marc Fisher

Introduction to Atherosclerosis

Atherosclerosis, involving the large extracranial arteries, is a common substrate for the development of ischemic stroke in the anterior or posterior cerebral circulations. Additionally, intracranial atherosclerosis may also be causally related to ischemic stroke, especially in non-white populations.[1] Many patients with large-vessel cerebral atherosclerosis harbor such lesions in other critical vessels, such as the coronary arteries, aorta, and lower extremity vessels.[2] Atherosclerosis is a ubiquitous problem in industrialized society, and although mortality secondary to acute myocardial infarction (MI) and ischemic stroke have declined, these twin scourges still cause over 600,000 deaths annually in the United States.[3,4] Atherogenesis is an insidious process that develops over decades and may go undetected or unrecognized until the appearance of a devastating MI or stroke. Much has been learned about the nature and pathogenesis of atherosclerosis.[5] These advances are beginning to be translated into therapeutic endeavors that can favorably affect the atherogenic process and its clinical consequences.

Atherosclerotic lesions were recognized in large vessels of the arterial tree by many nineteenth-century pathologists. Marchand in 1904 described the association between fatty degeneration and the stiffening of arteries.[6] Herrick ascribed the clinical manifestations of MI to coronary artery atherosclerosis and thrombosis in 1912.[7] Over the early decades of the 20th century, interest in coronary atherosclerosis heightened as the epidemic of myocardial ischemia increased in western societies. In the 1950s Fisher and colleagues began to explore the relationship between carotid atherosclerosis and the development of ischemic stroke and transient ischemic attacks.[8,9] Similarly, vertebrobasilar atherosclerosis was linked to the development of stroke in the posterior circulation.[10] The relationship of carotid atherosclerosis to ischemic cerebrovascular disease was an important advance in understanding the pathogenesis of stroke in many patients. This allowed for the development of medical and surgical interventions to try to reduce stroke incidence in patients with symptomatic and asymptomatic carotid artery lesions. Controversy surrounds these therapies, as outlined in other chapters, and it must be recognized that they are primarily directed at trying to prevent ischemic symptoms, not at impeding the atherogenic process directly.

Pathology of Atherosclerosis

The lesions of atherosclerosis have been well characterized by histopathologists. Their distribution within the arterial tree has also been identified. The earliest lesion of atherosclerosis is the fatty streak, which may be found in large elastic-muscular arteries in late childhood and early adolescence.[11] Fatty streaks are grossly visible yellowish areas on the intimal surface of these arteries (Fig. 2.1). They are more readily visible if a fat stain is applied to the specimen. Histologically, the fatty streak consists of cells whose cytoplasm is filled with lipid, predominantly cholesterol and its esters, but there is little evidence of extracellular lipid. These lipid-laden cells, or foam cells, have

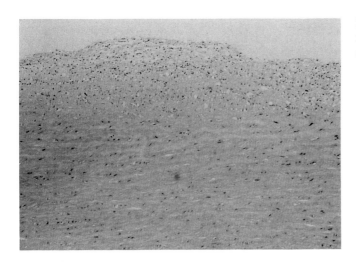

FIGURE 2.1. A fatty streak with numerous foam cells from a human aorta. (Courtesy of Dr. Isabelle Joris.)

been analyzed by the use of monoclonal antibody markers and have been demonstrated to consist primarily of monocyte-derived macrophages with a scattering of smooth muscle cells.[12] T lymphocytes are also observed in fatty streaks, but their significance is uncertain.

The most important pathological lesion of atherosclerosis is the fibrous plaque (Fig. 2.2). The intimal surface of the fibrous plaque usually consists of intact endothelium overlying a fibrous cap. The fibrous cap portion of the plaque contains many layers of smooth muscle cells that have migrated from the media, lymphocytes, and dense connective tissue. Under the fibrous cap lies a mixture of macrophages, smooth muscle cells, lymphocytes, and foam cells.[13] A central necrotic core is also frequently observed, and this region consists of cellular debris, extracellular lipid (predominantly cholesterol esters), and cholesterol crystals. Neovascularization from the adventitia is frequently observed at the edge of the lesion.[14] The percentage composition of lipid and fibrous constituents of the fibrous plaque is highly variable, and this will affect plaque consistency. As the fibrous plaque enlarges, it encroaches upon the lumen and may ultimately compromise arterial flow.

The final pathologic substrate of atherosclerosis is the complicated lesion.[15] This is a fibrous plaque that has accumulated calcium within the necrotic core. Ulceration or disruption of the luminal plaque surface may also occur. Intraplaque hemor-

rhage in association with plaque surface disruption may be seen. Plaque disruption and plaque hemorrhage appear to be related to symptom development in coronary and carotid arteries, and these events will be reviewed in detail.

An important controversy concerns the relationship of fatty streaks to the more advanced lesions of atherosclerosis.[16] Most authorities now agree that fatty streaks are a precursor for the development of fibrous plaques and complicated atheromatous plaques. There appears to be a slow progression and maturation from one lesion to another. This concept of plaque evolution is supported by animal models of atherogenesis in which serial sacrifice of animals at different time points demonstrated fatty streaks and then, at a later time, more advanced lesions at the same arterial sites.[17] Similarly, human autopsy studies demonstrate fatty streaks in the young at the same sites where fibrous plaques are seen in older patients.[18] Lesions that are intermediate in cellular and chemical composition between fatty streaks and fibrous plaques have been described in young adults.[19] Fatty streaks in the young are certainly more numerous than fibrous plaques, suggesting that only a small percentage of fatty streaks in certain arteries (coronary, carotid, abdominal aorta, etc.) undergo maturation.

The evolution of an atherosclerotic plaque in the cerebral or coronary circulation apparently can proceed for decades without detection by patient or physician. Suddenly, in most cases, a catastro-

FIGURE 2.2. A fibrous plaque beginning to expand into the arterial lumen. (Courtesy of Dr. Isabelle Joris.)

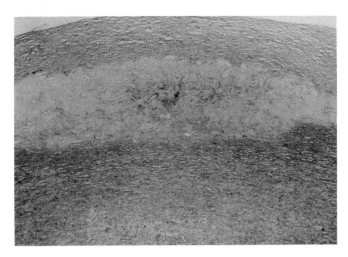

phic or even fatal clinical event—MI or ischemic stroke—occurs. What may have happened acutely to the plaque that led to the clinical event? This issue has been well studied in MI patients and to a lesser extent in patients with symptomatic carotid artery plaques. Complete coronary artery occlusion is commonly observed on angiography in MI patients.[20] At autopsy, patients with acute fatal MIs also frequently have luminal thrombosis superimposed upon a substantial degree of atherosclerosis.[21] Careful serial sectionings of the coronary artery tree in these patients have demonstrated that >90% of the luminal thrombi were directly associated with disruption, ulceration, or erosion of the plaque surface (Fig. 2.3).[21,22] Intraplaque hemorrhage was much less common and ascribed to dissection of blood from the surface into the plaque substance. It is widely accepted among cardiac pathologists that disruption of the luminal plaque surface is the most important initiating event in the development of coronary thrombosis and myocardial ischemia.

Pathologic examination of carotid arteries in relationship to cerebral ischemic symptoms has been much more limited than coronary artery studies. Carotid endarterectomy specimens have been the main source of pathologic specimens for studies that have attempted to correlate morphologic changes in plaques to the development of symptoms. Several investigators have implicated primary intraplaque hemorrhage as an important

event for the development of TIA or stroke.[23,24] According to this hypothesis, hemorrhage occurs within the plaque itself, then causes cerebral ischemic symptoms by acutely expanding the degree of luminal stenosis or by rupture of the plaque substance into the lumen, leading to thrombus formation and distal embolization. These suggestions were based primarily on gross inspection or imprecise histological evaluation of endarterectomy specimens. Several recent series have observed that plaque hemorrhage is frequently seen in highly stenotic endarterectomy specimens, but that plaque hemorrhages are just as common in plaques from asymptomatic patients as they are in symptomatic patients.[25,26] Additionally, there was no temporal relationship between the age of the plaque hemorrhage and the occurrence of symptoms. A significant relationship between luminal plaque surface disruption and intraplaque plaque hematoma was not described in these studies, nor did they incorporate serial sectioning at 100- to 200-µm intervals. Fisher and Ojemann did perform a study in which carotid artery endarterectomy specimens were sectioned at 8- to 10-µm intervals.[27] They observed hemorrhage in only 39% of transient ischemic attack (TIA) patients; and in over 90%, the hemorrhage could be traced to a surface disruption, where the blood had entered. Careful study of autopsy specimens from patients who die of acute carotid occlusion may be more helpful in trying to delineate whether

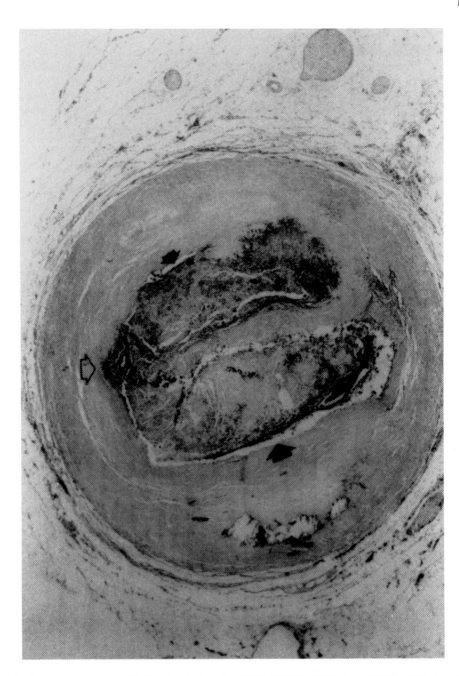

FIGURE 2.3. A coronary artery with intraluminal and intraplaque thrombus connected by a plaque fissure (open arrow). (Reprinted with permission from *Arch Neurol.* 1987;44:1086–1089. Copyright © 1987, American Medical Association.)

luminal plaque disruption or primary plaque hemorrhage is the more common mechanism for the development of acute destabilization of carotid artery atherosclerotic plaques. The issue remains unresolved, although it appears that primary intra-plaque hemorrhage may be less important, based upon recent studies and the experience in the coronary arteries.[28]

The presence of thrombi superimposed upon or within (plaque hemorrhages) atherosclerotic lesions are certainly important for the development of acute ischemic symptoms. Luminal thrombi can cause a clinical event within the cerebral or coronary arterial systems either by obstructing the artery, leading to distal hemodynamic failure, or by embolizing distally, so-called artery-to-artery embolization.[28] Both of these pathogenetic mechanisms are well documented in acutely symptomatic MI or stroke patients. Luminal thrombi are not always symptomatic and may contribute to asymptomatic enlargement of the underlying atherosclerotic plaque because thrombi can organize, and endothelial cells can then overgrow.[29] Fibrin, fibrinogen, and platelet antigens have been identified within plaques, suggesting that thrombosis may contribute to atherogenesis. This contribution is probably small, and thrombi appear to contribute mainly to the acute development of clinical symptoms.[15]

Animal Models

The slowly progressive nature of atherosclerotic plaque development makes it difficult to analyze longitudinally human atherogenesis. Atherosclerosis in humans may not be discovered until symptoms develop, and histological analysis can only be performed postmortem or after surgical removal of an offending plaque. For these reasons and many others, animal models of atherosclerosis have been widely employed to study atherogenesis.[30] Many different species, including rabbits, guinea pigs, fowl, swine and nonhuman primates, have been used for experimental models of atherosclerosis. A variety of mechanisms have been used to promote and enhance atherogenesis in these various species. The most common method for inducing experimental atherosclerosis is to render the animals hyperlipidemic by dietary manipulation.[31] Other animal models employ other nutritional, physical, chemical, or immunologic modifications, alone or in combination, to induce atherogenesis. Methodological criticisms have arisen, but in most models the atherosclerotic lesions are very similar to their human counterparts.

Animal models are helpful in the study of atherosclerosis in a variety of ways. Serial sacrifice of animals at different time points during an experiment has enabled investigators to study in detail cellular aspects of plaque progression, as well as where plaque progression occurs most commonly within the vascular tree.[17] The histochemical constituents of plaques can be analyzed in association with the study of cellular aspects of atherogenesis. Atherosclerosis in animal models can develop rapidly, over months rather than decades, allowing investigators to perform studies in a timely manner. Perhaps most importantly, animal models can serve as a testing vehicle to assess the effect of risk factor modification or pharmacologic intervention on the atherogenic process. Many of the presently employed or potentially useful therapies to inhibit progression or promote regression of atherosclerosis would not have been possible without the availability of appropriate animal models of atherosclerosis. These models will continue to be of great importance in adding to our knowledge about atherosclerosis and for the development of new treatment strategies.

The Pathogenesis of Atherosclerosis

Analyzing the pathological lesions of atherosclerosis has enabled investigators to gather clues about the cellular constituents of plaques. Animal models and human studies of plaque development have illuminated the sequence of cellular and histochemical events associated with plaque maturation. Initial hypotheses about how atherogenesis occurs were proposed in the 1800s, and the work of Virchow is most notable.[32] These early theories stressed the inflammatory nature of the cellular aspects of atherosclerotic plaques. An alternative proposal by Rokitansky emphasized organizing thrombi as the major mechanism for plaque enlargement.[29] In recent times, Russell Ross has widely espoused the "response to injury" hypothesis of atherogenesis, a modern adaptation of earlier suggestions about the inflammatory nature of atherogenesis.[33] This hypothesis has been extensively studied in experimental situations. As new knowledge has accrued, frequent updates have been added to the initial proposal.[5]

The response-to-injury hypothesis relies heavily upon the major cellular contributors to the atherogenic process—monocytes/macrophages, endo-

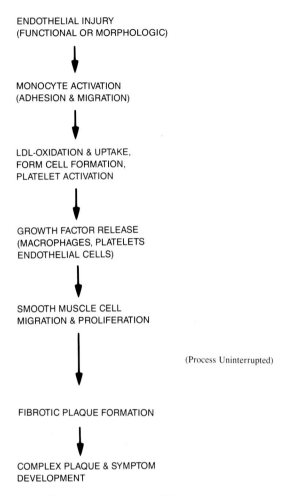

ENDOTHELIAL INJURY
(FUNCTIONAL OR MORPHOLOGIC)

↓

MONOCYTE ACTIVATION
(ADHESION & MIGRATION)

↓

LDL-OXIDATION & UPTAKE,
FORM CELL FORMATION,
PLATELET ACTIVATION

↓

GROWTH FACTOR RELEASE
(MACROPHAGES, PLATELETS
ENDOTHELIAL CELLS)

↓

SMOOTH MUSCLE CELL
MIGRATION & PROLIFERATION

(Process Uninterrupted)

↓

FIBROTIC PLAQUE FORMATION

↓

COMPLEX PLAQUE & SYMPTOM
DEVELOPMENT

FIGURE 2.4. A representation of the response-to-injury hypothesis.

thelial cells, smooth muscle cells, and platelets—in attempting to explain how atherosclerotic plaques develop. Additionally, information concerning how these cells interact with each other and the milieu of the plaque has been incorporated. The response-to-injury hypothesis, as recently updated, (Fig. 2.4) suggests that the initiating event for plaque development is endothelial cell injury, either functional or morphologic.[5] Endothelial injury can be induced by a wide variety of mechanical, biochemical, and physical agents, some of which, such as hemodynamic alterations related to hypertension, low-density lipoprotein (LDL) cholesterol, and cigarette smoke are widely recognized risk factors for atherosclerosis.[32] In response to the "injury," changes in endothelial cell function occur and monocytes/macrophages are recruited.

Platelets may begin to aggregate, and all three cells can release growth factors that promote smooth muscle cell migration from the adventitia to the intima.[34] Lipids gain access to the developing arterial lesion via enhanced endothelial transport. If the process continues because the favorable environment is not impeded, plaque maturation and enlargement can proceed, and ultimately symptoms occur. Obviously, the cellular aspects of atherogenesis are of great importance, and each of the major cellular contributors needs to be discussed in detail.

Monocytes/Macrophages

Circulating monocytes that gain access to the intima and become tissue macrophages have an important role in the early development of atherosclerotic plaques and their propagation.[35] Monocytes are noted to adhere to endothelial cells and to migrate into the intimal portion of the arterial wall very early in the course of both experimental and human atherosclerosis (Fig. 2.5).[36] The majority of foam cells that comprise the fatty streak are macrophage in origin, as identified by monoclonal antibody-based markers. Macrophages and derivative foam cells are also prominent constituents of fibrous plaques.

Macrophages are important inducers for plaque progression by a variety of mechanisms. They imbibe LDL-cholesterol to form foam cells, and this lipid species is taken up by at least two receptors: the native LDL receptor and the "scavenger" receptor.[37] The scavenger receptor avidly takes up LDL, modified by acetylation or oxidation. This receptor is much more potent than the native LDL receptor and is not down-regulated by increasing intracellular concentrations of LDL.[38] Therefore, the scavenger receptor is of primary importance for the generation of macrophage-based foam cells. Macrophages appear to release chemotactic factors that enhance the recruitment of additional circulating monocytes to the developing plaque.[39] Macrophages produce and release a large variety of cytokines, such as interleukin-1, tumor necrosis factor, leukotriene B_4, granulocyte-macrophage colony-stimulating factor, platelet-derived growth factor, and fibroblast growth factor.[40] Many of these cytokines have important effects upon other cells in the region of the developing plaque, both in an activating and in a recruiting mode. These substances contribute

FIGURE 2.5. A scanning electron micrograph of circulating monocytes adhering to the endothelium and beginning to migrate. (From *Am J Pathol.* 1983;113:341–358. Reprinted by permission.)

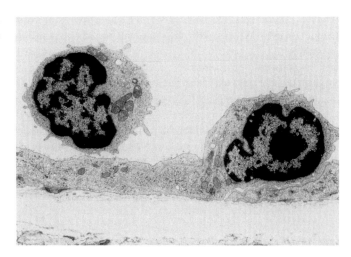

to the ability of the macrophage to induce inflammation, a state closely linked to atherogenesis.

Macrophages produce and release enzymes such as elastase and protease, which can degrade connective tissue, leading to formation of the core lesion seen in advanced plaques.[35] Macrophages release complement, which along with interleukin-1, can recruit lymphocytes. T lymphocytes are frequently found in early and developing plaques, and although their precise function is uncertain, they add further credence to the role of immunologically based inflammation as a factor in atherogenesis.[41] Free radical production by macrophages within plaques is a corollary observation.[42] The relationship of these toxic oxygen species to LDL-cholesterol modification and cytotoxicity will be detailed in another section. Finally, macrophages may have at least one beneficial effect on retarding plaque development. They participate in the reverse cholesterol transport system, which removes excess cholesterol from plaques.[43] High-density lipoprotein (HDL) cholesterol can enter tissue macrophages that may egress from the plaque and reenter the bloodstream. On balance, macrophages appear to be much more deleterious than beneficial and have a large number of increasingly recognized functions that relate to the promotion of atherogenesis.

Endothelial Cells

Endothelial cells are not passive bystanders that simply compose the luminal surface of developing atherosclerotic plaques. They are actively involved in plaque development by a variety of mechanisms.

As outlined, functional or morphologic endothelial cell injury induced by a multiplicity of mechanisms has been proposed as an early important step for the initiation of atherogenesis.[5] Endothelial cells serve as a conduit for plasma constituents to reach the arterial intima, and for many substances, transport is an active process.[44] Transport of lipid species such as LDL-cholesterol may be particularly important, and there is also evidence that endothelial cells can modify LDL-cholesterol, leading to enhanced uptake by the macrophage scavenger receptor.[45] Endothelial cells also release growth factors such as platelet-derived growth factor (PDGF), which can affect smooth muscle cell recruitment and function.[46] Heparin-like molecules released from endothelial cells inhibit smooth muscle cell proliferation, and inhibition of physiologic endothelial cell function may promote smooth muscle cell growth.[47]

Endothelial cells interact with the blood and its cellular constituents in a number of ways. Heparin, tissue plasminogen activator, proteins C and S, and antithrombin III are just a few endothelially derived substances that affect the formation and dissolution of fibrin thrombi associated with acute clinical events.[44] Platelet adhesion and aggregation are also affected by endothelial cell activity.

Smooth Muscle Cells

Smooth muscle cells (SMC) are important constituents of fibrous and advanced atherosclerotic plaques. In the normal arterial wall, SMC are found primarily in the medial layer and function primarily as contractile cells. In atherosclerotic plaques, migration of SMC into the intima has occurred, and the functional activity of these cells has been modulated to a more synthetic state.[48] Smooth muscle cells in the intima imbibe lipid and become a minority of the foam cells that typify fatty streaks.[41] Smooth muscle cells proliferate in this altered state, and become one of the predominant cellular constituents in fibrous plaques. They also form much of the connective tissue matrix observed in advanced plaques. Not only do SMC respond to growth factors and chemotactic agents produced by other cells within the milieu of the developing plaque, they can also produce a PDGF-like factor and oxidatively modify LDL-cholesterol.[45,49] Thus, SMC may contribute to their own migration and proliferation in an autocrine fashion. Smooth muscle cells contain receptors for native LDL, but, so far, "scavenger" LDL receptors have not been demonstrated.[32] Although SMC can modify LDL by oxidation, the lack of receptors for the more avidly imbibed, modified form of LDL may explain in part why foam cells are primarily derived from macrophages and not SMC.

Platelets

The role of platelets in atherogenesis has received widespread attention in the past.[33] It now appears that platelets are relative late contributors when a nondenuding functional endothelial injury is the predominant initiating and perpetuating mechanism for atherogenesis.[5] Animal studies of experimental atherosclerosis with serial observations of plaque growth have lent support to this proposal.[17] After structural denuding endothelial injury, platelets are early participants in plaque growth.[50] Denuding injury, such as that seen after coronary artery abrasion for angioplasty or associated with vascular grafts, are relatively special circumstances.

Earlier studies of platelets and atherosclerosis were important because they helped to identify the potent platelet-associated growth factor, PDGF. Platelet-derived growth factor was the first well-characterized growth factor, and its elucidation was an important step for understanding how cells within plaques interact with each other.[51] As mentioned, growth factors similar or almost identical to PDGF are produced by SMC, macrophages, and endothelial cells.[52] Although platelets are probably

not an important cellular contributor to initiation of atherosclerotic plaque development, in most circumstances PDGF activity derived from platelets and other cellular sources may be a key factor.

Growth Factors

The cellular aspects of atherogenesis as outlined imply a complicated series of interactions among the major cellular components of the process. Growth factors released by these cells appear to contribute substantially to atherogenesis.[34] Platelet-derived growth factor is the most widely studied growth factor associated with atherogenesis, but certainly not the only one. Other growth factors that have been identified, and cells that produce them, include: fibroblast growth factor (macrophages, endothelial cells, SMC), transforming growth factor, alpha and beta (platelets, macrophages, endothelial cells), and epidermal growth factors (platelets).[53] The various growth factors help to organize the events associated with atherogenesis by promoting transformation and proliferation of cells, affecting adhesion to endothelium and enhancing cellular migration.

Platelet-derived growth factor was originally identified in 1974 from platelets, but subsequently it has been found in many other cells.[52] It binds avidly to receptors upon fibroblasts, SMC, and other cells of mesenchymal origin, but not endothelial cells. Platelet-derived growth factor receptor binding leads to metabolic activation within the target cell, resulting ultimately in DNA synthesis and a proliferative response in the target cell.[46] Platelet-derived growth factor also activates membrane phospholipases, leading to arachidonic acid release and prostaglandin production.[54] Platelet-derived growth factor has chemoattractant capabilities, which aid in the migration of SMC from the arterial media to the intima. The amino acid sequence of PDGF has been characterized.[52] It contains two chains, and there is substantial homology (93%) between the B chain and a transforming protein associated with an oncogene from simian sarcoma retrovirus.[55] This homology implies a relationship between PDGF and cells transformed by viruses or other agents associated with neoplasia. The transformed cells may be able to express PDGF-like activity, which can then promote cellular proliferation. This interesting observation needs further exploration.

Fibroblast growth factor (FGF) is another growth factor associated with atherosclerosis that has been well studied.[53] Fibroblast growth factor is a potent SMC and fibroblast mitogen that also stimulates endothelial cell proliferation and angiogenesis. Heparin can stimulate FGF activity. Fibroblast growth factor is associated with cells involved in atherogenesis, and its ability to stimulate SMC and fibroblasts and promote vascular proliferation could contribute to plaque progression. The roles of other growth factors, such as transforming growth factor and epidermal growth factor, in atherogenesis remain to be established. Substances that can inhibit or modify growth factor activity, such as prostaglandin E_2, interleukin -1, and interferon, are produced by tissue macrophages.[32,40] Thus, a complex interaction of growth factor promoters and inhibitors probably leads to a dynamic cellular balance and also implies that growth-factor-mediated cellular aspects of atherogenesis potentially can be impeded or reversed.

Hemodynamic Factors

The distribution of advanced atherosclerotic plaques within the vascular tree is not random but occurs in reproducible areas of high predilection. The most common locations for human atherosclerosis include the proximal coronary arteries, descending thoracic aorta, femoral arteries, and, most importantly from the perspective of ischemic cerebrovascular disease, the proximal portions of the carotid and vertebral arteries.[56] Biochemical and systemic factors associated with atherogenesis would have a relatively uniform distribution within the vasculature, so what other factors may be implicated to explain the preferred sites of plaque development? An area of investigation that may, in part, offer an explanation is the effect of hemodynamic forces on atherogenesis.[57]

Fluid or blood flowing in a straight tube such as an artery will tend to follow a unidirectional, predictable path or a laminar flow pattern. It is mainly at branch points or in relationship to areas of vascular narrowing that laminar flow is disturbed and that vortices and recirculation zones form (Fig. 2.6).[57] The relationship of flow velocity to the arterial wall leads to the formation of wall shear stress, which tends to align endothelial cells and superficial arterial layers in the direction of flow.[58]

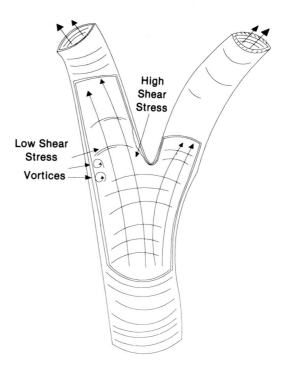

FIGURE 2.6. A schematic representation of laminar flow and vortices at the carotid bifurcation.

Tensile stress or circumferential pressure on the luminal surface of an artery is also exerted by the flowing blood.

The relationship of hemodynamic factors to the carotid bifurcation has been elaborately assessed. The outer wall of the internal carotid artery at the level of the carotid sinus is a region of low shear stress.[59] This region has been observed in experimental models to develop oscillations of flow direction and secondary vortices. This outer carotid wall is the region where intimal thickening and plaque formation develops first and to the greatest extent (Fig. 2.7).[60] The inner wall at the carotid bifurcation is a region of high shear stress, preserved laminar flow, and relatively meager plaque formation. These carotid artery observations related to hemodynamics are also relevant to the preferential formation of plaque at the origins of other major arterial branch points, such as those from the aorta, the left anterior descending coronary artery, and in the femoral arteries. The locations of plaque in other arteries are not as readily attributable to hemodynamic factors.

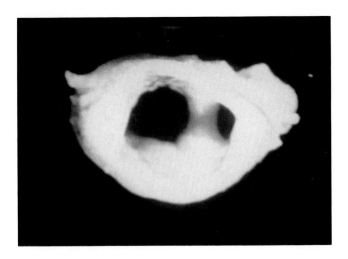

FIGURE 2.7. A carotid bifurcation seen from below with plaque development along the outer wall arrow.

Several physical and biochemical effects of hemodynamics may help to explain how these factors interact with the cellular aspects of atherogenesis. Endothelial cells elongate and align in the direction of blood flow and wall shear stress.[61] This alignment may lead to tighter intercellular junctions and reduced vascular permeability.[62] In areas of low shear stress, cells are not as well aligned and may therefore be more susceptible to leakage. Pulsatile flow enhances endothelial cell release of prostacyclin and endothelial relaxing factor, two substances that inhibit platelet aggregation.[60] Conceivably, this release may be reduced in areas of low shear stress, leading to enhanced tendency for platelet aggregation in these regions.

Clearance of particles in flowing blood is reduced in areas of low shear stress, such as the outer wall of the carotid bifurcation.[63] Therefore there is increased residence or exposure time of potentially deleterious materials contained in the blood, which could then promote endothelial cell or arterial wall injury. Animal experiments have shown that preferential dye staining occurs at arterial wall sites where plaques typically develop, an observation supportive of the notion of enhanced residence time.[64] Cellular elements of blood such as monocytes and platelets may also be affected by prolonged residence time. This may afford these cells a greater opportunity to interact with the arterial wall, promoting adhesion, migration, and release of cellular constituents into the arterial wall.[57] All of these factors are consistent with the previously outlined concepts related to the cellular aspects of plaque development.

Hemodynamic factors such as wall shear stress and tensile stress also affect the manner in which the artery modulates itself to adapt to the presence of an enlarging plaque.[65] The arterial wall reacts to the presence of a developing plaque by trying to maintain a round lumen. The outer arterial wall expands outward in an attempt to reduce luminal compromise and to maintain a concave luminal surface. Compensatory enlargement of the artery also occurs on the intact wall opposite to the developing plaque, perhaps related to increased flow velocity in a region of stenosis.[66] These compensatory changes may lead to an eccentric displaced, but round, lumen. However, there are limits to the compensatory mechanisms, and as the luminal cross-sectional area begins to decline when the plaque burden exceeds 40% of the area defined by the internal elastic lamina, this compensation becomes ineffective.

Risk Factors and Cellular Aspects of Atherosclerosis

Lipoproteins

There is substantial evidence demonstrating an association between elevated blood lipids, specifically, total and LDL-cholesterol, and atherosclerosis and atherothrombotic disorders. The observations linking cholesterol to atherosclerosis include pathological observation of cholesterol in plaques, experimental models in which atherosclerosis is induced by high cholesterol levels, epidemiological

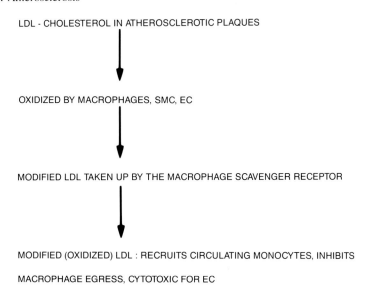

LDL - CHOLESTEROL IN ATHEROSCLEROTIC PLAQUES

OXIDIZED BY MACROPHAGES, SMC, EC

MODIFIED LDL TAKEN UP BY THE MACROPHAGE SCAVENGER RECEPTOR

MODIFIED (OXIDIZED) LDL : RECRUITS CIRCULATING MONOCYTES, INHIBITS

MACROPHAGE EGRESS, CYTOTOXIC FOR EC

FIGURE 2.8. LDL-cholesterol can be modified to an oxidized form that has a variety of physiological effects. EC = endothelial cells; SMC = smooth muscle cells.

associations between high cholesterol levels and human atherosclerotic coronary artery disease; and genetic factors that raise cholesterol levels are associated with premature atherosclerosis.[67] How elevated cholesterol levels promote the development of atherosclerotic plaques remains a matter of intense speculation. The lipid infiltration hypothesis initially proposed over a century ago suggests that elevated plasma cholesterol leads to an increased rate of lipid deposition in the artery wall.[66] Increased cholesterol within the arterial wall can then be accumulated or degraded by the cellular constituents in the environment. Lipoproteins may adversely affect endothelial cell function and could then initiate functional nonmorphologic injury.[69] The cascade associated with the cellular injury hypothesis of atherosclerosis would then be initiated.

A more complex interrelationship between LDL-cholesterol and the cellular aspects of atherogenesis has been proposed and studied, primarily by Steinberg and associates, as outlined in Figure 2.8.[70] Native LDL-cholesterol is taken up by macrophages at a relatively slow rate, but modified LDL-cholesterol is rapidly imbibed via the scavenger receptor, as previously described. Oxidation of LDL leads to the formation of just such a modified LDL species. LDL oxidation has been demonstrated to occur when LDL is incubated with macrophages, endo-

thelial cells, or smooth muscle cells, the key cellular contributors to atherogenesis.[71,72] Evidence has accumulated that supports the presence of oxidized LDL in vivo.[73] Thus, LDL reaching the arterial wall in greater abundance in patients with increased plasma levels can be oxidatively modified by several cells, leading to enhanced macrophage uptake and foam cell formation.

Oxidized LDL also has a number of other cellular effects that can influence the cellular contributors to atherosclerosis in a manner that may enhance plaque progression. Oxidized LDL is a powerful chemoattractant for the recruitment of circulating monocytes into the arterial wall.[74] Paradoxically, oxidized LDL inhibits motility of macrophages already residing in the arterial wall. Thus, oxidation of LDL can lead to the trapping of increased numbers of monocytes/macrophages at a site of plaque development. Oxidized LDL has highly cytotoxic properties and may promote nondenuding endothelial cell injury more vigorously than native LDL.[72] The implication of these effects is that interventions that inhibit LDL oxidation could be beneficial. Probucol, a drug with modest lipid-lowering potential but substantial antioxidant action, has been shown to inhibit atherogenesis in hyperlipidemic rabbits.[75] N-3 fatty acids have been observed to inhibit both animal and human atherogenesis and to reduce monocyte free radical production.[76] The effects of n-3 fatty acids on cellular aspects of atherosclerosis will be explored in detail.

Other Risk Factors

Hypertension is a well-recognized risk factor for the development of coronary artery disease and ischemic stroke. Hypertension may affect hemodynamic factors associated with atherogenesis but also has an impact upon cellular aspects of atherosclerosis. Hypertension can cause endothelial cell injury or affect metabolic function. Hypertension appears to enhance the atherogenic potential of hyperlipidemia in animal atherosclerosis models.[77] Pulsatile flow enhanced by hypertension may compress the vasa vasorum, leading to interference with arterial wall nutrition and clearance of lipids.[78]

Smoking is also a risk factor for atherothrombotic disorders with a variety of effects. Cigarette smoke stimulates platelet activity and elevates fibrinogen levels, factors that may enhance thrombosis in a region of arterial stenosis.[79] Smoking may damage the arterial intima and contribute to the cascade of cellular injury.[80] Lipoprotein levels, primarily HDL, are adversely affected by smoking, and this may also contribute to atherogenesis on that basis.[81]

The risks for atherothrombotic disorders associated with hypertension and smoking are both readily reversible with treatment or cessation. These observations suggest that these risk factors are primarily associated with ultimate development of clinical events and are only of secondary importance in the pathogenesis of atherosclerotic plaque.

Therapeutic Approaches

The traditional approach to treatment for atherosclerosis and associated atherothrombotic disorders such as MI and ischemic stroke has been to attempt modification of risk factors. Additionally, medications with an antithrombotic effect are frequently employed in high risk populations, such as patients suffering a transient ischemic attack or unstable angina, in an attempt to impede thrombus formation on an arterial lumen compromised by an atherosclerotic plaque. Lipid-lowering interventions, either by diet alone or in combination with a variety of medications, have been demonstrated to

reduce the risk of MI and to impede the development of coronary atherosclerosis.[82] The role of lipid-lowering therapy for the prevention of ischemic stroke remains uncertain. Ameliorating hypertension is clearly beneficial in reducing the risk of subsequent MI and ischemic stroke,[83] although direct benefits of this treatment on atherogenesis remain to be established. Stopping smoking[84] also reduces the risk for clinical events, but a direct relationship of this intervention to reducing progression or initiating regression of atherosclerotic lesions has not been demonstrated. Risk factor intervention has been a successful way to reduce the burden of atherosclerotic disorders, but there are inherent limits to patient motivation, compliance, and success. As knowledge of the cellular aspects of atherosclerosis has expanded, newer interventions that make use of this information have become possible.

N-3 Fatty Acids

Epidemiologic studies have revealed that populations such as Greenland Eskimos and coastal Japanese, who consume substantial quantities of n-3 fatty acids, have a markedly reduced rate of cardiovascular morbidity and mortality.[85]

Direct evidence that n-3 fatty acids reduce the extent of atherosclerosis within the coronary and cerebral vessels is still lacking but certainly is implied. Recently, a preliminary study showed that dietary n-3 fatty acid supplementation inhibited the extent of coronary artery restenosis after coronary angioplasty in comparison to aspirin.[86] This observation will need confirmation in larger trials, and these are in progress. Considerable data have been amassed concerning the effects of n-3 fatty acids on animal models of atherogenesis. Weiner et al. observed that dietary n-3 fatty acid supplementation markedly reduced the extent of coronary atherosclerosis in a swine hyperlipidemic model (Fig. 2.9).[87] This result was independent of any effects on serum lipid measurements. This observation of reduced atherogenesis in swine given n-3 fatty acids was confirmed by another group.[88] Total cholesterol levels were modestly reduced (816 mg/dl ±64 vs. 629 ±14) in this study, as were apolipoprotein B and E containing LDL molecules and LDL levels. Davis et al. reported that n-3 fatty acid dietary substitution reduced the extent of

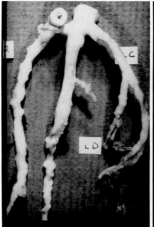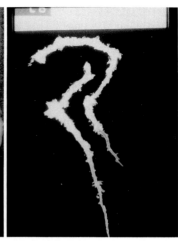

FIGURE 2.9. The coronary artery tree on the left is from a control animal, while the one on the right is from an animal that received dietary n-3 fatty acid supplementation.

aortic, femoral, and carotid atherosclerosis in a primate hyperlipidemic model.[89] All plasma lipoprotein fractions were reduced, but total cholesterol levels still remained >400 mg/dl, and HDL levels fell to 20 mg/dl. The concentration of apolipoprotein E was reduced. Microscopic examination of carotid atherosclerotic lesions revealed a reduced number of resident macrophages. Incubation of LDL with macrophages from the animals in vitro demonstrated a marked reduction in the uptake of lipoprotein isolated from the fish oil group as compared to controls.[90] Hollander et al. also observed that dietary n-3 fatty acid supplementation reduced the extent of aortic, coronary, and carotid atherosclerosis in another primate species, without significant changes in lipoprotein measurements.[91] These experiments strongly suggest that n-3 fatty acids can inhibit atherogenesis, at least in animal models that closely mimic human anatomy and pathology.

How n-3 fatty acids may inhibit atherogenesis remains uncertain. Their effects on lipids in animal models are variable, and even when reductions are noted, they are modest. In humans, total and LDL-cholesterol levels either remain stable or increase slightly when n-3 fatty acids are consumed by hyperlipidemic subjects.[92] Only triglyceride levels routinely fall, and the contribution of this lipid species to atherosclerosis remains speculative. Therefore, attention has begun to focus on the cellular and biochemical effects of n-3 fatty acids, outlined in Table 2.1, as the most likely mechanism for n-3 fatty acid-induced reduction of atherogene-

sis.[76] Inhibition of in vivo and in vitro platelet activity was the first cellular effect of n-3 fatty acids that was noted.[93] Platelets appear to be a relatively late and minor contributor to atherogenesis; so this effect may be more important for inhibiting arterial thrombi than reducing plaque development. Monocytes/macrophages are an early and important contributor to atherogenesis, and n-3 fatty acids have a variety of suppressant effects on these cells. Monocyte production of free radicals, interleukin-1, leukotriene B_4, tumor necrosis factor, and platelet activating factor were all reduced by n-3 fatty acids.[76] Monocyte chemotaxis is also inhibited.[94] These suppressant effects reduce the ability of monocytes to accrue, recruit, and act in a cytotoxic manner. The potential beneficial effects on atherogenesis are readily apparent. Production of a PDGF-like molecule by endothelial cells was

TABLE 2.1. Cellular and biochemical inhibitory effects of n-3 fatty acids.

Reduced production
Interleukin-1
Tumor necrosis factor
Toxic oxygen metabolites (free radicals)
Leukotriene by PDGF
Platelet activating factor
Cellular effects
Reduced monocyte chemotaxis
Monocyte recruitment into atherosclerotic plaque
Prolonged platelet survival
Prolonged bleeding time

reduced when these cells were incubated with n-3 fatty acids.[95] Production of endothelial-derived relaxing factor, a potent platelet antiaggregant and vasodilator, is increased by dietary n-3 fatty acid supplementation.[96] Thus, there is a wide variety of n-3 fatty acid effects on cellular aspects of atherogenesis, and it is likely that many others will be forthcoming. These changes are the probable mechanism of n-3 fatty acid inhibition of atherogenesis. This relatively safe and simple intervention may therefore serve as a paradigm for cellular intervention strategies directed at atherogenesis. However, until more definitive proof accrues in humans, it is too soon to recommend routine use of n-3 fatty acids for the prevention or amelioration of atherosclerosis.

Additional Potential Therapies

Calcium channel blockers have been evaluated in a variety of experimental models of atherosclerosis, primarily in hyperlipidemic rabbits.[97] Most of these studies demonstrated a reduction in the extent of early aortic atherosclerotic lesions. A preliminary study in primates with nifedipine also demonstrated a reduction in carotid atherosclerosis.[98] There are several reasons why calcium channel blockers might have an antiatherogenic effect. Calcium influx can lead to cell injury through mitochondrial damage, and calcium may affect platelet aggregation, PDGF release, and SMC proliferation.[99] Calcification is a hallmark of advanced plaque formation and may mechanically affect the plaque and vasa vasorum.

The potential beneficial activity of calcium channel blockers in atherosclerosis does not apparently relate to their effects on blood pressure or lipoprotein metabolism. Nicardipine reduces in vitro SMC migration, and isradipine inhibits proliferative lesions in mechanically injured carotid arteries.[100,101] Calcium channel blockers exert protective effects to prevent cell necrosis associated with intracellular calcium overload,[97] and are presently being evaluated in patients with asymptomatic carotid atherosclerosis and systemic arterial lesions.

Heparin is another medication that may positively affect the cellular aspects of atherosclerosis. For instance, it inhibits rat carotid artery SMC proliferation in response to endothelial injury.[102] In vitro heparin can inhibit smooth cell growth[103] and sup-presses SMC proliferation by competing for endoglycosidases.[104] Endoglycosidases released by platelets and leukocytes can break down SMC heparan sulfate, a compound that mediates growth factor effects on SMCs. Therefore, heparin inhibition of endoglycosidases reduces heparan sulfate activation and, ultimately, growth factor–induced proliferation. A trial of long-term low-molecular-weight heparin is presently under way in patients after coronary angioplasty, to assess the effects on the rate of restenosis. Heparin also possesses potent antithrombotic effects, as mediated by its activation of antithrombin III. When given long-term, it not only inhibits plaque proliferation but also prevents thrombus formation on unstable plaques.

Conclusion

Approaching the prevention of atherosclerosis at a cellular level is a new therapeutic approach with obvious appeal. A spectrum of new therapies directed at this concept will be studied in the near future, and some are already in clinical trial.

We may anticipate monoclonal antibodies directed at various growth factors, inhibition or competitive binding at growth factor receptors, antioxidant therapy, modulation of cytokines, and others, as new therapies directed at the cellular cascade of atherosclerosis.

As these therapies become available for clinical trials, the carotid arteries will be a fertile ground for evaluation because their lesions can be followed serially, accurately, and noninvasively to assess the effect of a given treatment. The era of primary inhibition and prevention of atherosclerosis may be shortly forthcoming.

References

1. Caplan LR, Gorelick PB, Hier DB. Race, sex and occlusive vascular disease: a review. *Stroke.* 1984; 17:648–655.
2. Hertzer NR, Young Jr, Beven EG, et al. Coronary angiography in 506 patients with extracranial cerebrovascular disease. *Arch Int Med.* 1985;145:849–852.
3. Arteriosclerosis. Report of the working group on arteriosclerosis of the National Heart, Lung and Blood Institute. vol 2. Washington, DC: U.S. Department of Health and Human Services; 1981.

4. Gillum RF. Cerebrovascular disease morbidity in the United States, 1970–1983: age, sex, region, and vascular surgery. *Stroke.* 1986;17:656–661.

5. Ross R. The pathogenesis of atherosclerosis: an update. *N Engl J Med.* 1986;314:488–500.

6. Long ER. The development of our knowledge of arteriosclerosis. In: Cowdry EV, ed. *Arteriosclerosis: A survey of the Problem.* New York, NY: Macmillan; 1933: pp 19–52.

7. Herrick JB. Clinical features of sudden obstruction of the coronary arteries. *JAMA.* 1912;58:2015–2020.

8. Fisher CM. Occlusion of the internal carotid artery. *Arch Neurol Psychiatry.* 1951;65:346–377.

9. Fisher CM. Observations of the fundus oculi in the transient monocular blindness. *Neurology.* 1959;9:333–347.

10. Fisher CM, Gore I, Okabe N, et al. Atherosclerosis of the carotid and vertebral arteries: extracranial and intracranial. *J Neuropathol Exp Neurol.* 1965;24:455–476.

11. Stary HC. Evolution and progression of atherosclerosis in the coronary arteries of children and adults. In: Bates SR, Gangloff EC, eds. *Atherogenesis and Aging.* New York, NY: Springer-Verlag; 1987: pp 20–36.

12. Azel NM, Ball RY, Waldman H, et al. Identification of macrophages and smooth muscle cells in human atherosclerosis using monoclonal antibodies. *J Pathol.* 1985;146:197–201.

13. Ross R, Wight TN, Strandness E, et al. Human atherosclerosis: I. Cell constitution and characteristics of advanced lesions of the superficial femoral artery. *Am J Pathol.* 1984;114:79–93.

14. Barger CA, Becuwkes R, Lainey LL, et al. Hypothesis: vasa vasorum and neovascularization of human coronary arteries. *N Engl J Med.* 1984;310:175–177.

15. McGill HC. The pathogenesis of atherosclerosis. *Clin Chem.* 1988;34:B33–B39.

16. McGill HC. Persistent problems in the pathogenesis of atherosclerosis. *Arteriosclerosis.* 1984;4:443–451.

17. Faggiotto A, Ross R. Studies of hypercholesterolemia in the non-human primate: II. Fatty streak conversion to fibrous plaque. *Arteriosclerosis.* 1984;4:341–356.

18. Montenegro MR, Eggen DA. Topography of atherosclerosis in the coronary arteries. *Lab Invest.* 1968;18:586–593.

19. Geer JC, McGill HC, Robertson WB, et al. Histologic characteristics of coronary artery fatty streaks. *Lab Invest.* 1960;18:565–570.

20. Deewood MA, Spores J, Notske R, et al. Prevalence of total coronary occlusion during the early hours of transmural myocardial infarction. *N Engl J Med.* 1980;303:897–902.

21. Falk E. Plaque rupture with severe pre-existing stenosis precipitates coronary thrombosis. *Br Heart J.* 1983;50:127–134.

22. Davies MJ, Thomas AC. Plaque fissuring: the cause of acute myocardial infarction, sudden ischemic death, and crescendo angina. *Br Heart J.* 1985;53:363–373.

23. Imparato AM, Riles TS, Mintzer R, et al. The importance of hemorrhage in the relationship between gross morphologic and cerebral symptoms in 376 carotid artery plaques. *Ann Surg.* 1983;197:195–203.

24. Persson AV. Intraplaque hemorrhage. *Surg Clin North Am.* 1986;66:415–420.

25. Lennihan L, Kupsky WJ, Mohr JP, et al. Lack of association between carotid plaque hematoma and ischemic cerebral symptoms. *Stroke.* 1987;18:879–881.

26. Bassiouny HJ, Davis H, Massama N, et al. Critical carotid stenosis: morphologic and chemical similarity between symptomatic and asymptomatic plaques. *J Vasc Surg.* 1989;9:202–212.

27. Fisher CM, Ojemann RG. A clinico-pathologic study of endarterectomy plaques. *Rev Neurol.* 1986;142:573–589.

28. Fisher M, Blumenfeld AM, Smith TW. The importance of carotid artery plaque disruption and hemorrhage. *Arch Neurol.* 1987;44:1086–1089.

29. Schwartz CJ, Valente AJ, Kelley JL, et al. Thrombosis and the development of atherosclerosis. *Semin Thromb Hemost.* 1988;14:189–195.

30. Vesselinovitch D. Animal models and the study of atherosclerosis. *Arch Pathol Lab Med.* 1988;112:1011–1017.

31. Gerrity RG, Naito HK, Richardson M, et al. Dietary induced atherogenesis in swine. *Am J Pathol.* 1979;95:775–792.

32. Munro MJ, Cotran RS. The pathogenesis of atherosclerosis: atherogenesis and inflammation. *Lab Invest.* 1988;58:249–301.

33. Ross R, Glomset JA. The pathogenesis of atherosclerosis. *N Engl J Med.* 1976;295:369–377, 420–425.

34. Duel TF. Polypeptide growth factors: roles in normal and abnormal cell growth. *Ann Rev Cell Biol.* 1987;3:443–492.

35. Mitchinson MJ, Ball RY. Macrophages and atherogenesis. *Lancet.* 1987;2:146–149.

36. Faggiotto A, Ross R, Harker L. Studies of hypercholesterolemia in the non-human primate: I. Changes that lead to fatty streak formation. *Arteriosclerosis.* 1984;4:323–340.

37. Steinberg D. Lipoproteins and the pathogenesis of atherosclerosis. *Circulation.* 1987;76:508–514.

38. Brown MS, Goldstein JL. Lipoprotein metabolism in the macrophage: implications for cholesterol deposition in atherosclerosis. *Annu Rev Biochem.* 1983;52:223-261.

39. Mazzone T, Jensen M, Chait A. Human arterial wall cells release factors that are chemotactic for monocytes. *Proc Natl Acad Sci.* 1983;80:5094-5097.

40. Nathan CF. Secretory products of macrophages. *J Clin Invest.* 1987;79:319-326.

41. Jonasson L, Holm J, Skalli O, et al. Regional accumulation of T cells, macrophages, and smooth muscle cells in human atherosclerotic plaques. *Arteriosclerosis.* 1986;6:131-138.

42. Cathcart MK, Morel DW, Chisholm GM. Monocytes and neutrophils oxidize low density lipoprotein making it cytotoxic. *J Leukocyte Biol.* 1985;38:341-350.

43. Yatsu FM, Alam R, Alam S. Scavenger activity in monocyte-derived macrophages from atherothrombotic strokes. *Stroke.* 1986;17:709-713.

44. Jaffe EA. Cell biology of endothelial cells. *Human Pathol.* 1987;18:234-239.

45. Morel DW, Dicorleto PE, Chisholm GM. Endothelial and smooth muscle cells alter low density lipoprotein in vitro by free radical oxidation. *Arteriosclerosis.* 1984;4:357-364.

46. Ross R, Raines EW, Bowen-Pope DF. The biology of platelet-derived growth factor. *Cell.* 1986;46:155-164.

47. Castellot JJ, Addonzio ML, Rosenberg R, et al. Cultured endothelial cells produce a heparin-like inhibitor of smooth muscle cell growth. *J Cell Biol.* 1981;90:372-379.

48. Campbell GR, Chamley-Campbell JH. The cellular pathology of atherosclerosis. *Pathology.* 1981;13:423-440.

49. Libby P, Warner SJC, Salomon RN, et al. Production of platelet derived growth factor-like mitogen by smooth muscle cells from human atheroma. *N Engl J Med.* 1988;318:1493-1498.

50. Goldberg ID, Stemerman MB, Handin RI. Vascular permeation of platelet factor 4 after endothelial injury. *Science.* 1980;209:611-612.

51. Ross R, Glomset JA, Kariya B, et al. A platelet-derived serum factor that stimulates the proliferation of arterial smooth muscle cells in vitro. *Proc Natl Acad Sci.* 1974;71:1207-1210.

52. Ross R. Platelet-derived growth factor. *Lancet.* 1989;1:1179-1182.

53. Klagsbrun M, Edelman ER. Biological and biochemical properties of fibroblast growth factors. *Arteriosclerosis.* 1989;9:269-278.

54. Habenicht A, Goerig M, Grulich J, et al. Human platelet derived growth factor stimulates prosta-glandin synthesis by activation and de novo synthesis of cyclooxygenase. *J Clin Invest.* 1985;75:1381-1387.

55. Doolittle RF, Hunkapiller MW, Hood LE, et al. Simian sarcoma virus onc gene, v-sis is derived from a tse gene (or genes) encoding a platelet-derived growth factor. *Science.* 1983;221:275-277.

56. Solberg LA, Strong JP. Risk factors and atherosclerotic lesions: A review of autopsy studies. *Arteriosclerosis.* 1983;3:187-198.

57. Glagov S, Zarins C, Giddens DP, et al. Hemodynamics and atherosclerosis. *Arch Pathol Lab Med.* 1988;112:1018-1031.

58. Friedman MH, Hutchins GM, Bargeron CR, et al. Correlation between intimal thickness and fluid shear in human arteries. *Arteriosclerosis.* 1981;39:425-431.

59. Zarins CK, Giddens DP, Bharadavaj BK, et al. Carotid bifurcation atherosclerosis: quantitation of plaque localization with flow velocity profiles and wall shear stress. *Circ Res.* 1983;53:502-514.

60. Reneman RS, van Merode T, Smeets FAM, et al. Velocity patterns and vessel wall properties in the carotid artery bulb in man−their relationship to atherosclerosis. In: Hennerici M, Sitzer G, Weger HD, eds. *Carotid Artery Plaques.* Basel; Karger; 1988: pp 143-162.

61. Lewis JC, Taylor RG, Normal BS, et al. Endothelial surface characteristics in pigeon coronary atherosclerosis. *Lab Invest.* 1982;46:133-138.

62. Nerum RM, Levesque MJ, Sato M. Mechanical properties of endothelial cells. *Biorrheology.* 1986;23:230.

63. Ku DN, Giddens DP. Pulsatile flow in a model carotid bifurcation. *Arteriosclerosis.* 1983;3:31-39.

64. Gerrity RG, Goss JA, Soby L. Control of monocyte recruitment by chemotactic factor(s) in lesion-prone areas of swine aorta. *Arteriosclerosis.* 1985;5:55-66.

65. Glagov S, Weisenberg E, Zarins CK, et al. Compensatory enlargement of human atherosclerotic coronary arteries. *N Engl J Med.* 1987;316:1371-1375.

66. Guyton JR, Hotley CJ. Flow restriction in one carotid artery in juvenile rats inhibits growth of arterial diameter. *Am J Physiol.* 1985;248:H540-546.

67. Roberts WC. Factors linking cholesterol to atherosclerotic plaques. *Am J Cardiol.* 1988;62:495-499.

68. Yatsu FM, Fisher M. Atherosclerosis: current concepts on pathogenesis and interventional strategies. *Ann Neurol.* 1989;26:3-12.

69. Lewis JC, Taylor RG, Jones ND, et al. Endothelial surface characteristics in pigeon coronary atherosclerosis. *Lab Invest.* 1982;46:123-138.

70. Steinberg D, Parthasarathy S, Carew TE, et al. Beyond cholesterol: modifications of low-density lipoprotein that increase its atherogenicity. *N Engl J Med.* 1989;320:915–924.

71. Mosel DW, DiCarleto PE, Chisolm GM. Endothelial and smooth muscle cells alter low density lipoprotein in vitro by free radical oxidation. *Arteriosclerosis.* 1984;4:357–364.

72. Hiramatsu K, Rosen H, Heinecke JW, et al. Superoxide initiates oxidation of low-density lipoproteins by human monocytes. *Arteriosclerosis.* 1987; 7:55–60.

73. Palinski W, Rosenfeld ME, Yla-Herttualla, et al. Low density lipoprotein undergoes oxidative modification in vivo. *Proc Natl Acad Sci USA.* 1984; 86:1372–1376.

74. Quinn MT, Parthasarathy S, Fong LG, et al. Oxidatively modified low density lipoproteins: a potential role in recruitment and retention of monocyte/macrophages during atherogenesis. *Proc Natl Acad Sci USA.* 1987;84:2995–2998.

75. Kita T, Nagano Y, Yokode M, et al. Probucol prevents the progression of atherosclerosis in Watanabe heritable hyperlipedimic rabbit, an animal model for familial hypercholesterolemia. *Proc Natl Acad Sci USA.* 1987;84:5928–5931.

76. Fisher M, Leaf A, Levine PH. N-3 fatty acids and cellular aspects of atherosclerosis. *Arch Int Med.* 1989;149:1726–1728.

77. Berry CL, Greenwald SE. Effect of hypertension on the static mechanical properties and chemical composition of the rat aorta. *Cardiovasc Res.* 1976; 10:437–451.

78. Sacks AM. The vasa vasorum as a link between hypertension and arteriosclerosis. *Angiology.* 1975; 26:385–390.

79. Fitzgerald GA, Oates JA, Nowak J. Cigarette smoking and hemostatic function. *Am Heart J.* 1981; 115:267–271.

80. Seiffert GF, Keown K, Moore SW. Pathologic effects of tobacco smoke inhalation on arterial intima. *Surg Forum.* 1981;32:353–359.

81. Mjos OD. Lipid effects of smoking. *Am Heart J.* 1988;115:267–271.

82. National Cholesterol Education Program Expert Panel on Detection, Evaluation, and Treatment of High Blood Cholesterol in Adults. Report. *Arch Int Med.* 1988;148:36–69.

83. Taguchi J, Freis ED. Partial reduction of blood pressure and prevention of complications of hypertension. *N Engl J Med.* 1974;291:329–331.

84. Shinton R, Beevers G. Meta-analysis of relation between cigarette smoking and stroke. *Br Med J.* 1989;298:789–794.

85. Goodnight SH, Fisher M, Fitzgerald GA, et al. Assessment of the therapeutic use of dietary fish oil in atherosclerotic vascular disease and thrombosis. *Chest.* 1989;95:19S–25S.

86. Dehmer GF, Popma JJ, Van den Berg EK, et al. Reduction in the rate of early restenosis after coronary angioplasty by a diet supplemented with n-3 fatty acids. *N Engl J Med.* 1988;319:733–740.

87. Weiner BH, Ockene IS, Levine PH, et al. Inhibition of atherosclerosis by cod liver oil in a hyperlipidemic swine model. *N Engl J Med.* 1986;315: 841–846.

88. Kim DN, Ho HT, Lawrence DA, et al. Modification of lipoprotein patterns and retardation of atherogenesis by a fish oil supplement to a hyperlipidemic diet for swine. *Atherosclerosis.* 1989;76: 35–54.

89. Davis HR, Bridenstine RT, Vesselinovitch D, et al. Fish oil inhibits development of atherosclerosis in rhesus monkeys. *Arteriosclerosis.* 1987;7:441–449.

90. Soltys PA, Massone T, Wissler RW. Effects of feeding of fish oil on the properties of lipoproteins isolated from rhesus monkeys consuming an atherogenic diet. *Atherosclerosis.* 1989;76:103–115.

91. Hollander W, Hong S, Kirkpatrick BJ, et al. Differential effects of fish oil supplements on atherosclerosis. *Circulation 70.* 1987; (suppl IV):313.

92. Harris WJ, Dujone CA, Zucker M, et al. Effects of a low saturated fat, low cholesterol fish oil supplement in hypertriglyceridemic patients. *Ann Int Med.* 1988;109:465–470.

93. Knapp HR, Reilly IA, Allessandrini P, et al. In vivo indexes of platelet and vascular function during fish oil administration in patients with atherosclerosis. *N Engl J Med.* 1986;314:939–942.

94. Schmidt EB, Pedersen JO, Ekelund S, et al. Cod liver oil inhibits neutrophil and monocyte chemotaxis in healthy males. *Atherosclerosis.* 1989;77:53–57.

95. Fox PL, DiCarleto PE. Fish oil inhibits endothelial cell production of a platelet-derived growth factor-like protein. *Science.* 1988;241:453–456.

96. Shimokawa H, Vanhoutte PM. Dietary ω-3 polyunsaturated fatty acids and endothelium-dependent relaxations in porcine coronary arteries. *Am J Physiol.* 1989;256:H968–H973.

97. Henry PD. Calcium antagonists as antiatherogenic agents. *Ann N Y Acad Sci.* 1988;522:411–419.

98. Vesselinovitch DJ, Mullan JF, Wissler RW, et al. Carotid atherogenesis inhibited by sympathectomy, propranolol and nifedipine in rhesus monkeys. *Arteriosclerosis.* 1986;6:516a.

99. Parmley WW, Blumlein S, Sievers R. Modification of experimental atherosclerosis by calcium channel blockers. *Am J Cardiol.* 1985;55:165B–171B.

100. Nakao J, Hideki I, Doyama T, et al. Calcium dependency of aortic smooth muscle cell migration induced by 12-L-hydroxy-5.8, 10, 14-eicostatetraenoic acid. *Atherosclerosis*. 1983;46:309–319.

101. Van Valen RG, Deacon RW, Farley C, et al. Antiproliferative effect of calcium channel blockers PN 200–110 and PY 108–068 in the rat carotid model of balloon catheterization. *Fed Proc*. 1985; 44:737.

102. Clones AW, Karnovsky MJ. Suppression by heparin of smooth muscle cell proliferation in injured arteries. *Nature*. 1977;256:625–626.

103. Castellot JJ, Beeler DL, Rosenberg RD, et al. Structural determinants of the capacity of heparin to inhibit the proliferation of vascular smooth muscle cells. *J Cell Physiol*. 1984;120:315–320.

104. Castellot JJ, Favreau LV, Karnovsky MJ, et al. Inhibition of vascular smooth muscle cell growth by endothelial cell-derived heparin—possible role of platelet endoglycosidase. *J Biol Chem*. 1982;257: 11256–11260.

3
Prevention of Atherothrombotic Brain Infarction: Role of Lipids

Frank M. Yatsu and Thomas J. DeGraba

Atherothrombotic brain infarction (ABI) is the primary cause of stroke both in the Western and Eastern worlds. The apparent successes of interventional measures in averting coronary atherosclerosis has fueled interest and optimism in applying these strategies to ABIs, both for primary and secondary prevention.[1] The magnitude of ABIs worldwide and the frustration in having no reliable or effective acute therapies to prevent ischemic brain injury have led to greater efforts to reduce the primary disease of atherosclerosis.[1] Therapeutic approaches in the past for ABI prevention have evolved behind those for coronary heart disease (CHD) and include surgical, medical, and "holistic" interventions through risk reduction. Surgical efforts to reduce strokes were undertaken with carotid endarterectomies for extracranial stenosis in patients with ipsilateral transient ischemic attacks (TIAs)[2,3] and the unsuccessful attempts with extracranial/intracranial (EC/IC) bypass surgery.[4] Medical advances were attempted with anticoagulation, still without confirmatory data, and more recently with the antiplatelet aggregation drugs, aspirin and ticlopidine, to prevent subsequent thrombotic strokes after TIAs.[5-8]

With a "holistic" approach to CHD, the identification and intervention of risk factors implicated hypertension, diabetes mellitus, smoking, elevated cholesterol (particularly low-density lipoprotein, LDL), obesity, stress, and sedentary life.[9-15] While the value of certain risk interventions are debated for ABIs, dramatic reduction of strokes over the past several decades in the United States is largely attributed to better surveillance and control of hypertension.[16,17]

Reduction of other risk factors, such as cholesterol, in decreasing CHD affects the cost/benefit ratio, although measurable reductions in CHD with these strategies are statistically significant.[18,19] Whether similar measures can be extended to ABIs, a temporal and spatial extension of CHD, is uncertain since this intervention has not been tested in a prospective, randomized study. Despite these arguments, it is prudent to attempt to minimize atherosclerosis risks, including reduction of blood cholesterol, to promote atheroma regression.

The essential reasons for this position are twofold. First, the atherosclerotic plaque is a harbinger of ABIs, and elimination or reduction of atheroma should decrease ABI occurrence. Second, attempts to lower elevated blood cholesterol and reduce CHD in otherwise healthy males has direct implications for ABIs.[18,19]

To provide background information to support these arguments for ABI prevention, this chapter will provide biochemical, cellular and molecular biological information on atherogenesis, particularly as it relates to the role of lipids and their association with ABIs. Epidemiological data on risk factors for stroke will be reviewed, including those implicating dietary and blood lipids, as well as studies correlating carotid atherosclerosis with lipid profiles.[20] Lipid and lipoprotein complexities will be discussed within the context of both CHD and ABIs, but especially to develop a foundation for current and future investigations on the fundamental aspects of lipids in atherosclerosis.

The basic studies on atherogenesis focus upon the following: the initial investigations implicating cholesterol; elaboration of lipid-carrying proteins, the lipoproteins; elucidation of their protein sub-classes, called apoproteins; and finally, a discussion of the molecular biological aspects of gene composition and regulation of these proteins and their membrane receptors. Studies supporting the value of cholesterol reduction, particularly the Lipid Research Clinic – Coronary Primary Prevention Trial (LRC-CPPT) and the Helsinki Heart Study, will also be reviewed.[18,19] Finally, a simplified approach to abnormal lipid management is provided as a guide for both primary and secondary ABI reduction.

Risk Factors for Atherothrombotic Brain Infarction

Data from epidemiological studies indicate that risk factors for ABIs are similar to CHD. These findings are not surprising; the underlying pathological process of atherosclerosis is similar histologically. Regular myocardial contractions impose mechanical stresses on coronary arteries, which accounts in part for their earlier manifestation of symptoms, but distinctions exist between intracranial and extracranial arteries, the former being more fibrous in composition. The risk factors for ABI include hypertension, diabetes mellitus, pre-existing CHD, and previous strokes or TIAs.[21-26] Smoking and lack of exercise are uncertain risk factors, but their contributory role was recently demonstrated, as in CHD.[27] With CHD, moderate alcohol consumption is protective.[28] Heavy or "binge" drinking is associated with strokes, but not ABIs.[29]

The most important factor accounting for the dramatic 50% decline in stroke occurrence over the past several decades is attributed to hypertension control, and although hypertension may be considered an independent risk, it can also aggravate and accelerate lipid accumulation in arterial endothelial cells and provoke experimental, diet-induced atherosclerosis.[30]

To focus on the role of lipid abnormalities in ABIs, studies demonstrating an association between abnormal serum lipid changes and ABIs will be emphasized. The older literature on stroke patients is somewhat misleading since there was no evidence of elevated serum cholesterol. Since cho-

lesterol levels stabilize or decrease with age, absolute values without comparison to the normal population may convey the erroneous view that cholesterol is irrelevant to ABIs.[31] With advances in knowledge of the pathophysiology of atherosclerosis, evaluation of lipoprotein patterns has proved to be a more sensitive means of identifying atherosclerosis-prone individuals.[32,33] A number of studies on ABIs now demonstrates either reduced serum high-density lipoprotein (HDL) or increased LDL/HDL ratios. In the future, identification of individuals at risk may be easier by:

1. Analysis of serum apoproteins, the self-contained protein components of the lipoproteins;
2. Analysis of the metabolism of lipoproteins, particularly LDL and HDL, to delineate synthesis and catabolism or fractional catabolic rates, or
3. Gene alteration, so-called gene polymorphism. Investigations on the value and predictive value of apoproteins in serum may necessitate quantitation of these parameters in the future and are discussed below.

Histopathology of Atheromas in Atherothrombotic Brain Infarction

Atheroma is essentially an intimal disorder, but the process involves a variety of cellular and biochemical reactions, both vascular and blood-element related. Histologically, the atheroma has four major features:

1. Abundance of lipids, particularly cholesterol and its ester;
2. Cellular proliferation, largely smooth muscle cells from media that migrate to the intima;
3. Increase in connective tissue elements, such as glycosaminoglycans and elastins; and
4. Macrophages laden with lipids, which appear foamy and hence are called "foam cells."

Each of these histological abnormalities has been a focus of investigative activities. The most promising areas of research are the roles of cholesterol and smooth cell proliferation; these two processes probably interact in provoking atherosclerosis.[34,35]

Elevated levels of LDL can injure arterial endothelium, causing endothelial damage and denudation, the exposed basement membrane provoking platelet adhesion and aggregation. In turn, platelets secrete a variety of substances during the "release reaction," which includes platelet derived growth factor (PDGF), one of a number of powerful growth factors that promote smooth cells in the media to proliferate and migrate to the intima. With elevated levels of LDL, the process of proliferation is sustained, leading eventually to necrosis, calcification, rupture and intraplaque hemorrhage. Since cholesterol is a prominent histological feature, emphasis on controlling cholesterol has caught the investigative imagination of those interested in preventing atherosclerosis.[36-41]

The possible role of reduced HDL in CHD was first suggested in 1975 when a negative correlation was demonstrated between serum HDL and CHD.[42] As early as 1978, Rossner et al. found that reduced HDL correlated with stroke in patients <55 years of age.[43] The following year Sirtori et al.[44] and Taggart and Stout[45] further substantiated the negative correlation of HDL with cerebrovascular disease (including TIAs and ABIs). Reduced levels of HDL in association with strokes is not a uniform finding. Noma et al., in 1979, reported a slight, though not statistically significant, decrease in HDL values in women >50 with strokes, whereas men of this age with strokes showed no changes in HDL levels.[46]

In 1981 Nubiola et al.[47] found a significant reduction of HDL in both men and women with strokes. In their study, 50 stroke patients aged 40 to 78, mean age 59, were compared to 65 control subjects, and the HDL cholesterol level of 41 $\pm$ 13 mg/dl was significantly lower than control values of 54 $\pm$ 16 mg/dl. Blood triglyceride levels were also statistically elevated at 167 $\pm$ 124 mg/dl versus 120 $\pm$ 78 mg/dl.

Subsequently, in 1981, Bihari-Varga et al.[48] and Murai et al.[49] found a negative correlation between stroke and HDL. With more recent clarification and perfection of isolation techniques for HDL, earlier findings and discrepancies may be in part due to technical factors. Also, racial differences may exist. More recently, Grotta et al.[20] (1989) reported their findings in 38 patients with carotid bifurcation stenosis and regular 2-month assessment by noninvasive testing of the bifurcation, lipid profile (LDL, HDL3, and HDL2), and platelet aggregation and coagulation parameters. This study indicates that progression of plaque, i.e., approximately 25% within a year's time or less, is associated with elevated levels of LDL and fibrinogen. There was also a correlation with low levels of HDL and high LDL/HDL ratio, suggesting that a single lipid parameter may not provide the total perspective on the multiple complexities of atherogenesis.

Furthermore, the concentrations of lipids, such as LDL or HDL, do not provide an index of the dynamic metabolic activities of these lipoproteins. Lipoprotein turnover sheds light on both synthesis and catabolism (so-called fractional catabolic rate) and may give a more powerful profile of deranged lipoprotein metabolism.[50]

The role of "foam cells" is controversial. One view is that macrophages protect against atherosclerosis by scavenging extraneous lipid debris in atheromas, but become overloaded. Another is that "foam cells" become the vehicle of self-destruction since they inadvertently release lysosomal enzymes during the process of lipid endocytosis and cause local tissue damage and necrosis, exacerbating the atherosclerotic process. On the basis of our studies on monocyte-derived macrophages from ABI patients and controls, we believe that macrophages play a protective role in promoting atheroma regression. We demonstrated defective "scavenging" of modified LDL, through the so-called "scavenger receptor," a process that can account for atherogenesis since modified LDL is believed to be atherogenic.[51-54]

Cholesterol-loaded macrophages linearly upregulate HDL3 receptors to enhance HDL3 endocytosis. Intracellularly, HDL3 adsorbs both cholesterol and apoprotein E to form a particle identical with HDL2. We believe this lipoprotein subfraction is earmarked for hepatic receptor recognition and uptake for bile transformation. This transformation is the terminal process of "reverse cholesterol transport" with delivery of cholesterol from the periphery, such as vessel wall, to liver for cholesterol disposal.

In summary, the histopathology of atheromas has emphasized its multifactorial characterization, although in initial investigations cholesterol played a central and prominent role in explaining pathogenesis. While CHD is characterized by elevated LDL primarily, with probable secondary reduction in HDL, ABIs are associated with reduced HDL primarily or increased LDL/HDL ratios. To understand more fully the scientific basis implicating lipoproteins, particularly HDL in ABIs, and how these changes are subject to correction with interventional steps to reduce ABIs, the following sections will discuss in greater detail investigations supporting the lipid hypothesis for atherosclerosis.

The Lipid Theory of Atherogenesis

The lipid theory has evolved considerably since its inception, reflecting technological advances for particle isolation and molecular biology. Stages in lipid theory development were:

1. Animal studies;
2. Human investigations;
3. Cholesterol subfractionation into lipoprotein classes;
4. Apoprotein determination;
5. Molecular biological investigations on gene abnormalities or polymorphisms.[55]

Animal Studies

A large number of animal investigations using diets high in cholesterol collectively demonstrate a correlation between high-plasma cholesterol and atheroma. Atherosclerosis is usually found in the coronary circulation or aorta, although some species are resistant and require the additional stress, such as chemically induced hypothyroidism, to produced atheromas. The histological features of atheromas in animals differ from those in humans, such as in the absence of a fibrous "cap" in animal models. Perhaps the model most closely simulating the human condition is diet-induced atherosclerosis in subhuman primates.[56] Diet-induced atheromas reverse with low-cholesterol diets, suggesting a similar role in the human condition.[57] Although diet-induced experimental disease differs from the human condition (particularly in the role of factors other than elevated LDL), the reduction of experimental atherosclerosis by diet suggests a possible relevance to atheroma regression in humans.

Human Investigations

No study similar to experimental, diet-induced atherosclerosis has been undertaken in humans, but both "experiments in nature" and natural history provide evidence supporting the lipid theory for atherosclerosis. For example, in North Karelia, Finland, a diet high in saturated fats and cholesterol is believed to be responsible for accelerated rates of atherosclerosis, particularly CHD.[58] Conversely, while multiple risk-factor intervention was undertaken, dietary intervention is believed to be partly responsible for the reduced incidence of CHD.[59] The CHD rate of 467 per 100 000 population (one of the highest in the world) fell significantly, with a 38% and 50% reduction in stroke occurring in men and women, respectively.[58] Other similar studies in various areas of the world with high incidences of atherosclerosis have implicated increased dietary cholesterol and fat in causing early symptomatic atherosclerosis. Diets low in cholesterol and saturated fats are accompanied by low incidences of symptomatic atherosclerosis. This was seen in World War II, with limited food supplies in Europe, or in vegetarians and lacto-vegetarians, as in certain religious sects, such as the Mormons and Seventh Day Adventists.[59] Disturbingly, and as yet inexplicably, certain forms of cancer are inversely related to dietary lipids.

As an experiment in nature, familial hypercholesterolemia (FH) provided the most dramatic evidence that elevated LDL was a cause of symptomatic atherosclerosis. Studies by Brown and Goldstein into the molecular biology of FH led to the most fundamental breakthroughs in understanding the disease process, particularly receptor-mediated endocytosis and even "reverse cholesterol transport."[60]

In summary, worldwide epidemiological studies, such as that of Keys and his seven-nation study,[61] have demonstrated the relationship between dietary or plasma cholesterol and CHD and have provided powerful proof of the role of cholesterol in atherogenesis.

Cholesterol Subfractionation

Since the 1950s, a great deal of information has been gained on the particles carrying cholesterol in blood. Advances in knowledge coincided with greater sophistication in separation techniques, such as ultracentrifugation and electrophoretic methods. Because lipids such as cholesterol are insoluble in aqueous solutions such as plasma, cholesterol must be packaged in a hydrophilic protein envelope. With ultracentrifugation, classes of protein-carrying lipids (lipoproteins) were isolated and identified. Initial characterizations were based upon relative densities to serum, which is approximately 1.006. Thus, separate lipoproteins, having varying quantities of lipid, which makes the particle less dense, and protein, making it more dense, were identified. Low-density lipoprotein, very low density lipoprotein (VLDL), and HDL are the major subfractions for the cholesterol-carrying proteins in blood.[62]

With advances in the chemical and structural analyses of lipoproteins, both their metabolic fate and composition were determined. Both in vivo and in vitro studies demonstrated that liver synthesized cholesterol and exogenous dietary cholesterol, are both packaged in the protein, VLDL, which has a large amount of triglyceride. This particle has a diameter of 50–80 Å and a half-life of several hours and becomes converted to an intermediate density lipoprotein (IDL) after losing triglycerides to muscle and adipose tissues. Triglycerides are an energy source in muscle and an energy storage form in adipose tissues. Because of apoprotein B100 on IDL, it is taken up by the liver, but a fraction remains for conversion to the final form, LDL. Low density lipoprotein delivers cholesterol to all cells through the LDL receptor after receptor binding with its single apoprotein B100. Low-density lipoprotein is 200 Å in diameter and has a half-life in the circulation of nearly 3 days. Because LDL is composed primarily of cholesterol and its ester, it makes up approximately two thirds of the total plasma cholesterol concentration. For reasons not clearly understood, but related to its elevated level, increases in LDL are associated with accelerated atherosclerosis, presumably because it has a damaging effect on vascular endothelium.[1]

A closely related compound to LDL is lipoprotein (a) or LP(a), implicated as a risk factor in atherosclerosis. The compound is well characterized and is essentially a LDL with a long protein molecule linked through sulfhydryl bonds on apoprotein B.

Lipoprotein (a) has been sequenced and cloned. It is not known whether it is linked independently to atherosclerosis. However, the unusual structure and its close link to LDL suggest it is a paraphenomenon; its fragile nature is suggested by its ready dissociation with a reducing agent.[63,64]

High-density lipoprotein is relatively dense compared to plasma, largely because of high protein and low lipid content. On centrifugation or electrophoresis, two or more HDLs are separated, representing a continuum of both interchange and metabolism. On the basis of epidemiological studies on the inverse relationship between HDL and CHD, HDL operates to deliver cholesterol from the periphery to liver for bile transformation, or the so-called reverse cholesterol transport.

These theoretical assumptions made from epidemiological associations were strengthened by in vitro studies demonstrating that cholesterol-loaded cells released cholesterol primarily and selectively to HDL that had a high affinity to hepatic receptor cells. More recently, on the basis of injected acetylated-LDL in animals subsequently given HDL, clear evidence of in vivo documentation of reverse cholesterol transport with HDL exists.[65] In our studies using monocyte-derived macrophages, HDL3 is taken up by cholesterol-loaded macrophages that express HDL3 receptors in response to intracellular cholesterol, and the endocytosed HDL3 is serially associated with cholesterol and apoprotein E and then exocytosed with little lysosomal catabolism. We believe these findings support a receptor-regulated control of HDL3 to HDL2 conversion, and that by participating in this activity, macrophages operate to reduce atherogenesis.[66]

Apoprotein Determination

With increased technical and chemical sophistication for particle separation and protein analyses, the protein structure of lipoproteins was determined. When the lipoproteins were subjected to peptic digestion, the remaining larger fractions were analysed and characterized. Alphabetical nomenclature identifies these large fragments, and most apoproteins have been studied with molecular biological techniques to identify the exact genomic sequences regulating apoprotein synthesis. For example, the major protein for LDL is apoprotein B100, synthesized in the liver (B48 is synthesized in the gut). High-density lipoprotein's major apoproteins are AI, AII and CII. Plasma determination of apoproteins may be a more precise means of defining atherosclerosis risk, but since apo B is primarily associated with LDL and apo AI and AII are with HDL, the apoprotein quantitation should reflect primarily their parent lipoprotein.[67-69]

Molecular and Cellular Biology and the Dynamic Metabolism of Lipoproteins

The insightful studies of Brown and Goldstein on the regulation of cholesterol synthesis in FH led to their defining receptor-mediated endocytosis and sequencing the LDL receptor. They received the Nobel Prize in medicine for this work in 1985.[61] The simple observation that fibroblasts from FH would not down-regulate endogenous cholesterol synthesis with increasing concentrations of LDL in the media, unlike normal controls, suggested that a membrane property or receptor regulated the entrance of LDL to the cytoplasm. This led to the definition of the important cellular processes of endocytosis and to molecular biological insights into atherogenesis by defining specific gene defects accounting for abnormalities in the receptor structure.

While specific structural defects do not account for symptomatic atherosclerosis in the general population, the consistent abnormality in these patients is elevated LDL, which translates to cholesterol overload. But in addition to the cholesterol overload, cholesterol efflux is clearly an important factor in the continuum of cholesterol metabolism and homeostasis. With a clearer definition of HDL and its functions in reverse cholesterol transport, evaluation of studies on atherosclerosis suggests that low plasma concentrations of HDL may be a more crucial feature in provoking atherosclerosis.

To gain further insights into the molecular and cellular biological aspects of HDL in ABIs, we have undertaken studies on the synthesis and fractional catabolic rates of HDL and ABI patients and controls. These investigations involve the isolation and purification of an individual's HDL, followed by iodination with 125-Iodine. After it is tested to exclude contaminants, the compound is injected

into the same subject after oral dosing of potassium iodide to protect the thyroid from irradiation. After an equilibrium period, blood is drawn daily for 10 days. On the basis of an analysis of synthesis rate, derived from the HDL3's specific activity, and fractional catabolic rate, calculated from the daily decline in radioactivity, patients and controls can be compared. From our preliminary data, ABI patients show both a more rapid catabolism compared to controls of HDL3 and a poor conversion to HDL2, suggesting that HDL3 is poorly utilized for reverse cholesterol transport. LDL is more slowly catabolized than controls. In addition to identifying individuals at risk for ABI on the basis of their dynamics of HDL metabolism we believe that anti-atherogenic therapies can be objectively evaluated.

Since abnormal protein structure of the major apoprotein of HDL3 may be present, namely, of apoprotein AI, we are comparing individuals at risk for ABI — either with TIAs, strokes, or carotid stenosis — with controls. With a 2.2 kb probe for apoprotein AI, kindly given to us by Professor Karathanasis of Harvard Medical School, we have probed the leukocyte genome of 3.3 billion base pairs in > 100 patients and controls. Our preliminary findings indicate that gene polymorphism with the restriction enzyme SacI and PstI are present in stroke-prone individuals, but particularly of SacI plus hypertriglyceridemia with ABIs. Further studies are needed to determine the degree, importance, and frequency of this finding in predicting accelerated atherosclerosis and ABIs, but, possibly, ABI risk can be determined using powerful molecular biological techniques identifying gene alterations or polymorphisms.[70,71]

Clinical Disorders Associated with Accelerated Atherosclerosis

A variety of diseases is associated with accelerated atherosclerosis, but since CHD is symptomatic at an earlier age than ABIs, it has dominated their clinical presentation. For example, the familial hyperlipidemias, types IIa and IIb, including FH, III, and IV, are associated with accelerated atherosclerosis of the carotid bifurcation, but it is symptomatic later than potentially fatal CHD. Nonetheless, because of the risk of ABIs in these patients, the carotid bifurcation should be assessed with noninvasive tests and used to monitor the effectiveness of cholesterol-lowering therapies.[72]

Diabetes mellitus is particularly prone to accelerated atherosclerosis, and while the exact mechanism for this is not clear, elevated cholesterol and LDL may play a contributory role. Because of this possibility, elevated levels of LDL warrant aggressive therapy, including the use of cholesterol-lowering agents, such as lovastatin or gemfibrozil.[73,74]

In our study mentioned above, organized by Dr. James C. Grotta, 38 individuals with asymptomatic carotid stenosis were followed at 2-month intervals for 2 years with noninvasive tests of the bifurcation, lipid profiles (cholesterol, LDL, HDL3 and HDL2), platelet aggregation, and coagulation parameters. Eight patients demonstrated progression, gauged as nearly 25% increase in focal stenosis in <1 year, and these patients demonstrated concomitantly high levels of LDL and fibrinogen. In addition, there was a strong correlation between low levels of HDL (<30 mg/dl) and high ratios of LDL/HDL, with the rate of carotid stenosis. The data were not enough to reach statistical significance, but the findings suggest that in patients with ABI, critical reductions of HDL (or increased ratios of LDL/HDL) require aggressive intervention to normalize their lipid profile using strategies outlined below.[20]

Prevention of Symptomatic Atherosclerosis by Correction of Abnormal Lipoprotein Patterns

Although the Multiple Risk Factor Intervention Trial (MRFIT)[75] did not display any convincing reduction in symptomatic atherosclerosis by correcting the risk factors for atherosclerosis, two other highly targeted studies did demonstrate improved outcome by reducing elevated serum cholesterol. These were the Lipid Research Clinic -Coronary Primary Prevention Trial (LRC-CPPT)[18] and the Helsinki Heart Study,[19] in which asymptomatic males in the middle years with elevated cholesterol (>260 mg/dl) were treated in a randomized, double-blind fashion to determine the effects of cholesterol reduction on primary and secondary end points for CHD. In the LRC-CPPT

study, nearly 7000 males were randomly assigned to a low-cholesterol diet and placebo or that diet plus the bile-sequestrant cholestyramine. In >7 years' average follow-up, significant reductions in CHD end points began after 2 years.

Recent arguments have surfaced in both the lay and medical press on the significance of these findings in terms of "real" numbers or cost/benefit.[76,77] Despite the uncertainty in predicting response and the relatively small numbers benefiting, improvement is a powerful reason to continue interventions. It also underscores the need to define more precisely those who may benefit from interventional therapies.[78]

Preventive Management of Hyperlipidemias in Stroke-Prone Individuals

Preventing strokes in patients at risk requires management of risk factors such as reduction of serum cholesterol, specifically, to reduce LDL and increase HDL. For hypertension, diabetes mellitus, smoking, sedentary lifestyle, stress, and obesity, control should be achieved as soon as possible. Successful intervention requires a highly motivated patient and the physician's involvement in instructing patients on the importance of changing their lifestyle. Also, patients with TIAs should be treated with medical or surgical prophylaxis.

Strategies to decrease LDL and raise HDL involve two sequential steps. The first is to institute a diet low in cholesterol (<300 mg/d), low in saturated fats (<30% of the total dietary fats, which should represent no >30% of the entire dietary calories), and high in polyunsaturated fats. Controversies remain as to the additional benefits obtained from diets high in monounsaturated fatty acids.[79,80] Diets compatible with this regimen are low in red meat, high in fish and fowl, low in butter and milk, and low in eggs. In our experience, the most crucial feature in implementing this so-called Prudent Diet of the American Heart Association is the patient's motivation to change his or her lifestyle. Unless this attitude is established through interaction with the physician, lectures, seminars, and consultation with dieticians are not successful.[81]

According to the Consensus Panel on Cholesterol[82] as well as the American Heart Association[83] and the European Heart Association,[84] plasma cholesterol >240 mg/dl should be lowered. Levels between 200 and 240 mg/dl are borderline, and attempts to reduce the levels further must be taken within the context of the medical condition of the patient. For lipoprotein levels, HDL concentrations <30–35 mg/dl are low, and for LDL, levels >150–160 mg/dl are high. These values are generic and risks differ: adjustments are needed according to age and sex.[85]

Drug therapy is indicated for cholesterol elevations not responding to conservative management with diet, exercise, weight reduction, and stress management. These include bile sequestrants, drugs that reduce cholesterol synthesis or increase HDL concentrations.

Bile sequestrants such as cholestyramine or colestipol are used first since they are relatively benign. They may cause nausea and should be taken with a vehicle such as orange juice, but nausea may cause patients to discontinue therapy.[73]

Dramatic advances in the medical therapy of hypercholesterolemia have resulted from the use of cholesterol-lowering agents, such as the fungi-derived enzymes lovastatin or mevinolin. These inhibit the rate-limiting enzyme for cholesterol synthesis, HMG CoA reductase, plus increase hepatic LDL receptors. Gemfibrozil, 600 mg twice daily, will lower LDL and increase HDL[18,19] in patients with low HDL, particularly with levels <30–35 mg/dl.

lipoprotein synthesis, catabolism, receptor activity, intracellular processing, or other as yet unknown vascular or lipid factors that require precise intervention. For example, on the basis of our unpublished studies on lipoprotein receptor activity in macrophages and their response to a variety of calcium channel blockers, patients with specific receptor impairment may benefit from the action of certain calcium channel blockers to optimize receptor activity for HDL and LDL.[86–89]

Until these strategies for specific intervention for lipid abnormalities are developed, intervention in conditions (such as progressing carotid stenosis or stroke patients with abnormal lipid profiles) must be simple and effective. First, reduce all known risk factors and optimize the lipid profile, specifically lowering LDL and increasing HDL concentrations. Initial attempts should be dietary control combined with weight loss and exercise, but if these fail after a trial of at least several months, drug therapy should be instituted to optimize the LDL and HDL concentrations.

While no prospective study has yet been instituted on the value of lowering cholesterol (or decreasing the LDL/HDL ratio) in averting ABIs, the extension of interventions to reduce coronary heart disease will likely prevent strokes due to ABIs.

Acknowledgments. This study was supported by the Clayton Foundation for Research, Houston, Texas, USA. This report is dedicated to Professor Carlo Loeb of Genoa, Italy, on the occasion of his retirement.

Future Strategies to Optimize the Lipoprotein Profile of Stroke-Prone Individuals

Future strategies to reduce stroke risk will depend on more precise measurements of impaired lipoprotein metabolism due to receptor activities, both LDL and HDL, as well as genetic factors predisposing to ABIs. This is suggested by preliminary studies on the restriction fragment length polymorphisms (RFLP) on the major apoprotein of HDL, apoprotein AI. It is predicted that future interventions will be multifactorial, guided by specific knowledge of metabolic defects, such as

References

1. Yatsu FM, Fisher M. Atherosclerosis: current concepts on pathogenesis and interventional therapies. *Ann Neurol.* 1989;26:3–12.
2. Grotta JC. Current medical and surgical therapy for cerebrovascular disease. *N Engl J Med.* 1987;316: 1505–1516.
3. The Asymptomatic Carotid Atherosclerosis Study Group. Study design for randomization prospective trial of carotid endarterectomy for asymptomatic atherosclerosis. *Stroke.* 1989;20:844–849.
4. The EC/IC bypass Study Group. Failure of extracranial-intracranial arterial bypass to reduce the risk of ischemic stroke: results of an international randomized trial. *N Engl J Med.* 1985;313:1191–1200.

5. Fields WS, Lemak NA, et al. Controlled trial of aspirin in cerebral ischemia. *Stroke.* 1977;8:301–316.

6. The American-Canadian Co-operative Study Group. Persantine aspirin trial in cerebral ischemia, part II. Endpoint results. *Stroke.* 1985;16:406–415.

7. UK-TIA Study Group. United Kingdom transient ischemic attack (UK-TIA) aspirin trial: interim results. *Br Med J.* 1988;296:316–320.

8. Hass WK, Easton JD, Adams HP, et al. A randomized trial comparing Ticlopidine Hydrochloride with aspirin for the prevention of stroke in high-risk patients. *N Engl J Med.* 1989;321:501–507.

9. Grundy SM, Greenland P, et al. Cardiovascular and risk factor evaluation of healthy American adults–a statement for physicians by an ad hoc committee appointed by the steering committee, American Heart Association. *Circulation.* 1987;75:1340A–1362A.

10. Kannel WB, McGee DC. Diabetes and cardiovascular disease: the Framingham study. *JAMA.* 1979;241:2035–2038.

11. Strategies for the prevention of coronary heart disease: a policy statement of the European Atherosclerosis Society. *Eur Heart J.* 1987;8:77–88.

12. Castelli WP, Garrison RJ, et al. Incidence of coronary heart disease and lipoprotein cholesterol levels: the Framingham study. *JAMA.* 1986;256:2835–2838.

13. Lipid Research Clinics Program. The lipid research clinics coronary primary prevention trial results: II. The relationship of reduction in incidence of coronary heart disease to cholesterol lowering. *JAMA.* 1984;251:365–374.

14. Leon AS, Connett J, et al. Leisure-time physical activity levels and risk of coronary heart disease and death: The multiple risk factor intervention trial. *JAMA.* 1987;258:2388–2395.

15. Kannel WB, Wilson P, Blair SN. Epidemiological assessment of the role of physical activity and fitness in the development of cardiovascular disease. *Am Heart J.* 1985;109:876–885.

16. Hypertension Detection and Follow-up Program Cooperative Group. Five-year findings: III. Reduction in stroke incidence among persons with high blood pressure. *JAMA.* 1982;247:663–683.

17. Whelton PK. Declining mortality from hypertension and stroke. *South Med J.* 1982;75:33–38.

18. The Lipid Research Clinics Coronary Primary Prevention Trial results. I. Reduction in incidence of coronary heart disease. II. The relationship of reduction in incidence of coronary heart disease to cholesterol lowering. *JAMA.* 1984;251:351–364.

19. Frick MH, Elo O, Haapa K, et al. Helsinki Heart Study: Primary prevention trial with gemfibrozil in middle-aged men with dyslipidemia: safety of treatment, changes in risk factors and incidence of coronary heart disease. *N Engl J Med.* 1987;317:1237–1245.

20. Grotta JC, Yatsu FM, et al. Prediction of carotid stenosis progression by lipid and hematological measurements. *Neurology.* 1989;39:1325–1331.

21. Yatsu FM, Becker C, McLeroy KR, et al. Community hospital based stroke programs: North Carolina, Oregon and New York: I. Goals, objectives and data collection procedures. *Stroke.* 1986;17:276–284.

22. Abbott RD, Donahue RP, et al. Diabetes and the risk of stroke: the Honolulu heart program. *JAMA.* 1987;257:949–952.

23. Kannel WB, Wolf PA, McGee DL, et al. Systolic blood pressure, arterial rigidity and risk of stroke: the Framingham study. *JAMA.* 1981;245:1225–1229.

24. Price TR, Dambrosia J, et al. Early determination of prognosis for 30 day and 1 year survival in ischemic infarction. The NINCDS stroke data bank. *Neurology.* 1985;35 (suppl 1):212.

25. Sacco RL, Foulkes MA, Mohr JP, et al. Determinants of early recurrence of cerebral infarction: stroke data bank. *Stroke.* 1988;19:144.

26. Dexter DD Jr, Whisnant JP, et al. The association of stroke and coronary heart disease: a population study. *Mayo Clin Proc.* 1987;62:1077–1083.

27. Abbott RD, Yin Y, Reed DM, et al. Risk of stroke in male cigarette smokers. *N Engl J Med.* 1986;315:717–720.

28. Stampfer MJ, Colditz GA, et al. A prospective study of moderate alcohol consumption and the risk of coronary disease and stroke in women. *N Engl J Med.* 1988;319:267–273.

29. Gill J, Zezuika, AV, et al. Stroke and alcohol consumption. *N Engl J Med.* 1986;315:1041–1046.

30. Fry DL, Manley RW, Oh SY, Smyt CR. Aortic transmural serum protein transport: effect of concentration time and location. *Am J Physiology.* 1981;241:1454–1461.

31. Gordon, T. The Framingham diet study: diet and the regulation of serum cholesterol. In: Kannel WB, Gordon T, eds. *Framingham Study: An Epidemiological Investigation of Cardiovascular Disease.* Section 24. Washington, DC: Government Printing Office; 1970.

32. Steinberg D. Lipoproteins and the pathogenesis of atherosclerosis. *Circulation.* 1987;76:508–514.

33. Mahley RW. Atherogenic hyperlipoproteinemia. The cellular and molecular biology of plasma lipoproteins altered by dietary fat and cholesterol. *Med Clin North Am.* 1982;66:375–400.

34. Ross R. The pathogenesis of atherosclerosis—an update. *N Engl J Med*. 1986;295:369–377.

35. Jonasson L, Holm J, Skalli O, et al. Regional accumulation of T cells, macrophages and smooth muscle cells in the human atherosclerotic plaque. *Arteriosclerosis*. 1986;6:131–138.

36. Ross R, Glomset J, Kariya B, et al. A platelet-dependent serum factor that stimulates the proliferation of arterial smooth muscle cells in vitro. *Proc Natl Acad Sci USA*. 1974;71:1207–1210.

37. Joris I, Zand T, Nunnari JJ, et al. Studies on the pathogenesis of atherosclerosis: I. Adhesion and emigration of mononuclear cells in the aorta of hypercholesterolemic rats. *Am J Pathol*. 1983;113:341–385.

38. Brown MS, Goldstein JL. Lipoprotein metabolism in macrophages: implications for cholesterol deposition in atherosclerosis. *Annu Rev Biochem*. 1983;52:223–261.

39. Fielding CJ, Fielding PE. Cholesterol transport between cells and body fluids. *Med Clin North Am*. 1982;66:363–373.

40. Schmitz G, Niemann R, Brennhausen B, et al. Regulation of high density lipoprotein receptors in cultured macrophages: role of acyl-CoA: cholesterol acyltransferase. *EMBO J*. 1985;4:2773–2779.

41. Stein O, Halperin G, Stein Y: Cholesteryl ester efflux from extracellular and cellular elements of the arterial wall. *Arteriosclerosis*. 1986;6:70–78.

42. Miller GM, Miller NE. Plasma high density lipoprotein concentration and development of ischaemic heart disease. *Lancet*. 1975;1:16–18.

43. Rossner S, Kjellin KG, Mettinger KL, et al. Normal serum cholesterol but low high density lipoprotein cholesterol concentrations in young patients with ischaemic cerebrovascular disease. *Lancet*. 1978;1:577–579.

44. Sirtori CR, Gainfrancheschi G, Gritti I, et al. Decreased levels of high-density lipoprotein cholesterol levels in male patients with transient ischemic attacks. *Atherosclerosis*. 1979;30:205–211.

45. Taggart H, Stout RW. Reduced high density lipoprotein in stroke: relationship with elevated triglyceride and hypertension. *Eur J Clin Invest*. 1979;9:219–221.

46. Noma A, Matshushita S, Komori T, et al. High and low density lipoprotein cholesterol in myocardial and cerebral infarction. *Atherosclerosis*. 1979;32:327–331.

47. Nubiola AR, Masana L, Masdeu S, et al. High density lipoprotein but low high density lipoprotein cholesterol concentrations in young patients with ischaemic cerebrovascular disease. *Lancet*. 1978;1:577–579.

48. Bihari-Varga M, Szekely J, Gruber E. Plasma high density lipoproteins in coronary, cerebral and peripheral vascular disease: the influence of various risk factors. *Atherosclerosis*. 1981;40:337–345.

49. Murai A, Tanaka T, Miyahara T, Kameyama M. Lipoprotein abnormalities in the pathogenesis of cerebral infarction and transient ischemic attack. *Stroke*. 1981;12:167–172.

50. Brinton, EA, Eisenberg S, Breslow JL. Elevated high density lipoprotein cholesterol levels correlate with decreased apolipoprotein A-1 and A-II fractional catabolic rate in women. *J Clin Invest*. 1989;84:262–269.

51. Yatsu FM, Alam R, Alam S. Scavenger activity in monocyte-derived macrophages from atherothrombotic strokes. *Stroke*. 1986;17:709–713.

52. Hartung HP, Kladetzky RG, Melnik B, et al. Stimulation of the scavenger receptor on monocyte-macrophage evokes release of arachidonic acid metabolites and reduced oxygen species. *Lab Invest*. 1986;55:209–216.

53. Gerrity RG. The role of the monocyte in atherogenesis: I. Transition of blood-borne monocytes into foam cells in fatty lesions. *Am J Pathol*. 1981;103:181–190.

54. Van Lenten BJ, Fogelman AM, Jackson RL, et al. Receptor-mediated uptake of remnant lipoproteins by cholesterol-loaded human monocyte-macrophages. *J Biol Chem*. 1985;260:8783–8788.

55. Wissler RW. Principles of the pathogenesis of atherosclerosis. In: Braunwald E. ed. *Heart Disease*. Philadelphia, PA: W.B. Saunders Co.; 1980: pp 1221–1245.

56. Faggiotto A, Ross R, Harker L: Studies of hypercholesterolemia in the nonhuman primate: II. Fatty streak conversion to fibrous plaque. *Arteriosclerosis*. 1984;45:341–356.

57. Malinow MR, Blaton V. Regression of atherosclerotic lesions. *Arteriosclerosis*. 1984;4:292–295.

58. Salonen JT, Puska P, Mustaniemi H. Changes in morbidity and mortality during comprehensive community programme to control cardiovascular diseases during 1972–77 in North Karelia. *Br Med J*. 1979;2:1178–1183.

59. West RO, Hayes OB. Diet and serum cholesterol levels: a comparison between vegetarians and non-vegetarians in a Seventh Day Adventist group. *Am J Clin Nutr*. 1986;21:853.

60. Brown MS, Goldstein JL. A receptor-mediated pathway for cholesterol homeostasis. *Science*. 1986;232:34–47.

61. Keys A. Coronary heart disease in seven countries. *Circulation*. 1970;41 (suppl 1):1–8.

62. Havel RJ. Classification of hyperlipidemias. *Ann Rev Med*. 1977;28:195–209.

63. Scanu AM. Lipoprotein (a): A potential bridge between the fields of atherosclerosis and thrombosis. *Arch Pathol Lab Med*. 1988;112:1045–1047.

64. Zenker G, Koltringer P, Bone G, et al. Lipoprotein (a) as a strong indicator for cerebrovascular disease. *Stroke*. 1986;17:942–945.

65. van Berkel JC, Bakkeren HF, Kuipers F, et al. In vivo evidence for reverse cholesterol transport from liver endothelial cells to parenchymal cells and bile by high density lipoproteins. Tenth International Symposium on Drugs Affecting Lipid Metabolism; November 8–11, 1989:47. Abstract 223.

66. Alam R, Yatsu FM, Tsui L, Alam S. Receptor-mediated uptake and "retroendocytosis" of high-density lipoproteins by cholesterol-loaded human monocyte-derived macrophages: possible role in enhancing reverse cholesterol transport. *Biochimica et Biophysica Acta*. 1989;1004:292–299.

67. Brunzell JD, Sniderman AD, Albers JJ, et al. Apoproteins B and A-I and coronary heart disease. *Arteriosclerosis*. 1984;4:79–83.

68. Wallentin L, Sundin B. HDL2 and HDL3 lipid levels in coronary heart disease and other causes. *Atherosclerosis*. 1986;59:3–104.

69. Norum RA, Lakier JB, Goldstein S, et al. Familial deficiency of apolipoprotein A-I and C-III and precocious coronary heart disease. *N Engl J Med*. 1986; 306:1513–1519.

70. Karathanasis SK, Zannis VI, Breslow JL. A DNA insertion in the human apoprotein A-I gene locus related to the development of atherosclerosis. *Nature*. 1983;301:718.

71. Rees A, Stocks J, Sharpe CR, et al. DNA polymorphism in the apoprotein A-I-CIII gene cluster. *J Clin Invest*. 195;76:1090–1095.

72. Roederer GD, Langlois YE, Jagar KA, et al. The natural history of carotid arterial disease in asymptomatic patients with cervical bruits. *Stroke*. 1984; 15:605–613.

73. Garg A, Grundy SM. Lovastatin for lowering cholesterol levels in non-insulin-dependent diabetes mellitus. *N Engl J Med*. 1988;318:81–86.

74. Bilheimer DW, Grundy SW, Brown MS, et al. Mevinolin and colestipol stimulate receptor-mediated clearance in familial hypercholesterolemia heterozygotes. *Proc Natl Acad Sci USA*. 1983;80: 4124–4128.

75. Multiple Risk Factor Intervention Trial Research Group. Risk factor changes and mortality results. *JAMA*. 1982;248:1465–1477.

76. Moore, TJ. The cholesterol myth. *Atlantic Monthly*. September 1989. pp 37–70.

77. Brett A. Treating hypercholesterolemia – how should practicing physicians interpret the published data for patients? *N Engl J Med*. 1989;321:676–680.

78. Leaf A. Management of hypercholesterolemia – are creative interventions advisable? *N Engl J Med*. 321:680–684.

79. Mensink RP, Katan MB. Effects of a diet enriched with monounsaturated or polyunsaturated fatty acids on levels of low-density and high density lipoprotein cholesterol in healthy women and men. *N Engl J Med*. 1989;321:436–441.

80. Mattson FH, Grundy SM. Comparison of effects of dietary saturated, monounsaturated and polyunsaturated fatty acids on plasma lipids and lipoproteins in man. *J Lipid Res*. 1985;26:194–202.

81. AHA Special Report. Recommendations for the treatment of hyperlipidemia in adults: a joint statement of the Nutrition Committee and the Council on Arteriosclerosis. *Circulation*. 1984;69, 1065A.

82. Consensus Conference. Lowering blood cholesterol to prevent heart disease. *JAMA*. 1985;253:2080–2086.

83. American Heart Association Committee Report. Rationale of the diet-heart statement of the American Heart Association. *Circulation*. 1982;65:839–854.

84. Strategy for the Prevention of Coronary Heart Disease. A policy statement of the European Atherosclerosis Society. *Eur Heart J*. 1987;8:77–88.

85. Hoeg JM, Gregg RE, Brewer HBV Jr. An approach to the management of hyperlipoproteinemias. *JAMA*. 1986;255:512.

86. Yatsu FM, Alam R, Alam S. Enhancement of cholesteryl ester metabolism in cultured human monocyte-derived macrophages by Verapamil. *Biochim Biophys Acta*. 1985;847:77–81.

87. Kramsch DM, Aspen AJ, Apstein CS. Suppression of experimental atherosclerosis by the calcium antagonist lanthanum. Possible role of calcium in atherogenesis. *J Clin Invest*. 1980;65:967–981.

88. Parmley WW, Blumlein S, Sievers R. Modification of experimental atherosclerosis by calcium channel blockers. *Am J Cardiol*. 1985;55:165B–171B.

89. Betz E, Hammerle H, Strohschneider T. Inhibition of smooth muscle cell proliferation and endothelial cell permeability with Flunarizine in vitro and in experimental atheromas. *Res Exp Med*. 1985;185: 325–340.

4
Regression of Atherosclerosis

Michael G. Hennerici

Several studies carried out on animal models indicate regression of experimental atherosclerosis after the return to a normal or hypocaloric diet, either alone or in combination with various drugs.[1-6] However, pathoanatomic, epidemiologic, and clinical studies in man on this subject are not unanimous.[7-10] Arguments in favor of regression of atherosclerosis in man are:

1. The capacity of arteries to adapt and to recover from previous lesions;
2. The inflammatory rather than degenerative nature of atherosclerosis;
3. The slow and variable course of the disease from its onset in early infancy to senescence;
4. The encouraging results of animal experiments and, recently, of plasmapheresis in homozygous and heterozygous patients with low-density lipoprotein (LDL) receptor abnormalities.

However, there are several problems in evaluating regression, namely,

1. The inaccessibility of the lipid material and cell detritus in the core of the plaque to humoral and cellular recovery mechanisms;
2. The lack of methods to monitor accurately the course of the disease in vivo, as well as the limited usefulness of criteria to establish regression in man; and
3. Extrapolation of results of animal studies to man.

This chapter reviews experimental models of atherosclerosis regression in nonprimate and primate animals as well as recent attempts to document similar developments in man. Most of the material reported deals with the aorta[11,12] and the coronary arteries[13] so that the few available data on carotid and cerebral arteries are of particular interest.[14-17]

Many studies have concentrated on mechanisms such as the balance of cellular uptake of lipoproteins versus the removal of cholesterol esters,[18-20] both of which have been major strategies for diet and drug regimens. Similarly, mechanisms influencing the eicosanoid balance, the metabolism of essential fatty acids (e.g., eicosapentaenoic acid) to prevent thrombosis and atherosclerosis, and the role of calcium and calcium antagonists[21,22] have been investigated in experimental and clinical trials.[23]

The potential clinical implication of much of this work is uncertain, and few studies relate to the significance of hemostatic variables and calcium flux for atherosclerotic regression.[24] Differences in the extent and type of atherosclerosis in different species[25] and vascular territories are also discussed, since the etiology and duration of atherogenesis varies considerably among nonprimate animals, primate models, and man, and the studies reported also vary widely in methodology and design.

Stages of Atherogenesis

The classification of atherogenesis is briefly described with special reference to the terminology used in many angiographic and ultrasound studies (Table 4.1).[26,27]

TABLE 4.1. Classification of atherogenesis and suggested mechanisms of regression.

Stages	Pathology	Mechanisms involved
Initial phase	Fatty streaks	cholesterol depletion
		Inhibition of immunomediated processes
	Lipid plaques	Endothelial recovery
		Reduction of macrophage/monocyte generating toxic metabolites
		Lipid elimination from SMC and macrophages
		Inhibition of platelet function
	Fibrous plaques	SMC atrophy and loss of proliferation
		Intimal thinning
		Cholesterol efflux and transport
		Restructuring with loss of foam cells
		Lipophagocytosis
Advanced phase	Soft plaques	Disintegration of cells
		Breakdown of extracellular space
		Resolution of cell necrosis
		Monocyte enzyme activity
		Lipolysis
		Loss of foam cells
	Hard plaques	Vessel ectasia and dilatation
Complications	Plaque hemorrhage	Intraplaque hemorrhage resolution
		Plaque disrupture and reendothelialization
	Thromboembolism	Eicosanoid activity and fibrinolysis

Lipoid Lesions

A fatty streak is an intimal fatty lesion without other underlying changes. These lesions are flat, and since there is no luminal narrowing, they are difficult to identify in vivo either by angiogram or ultrasound. Lipid-laden macrophages in the aorta of cholesterol-fed rabbits were first described by Anitschkow and Chalatow.[28] Later observations in nonhuman primates, pigs, and genetically hyperlipidemic rabbits indicated that attachment of monocytes to the endothelial surface is one of the earliest cellular events. Macrophages can penetrate between endothelial cells and enter the subendothelial space. Identification of the cell types involved at this stage of atherogenesis has greatly improved with the development of immunocytochemical techniques, which use antibodies specific for macrophages and smooth muscle cells (SMC). Both are major cellular components of the atheromatous lesion. Recent immunohistochemical analyses have demonstrated activated macrophages and T lymphocytes in the fatty streaks. A cell-mediated immune response is considered important in the pathogenesis of human atherosclerosis.[29]

Fibrous Lesions

A fibrous plaque is characterized by SMC proliferation, probably mediated by the platelet-derived growth factor (PDGF) released from platelets, macrophages, endothelial cells, and SMC, and the accumulation of lipid in the SMCs and the macrophages.[30]

Developed Lesions

These plaques usually contain a core of extracellular fat and/or debris of varying amount. Although not detectable by angiography, the flat nonstenosing plaque may be diagnosed by high-resolution echotomography; it is classified according to its homogeneous or heterogeneous echostructures ("soft plaques").

Complicated Advanced Lesions

Hemorrhage, surface ulceration, and thrombosis of the atherosclerotic plaque, or calcification ("hard plaques"), characterize the advanced stage of atherogenesis. Complex interactions between the vessel wall and blood constituents occur in both the initiation of atherosclerotic plaques and the pathogenesis of thrombotic complications. Endothelial cells are the center of these processes.[31]

Details of these interactions are well known, but in human disease the diagnosis and natural history are still difficult to establish. The following factors remain uncertain:

1. The influence of platelet-mediated endothelial destruction or intimal proliferation;
2. Transport function in the presence of altered endothelium permeability;
3. The controlled release of platelet, endothelial cell, or macrophage/monocyte/derived growth factors (PDGF, ECDGF, MDGF, respectively).

These are important factors in the initiation of the atherosclerotic lesion and its progression and in regression; yet they have scarcely been investigated. However, the interaction of blood cells, platelets, thrombotic and fibrinolytic components for the promotion and limitation of thrombus formation is much better understood and forms the basis of strategies for treatment.[32]

Reports on the reliability of in vivo diagnoses for the identification and the composition of these lesions are inconclusive. Much of the present controversy derives from the different methods used, the designs selected for image analysis, and the varying technical experience of individual investigators.

Models of Atherogenesis

Three models exist demonstrating the evolution of atherogenesis: nonprimate, primate, and human.

Nonprimate Animal Models

Many studies have shown that regression of atherosclerotic plaques occurs after withdrawal of a hypercholesterol diet or with certain medical treatment.

At the turn of the century Anitschkow and Chalatow[28] studied reversible arterial and hepatic lesions in the hypercholesterolemic rabbit. Four months after the withdrawal of the hypercholesterol diet, hypercholesterolemia and hepatic steatorrhea rapidly disappeared, while the diminution of lipid material and enrichment of collagen and calcium were associated with a slow regression of atheromatous deposits in the aorta. More recently, Adams and Morgan[11] noted an exponential time course from experiments in the vegetarian rabbit with immediate recovery of hyperlipidemia but longer lasting plaque repair. Okamoto et al.[12] found a positive effect of oxygen on plaque regression in the spontaneously hypercholesterolemic Watanabe rabbit, and Sterne[33] showed that antiatherosclerotic (not lipid-lowering) drugs, such as metformin, produced a strong inhibitory effect on the progression of atherosclerotic lesions.

Others investigated the pigeon and the pig, which, although phylogenetically quite different from man, are probably more closely related to human atherosclerosis.[25] Horlick and Katz[34] and Wagner and Clarkson[35] reported the disappearance of induced fatty streaks and lipid-laden cells in aortic lesions of the chicken and the pigeon, if hypercaloric and normal diets were changed intermittently. In addition, Wagner and Clarkson[35] showed a positive effect of calcium-blocking agents for cholesterol efflux from aortic plaques.

Coronary artery regression was associated with a reduction in myocardial infarction related to the regression of obstructive arterial lesions,[36] and the more advanced the lesions, the less frequently they regressed. Rats and cats rarely develop atherosclerosis. The pig is the best model, where aortic lesions, including plaque complications (thrombosis, hemorrhage, and necrosis), occur spontaneously or may be induced by the same factors as in human atherosclerosis. Daoud et al.[37] studied such lesions 14 months after the withdrawal of hypercholesterol diet and reported reduced calcium deposits and necrosis in the absence of hemorrhage and thrombosis. Fisher et al.[38] reported the favorable lipid-lowering effects of fish oil on coronary atherosclerosis in the pig model. Other mechanisms include suppression of platelet function, reduction of monocyte/macrophage generation of inflammatory leukotriene B4[39] and the release of other toxic oxygen metabolites.[40,41] Similar results reported by Davis et al.[42] confirmed the protective effect of fish-oil diet on the progression of atherosclerosis during severe atherogenic stimuli. After 6 months of hypercholesterol diet followed by normal diet for 3 months, Hadjiisky et al.[43] demonstrated diminished lipoidosis in the aorta restricted to the intima only, with preservation of medial deposits even after 14 months.

Primate Models

The development of fibrous plaques from fatty streaks to complicated lesions takes years in rhesus and cynomologous monkeys,[44,45] the favorite primate models.[46,47] They have a close phylogenetic relationship to man, with similarities between experimentally induced changes in lipid metabolism and lesion distribution, and composition and complications in the human disease process. These nonhuman primates are the most important animal group for the study of cerebral artery occlusion and cerebral infarction.[15]

Regression from lipid to fibrous plaques occurred in the aorta of rhesus monkeys after withdrawal of 20 to 40 months' hypercholesterol diet. Resting hypercholesterolemia, the extent of the induced atherosclerotic plaque, and the duration of exposure to atherogenic diet determine the intensity of the regression.[46] The influence of medical treatment was tested either during the period of atherogenic diet or in the subsequent vegetarian state. Beta-blockers and antiplatelet agents (e.g., propranolol, minoxidil, dipyridamole, and aspirin)[48] failed to produce consistent improvement, and clofibrate and cholestyramine had only a mild effect.[3,47]

Weber et al.[17] found that carotid plaques produced by an atherogenic diet in cynomologous monkeys were markedly modified after cholestyramine treatment, even though the monkeys continued the same diet. The lesions shrunk and were covered by regenerated endothelial cells with less cell and lipid accumulation, though there was a marked increase in collagen and elastin fibers in the intracellular matrix; thus these lesions healed rather than regressed.

Different species of primates regress differently. For instance, two macaque species (*M. mulatta* and *M. fascicularis*) were compared using identical induction and treatment regimens.[49] In *M. fascicularis* a severe transmural concentric type of lesion developed, with signs of healing but without significant regression following therapy. In contrast, in *M. mulatta* the lesions predominantly involved the intima and did show regression. Thus little is known about the repair mechanisms involved, and the real nature of regression remains obscure.

Human Studies

The concept of regression of atherosclerosis began with postmortem observations in dystrophic, starving, and cachectic patients.[50-53] Drug prevention trials, in which the clinical event represents the end point of the study, have indirectly supported atherosclerotic regression but are unable to provide any evidence of the state of the arteries. This also applies to studies correlating risk factors with the final development of atherosclerosis.

Solberg and Strong[54] reviewed autopsy studies in which information about risk factors was available and found that elevated serum cholesterol and blood pressure were significantly associated with atherosclerotic plaques. In the Oslo Study,[16] the largest of the few prospective series dealing with data from cerebral arteries (129 cases from a cohort of 16 232 during a 7-year follow-up), raised serum cholesterol and hypertension were associated with advanced coronary and cerebral artery lesions. In contrast, high-density lipoprotein (HDL) cholesterol showed an inverse association with advanced atherosclerosis in coronary but not in cerebral arteries. Notably, atherogenesis differs in different segments of the vascular tree and develops later in the cerebral arteries than in the carotid or coronary arteries.[14,55,56]

In vivo studies have been limited to angiographic investigations in patients with clinical deterioration, or to the history and physical examination in untreated "controls" at follow-up, in whom surgical or medical treatment was not recommended. Serial examinations at best consist of repeat angiograms of the coronary or femoropopliteal arteries carried out often for different reasons.

Malinow[57] reviewed 1675 patients treated with hypolipid drugs: 5.1% showed reperfusion of the coronaries and 23% of the femoral arteries in a second arteriogram. However, reperfusion does not necessarily imply regression of atherosclerosis but occurs due to unrelated mechanisms such as thrombolysis, the relaxation from spasm, or from ectasia. In combination with an increasing efficacy of collateral pathways and changing metabolic demands, these mechanisms may cause an improvement in the clinical signs and symptoms. To rely on such parameters alone may lead to different and sometimes misleading interpretations.

Experimental atherosclerosis differs from human atherosclerosis in several ways. In man, the disease evolves slowly from early childhood to senescence and is usually multifactorial. Also, different stages of plaque development exist side by side, each characterized by a rather heterogeneous mixture of progressive and repair stages, the sequence of which is unknown. Interventional regimens interfere with a series of ongoing atherogenic mechanisms and may have quite heterogeneous or contradictory results.

Mechanisms of Regression

Biochemical Factors

In an experiment lasting >7 years, investigators at the Arteriosclerosis Research Center of the Bowman Gray School of Medicine in Winston-Salem studied mechanisms associated with regression in the coronary arteries of rhesus monkeys.[58,59] Arteries were fixed in situ by standard perfusion pressures, and computer-assisted morphometry was used for the calculation of plaques and vessels. Hypercholesterol diet (800 mg/dl) produced fatty streaks in the intima during the initial observation period of 19 months, but this diminished after a further 19-month interval, when collagen-containing plaques, extracellular lipid, and medial damage predominated. Then, cholesterol levels were reduced to either 200 or 300 mg/dl (but not <150 mg/dl as achievable in man), and the animals were followed up for another 2 or 4 years.

During the subsequent observations coronary artery size increased, especially in arteries with more atherosclerosis. This was mainly because of arterial wall dilatation rather than plaque regression.[58-61] There was also restructuring of the lesion accompanied by a loss of foam cells and lipid, an increase in collagen, and sometimes a decrease in size.[4,5]

Fatty streaks dispersed completely without collagen transformation within a year after the monkeys' diet was changed to low-cholesterol food.[62]

If regression also occurred in man when there is only moderate serum cholesterol elevation it would be critical, since carotid stenosis is frequently diagnosed at the asymptomatic stage of the disease[63-65] or when symptoms first occur. Possibly massive intimal lipid accumulation seen in patients with severe familial hypercholesterolemia is similar to this type of atherosclerosis and might regress with modern lipid-lowering drugs and plasmapheresis.[66,67]

This hypothesis is supported by recent studies using new methods for arterial imaging.[26,68,69]

Cellular Factors

Plaque shrinkage may result from death of the foam cells, disintegration of the cells, and breakdown of the extracellular space of lipid and debris derived from dead cells. Macrophages may play an important (although counteractive) role in this process. Among their beneficial functions is the ability to phagocytize and remove cellular and extracellular debris from the arterial wall. This is enhanced by the secretion of fibronectin and hydrolytic enzymes, which renders them diffusible, as well as the secretion of SMC mitogen and components of the vessel wall.[70] Macrophages may, however, be detrimental to regression if excess secretion of the same hydrolytic enzymes is directed to the normal or healing arterial wall.[40,70-74]

Little is known about the mechanisms and sequence of changes in the structure of larger, complicated plaques. Animal experiments do not easily reproduce such lesions and fail to induce surface platelet and fibrin deposits on collagenous plaques, particularly in nonhuman primates with experimental atherosclerosis.

Hemodynamic Factors

Regression of atherosclerosis may be associated with important hemodynamic sequelae. Armstrong et al.[75] studied limb, coronary, and cerebral hemodynamics in cynomologous monkeys given either an atherogenic diet for 20 months or a regression diet for an additional 18 months. Lesions of moderate

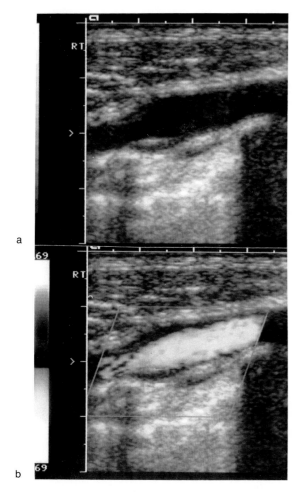

a

b

FIGURE 4.1. Echotomogram (a) and color-coded duplex sonogram (b) of the common and internal carotid arteries at the bifurcation. There is normal laminar flow near the re-endothelialized, formerly ulcerative plaque at the carotid bulb. This figure is also reproduced in color.

severity (50–60% stenosis) were induced and regressed with luminal enlargement and increased fibrosis. Blood flow measurements with microspheres indicated that vascular resistance decreased inconsistently in the coronary (-19%) but significantly in the cerebral territories (-44%), indicating considerable hemodynamic improvement with restoration of the dilator capacity. The mechanisms contributing to these effects are still obscure but may probably involve alterations in the response of the vasa vasorum to vasoactive stimuli.[76]

Plaque Restructuring

Human atherogenesis is less well understood (Table 4.1).[6] A plaque becomes "safer" when there is depletion of lipids, cell numbers, and extracellular material, such as fiber proteins and calcium. Condensation and reorientation of collagen or elastin, as well as loss of migration capacity of SMCs and healing of endothelial damage, also contribute (Fig. 4.1. See the color plate.)

Control of the phospholipid-free cholesterol ratio in blood and artery wall is also important. Excluding abnormal circumstances such as familial hypercholesterolemia, reduction of excessive dietary intake of calories, saturated fats, and cholesterol is mandatory. Because of delivery of fat to the liver, very-low-density lipoprotein (VLDL) production and LDL conversion occurs, and the level of circulating plasma LDL cholesterol increases. Saturation of the LDL receptors causes a significant decrease in the phospholipid-free cholesterol ratio in the blood, a parameter associated with atherosclerosis.[77] Cholesterol and other lipids move from the blood into the arterial wall, causing fatty streaks and lipid plaques. The transfer of fats stops when the phospholipid-free cholesterol ratio is equal in blood and vessel wall, and so regression of plaques occurs only when this ratio increases in the blood.

Arterial Enlargement and Plaque

Hort et al.,[78] Glagov et al.,[79] and Zarins et al.[61] confirmed that arterial dilatation is important in the restructuring of plaques. They studied the relationships between intimal plaque area, lumen area, and artery size in 481 sections of the left anterior descending coronary artery taken at different standard sampling sites in 125 pressure-perfusion-fixed postmortem adult human hearts.

Artery size correlated significantly with intimal plaque area. In *proximal segments* the most severely diseased arteries increased 62% in size, but lumen area decreased 25%. In the most severely diseased *distal segments* there was a fourteenfold increase in size and a twofold increase in lumen. If no enlargement occurred, the most severely diseased arteries in the proximal segments would have developed a 92% stenosis rather than the observed 25%, and in the distal segments there would have been a 65% stenosis rather than the 85% increase in lumen area that was found. This suggests arterial enlargement in response to increasing atherosclerotic plaques to prevent narrowing of the lumen,[61] or plaque formation in proportion to the size of the artery[80]; so small plaques formed in small arteries and larger ones in large arteries. The interpretation was based on the relationship between flow disturbances and plaque formation.[81] Flow separation occurs in proportion to the size of the vessel, with larger arteries having larger areas of flow separation and larger plaques. During early atherogenesis small flow separation zones, such as usually occur in the carotid bulb, may cause small plaque formation in small vessels. Enlargement of the arterial wall with increasing plaque size may cause extended flow separation zones and plaque progression. Progression of atherogenesis might be misinterpreted as regression if only the size or hemodynamics within the arterial lumen were observed.

There are serious technical problems in determining the sequence of events during plaque progression and regression using arteriography or ultrasound. Surface events such as platelet aggregation or thrombosis are difficult to evaluate. Reduction in plaque size may be due to shrinkage of the plaque (as in animal regression) or to other processes, such as thrombolysis, release of spasm, or arterial dilatation due to ectasia. The recent introduction of color-coded duplex-sonography facilitates the display of fresh thrombus in arterial zones without blood flow and in the absence of echostructures, suggesting plaque or vessel wall tissue (Fig. 4.2. See the color plate).[82] In prospective studies of the morphologic and hemodynamic effects of atherogenesis, the natural history of the disease and repair mechanisms should be investigated further. Unfortunately, application of this technique is still limited to a few segments of the human vascular tree.

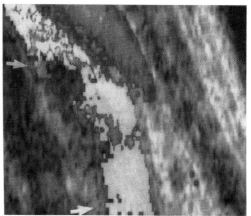

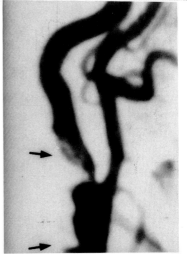

FIGURE 4.2. Color-coded duplex sonogram (a) and angiogram (b) of an internal carotid artery stenosis with adherent thrombus formation. Echodensity is reduced at the site of the thrombus formation but can easily be detected by the absence of flow velocity. At the site of stenosis, flow velocity is increased (white) with marked flow reversal zones (blue). This figure is also reproduced in color.

Angiographic Studies in Man

Angiography is now safer, making it easier to study the evolution of atherosclerosis with this method. However, most reported data deal with the coronary rather than the cerebral arteries. The poor quality of digital subtraction angiography has produced difficulties in data interpretation, and the criteria for regression vary among investigators. Even with optimal quality, readings based on "percent stenosis" are misleading, when stenotic segments are compared with proximal segments considered free of disease. If progression occurs in the proximal segment, the distal segment may appear to regress, although actually no change has occurred.

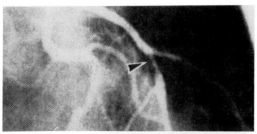

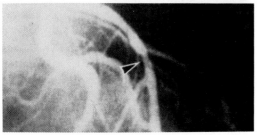

FIGURE 4.3. Regression of coronary atherosclerosis demonstrated by serial arteriograms. In the upper film, a moderate stenosis in the midleft anterior descending coronary artery is displayed (arrow). Two years later the stenosis is reduced and the diameter of the artery has increased (lower film). (From Waters and Lespérance *Drugs* 1988;36(suppl):37–41.)

Visual interpretation of coronary arteriograms is further affected by the high degree of inter- and intraobserver variability.[83] Changes of $\geq 20\%$ in the diameter of a stenosis at angiography can be detected with confidence, but smaller changes (especially small plaques, which have a special tendency to regress) are affected by technical and observer variability.[10] The reproducibility of repeat measurements is improved by recently developed quantitative, digitized, coronary arteriography using photodensitometry and image-border information.[84,85] However, remodeling or lysis of thrombi are still not distinguishable from regression of an atherosclerotic plaque, and so the proportion of "true" regression compared to spontaneous thrombolysis is difficult to estimate. "Progression" from a superimposed thrombus cannot be distinguished from worsening atherosclerosis.

Malinow[57] evaluated 24 studies of progression and regression in 1675 patients based on serial angiography. In 10 *retrospective studies* progression occurred in 53% and regression in 2%. In 8 *prospective studies*, where repeat angiography was performed in a standard manner, progression occurred

in about 50% and regression in 20%. This high rate of regression may represent selection bias, reflecting preference given to patients with successful reduction of risk factors, such as hyperlipidemia and blood pressure control. Also, most instances of regression were cases of arterial occlusion reverting to subtotal stenosis, which may reflect thrombolysis in the absence of lipid-lowering treatment. Until recently, diet and medical therapy could not reduce cholesterol levels by more than 25%; so lesion stasis occurred rather than regression.

Treatment Strategies Available

Lipid-Lowering Drugs

Diet, colestipol, and nicotinic acid lowered the LDL cholesterol levels by 43% and raised the HDL levels by 37%. This reduction of the total/HDL cholesterol ratio is in the range where in animal experiments regression occurs.[86,87] Patients in the Cholesterol Lowering Atherosclerosis Study benefited from this treatment even if their plasma cholesterol concentrations were normal. With the administration of newly developed substances such as HMG Co A reductase-inhibitors that reduce cholesterol concentrations by 70%, regression of atherosclerosis can be confidently expected.[88,89]

Calcium Antagonists

In an ongoing trial 383 patients were enrolled in a prospective, randomized double-blind treatment of nicardipine.[90] Repeat quantitative coronary angiography was performed after 2 years. Results from the first 75 patients indicate regression in 24% using a minimum diameter change of $> .4$ mm and in 33% using a $> 10\%$ stenosis as criteria (Fig. 4.3).

Ileal Bypass

The clinical course and appearance of coronary angiograms in patients with hypercholesterolemia suggested a decrease in plaque size 2 years after ileal-bypass surgery.[91,92] The effect of serum-lipid-lowering drugs on the development of femoral artery atherosclerosis appears promising.[93,94] Computerized image analysis of repeat femoral arteriograms showed regression in 16% of treated patients.[93,94]

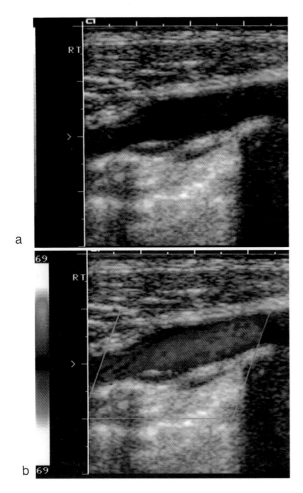

a

b

FIGURE 4.1. Echotomogram (a) and color-coded duplex sonogram (b) of the common and internal carotid arteries at the bifurcation. Note the normal laminar flow (red color-coded) nearby the reendothelialized, formerly ulcerative plaque at the carotid bulb.

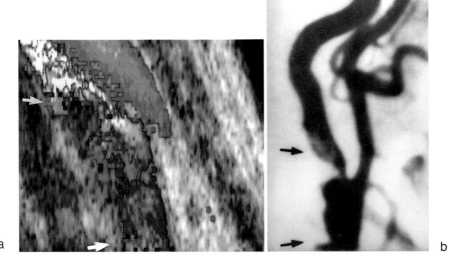

a   b

FIGURE 4.2. Color-coded duplex sonogram (a) and angiogram (b) of an internal carotid artery stenosis with adherent thrombus formation. Echodensity is reduced at the site of the thrombus formation but can easily be detected by the absence of flow velocity. At the site of stenosis, flow velocity is increased (white), with marked flow reversal zones (blue).

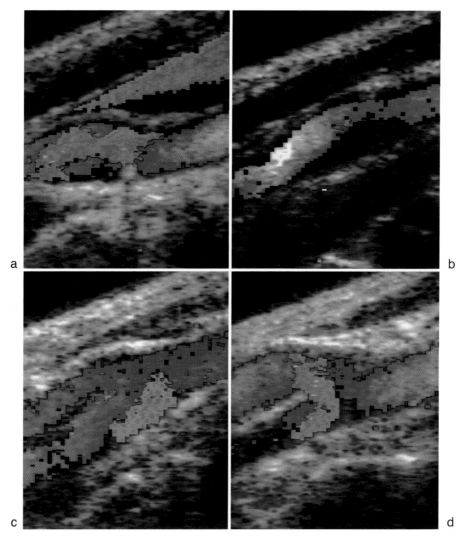

a   b

c   d

FIGURE 4.4. Color-coded duplex sonograms of four carotid systems in the neck. There is flow reversal or separation (blue) in the carotid bulb originating from a small homogeneous plaque at its entry on the opposite side (a) in contrast to the orthograde flow (red) along the echolucent, thrombotic mass, with absent flow signals adjacent to the posterior wall (b). Examples of physiological flow reversal are displayed at the origin of the external carotid artery in (c) and horse-shoe shaped extending in both the internal and external carotid arteries in (d) in the absence of atherosclerotic lesions.

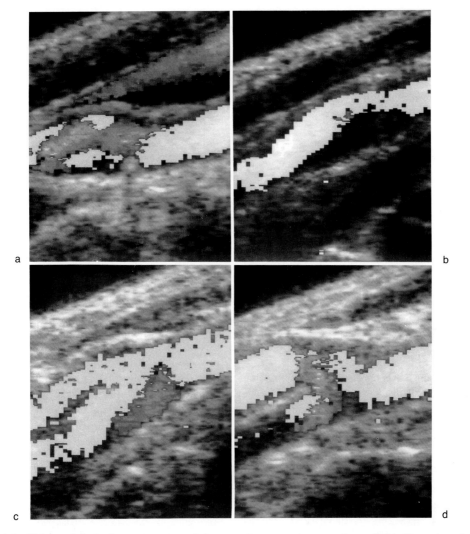

a
b
c
d

FIGURE 4.4. Color-coded duplex sonograms of four carotid systems in the neck. There is flow reversal or separation (blue) in the carotid bulb originating from a small homogeneous plaque at its entry on the opposite side (a) in contrast to the orthograde flow (red) along the echolucent, thrombotic mass, with absent flow signals adjacent to the posterior wall (b). Examples of physiological flow reversal are displayed at the origin of the external carotid artery (c) extending into both the internal and external carotid arteries in (d) in the absence of atherosclerotic lesions. This figure is also reproduced in color.

Repeat Plasma Exchange

Heterozygous or homozygous forms of familial hypercholesterolemia respond dramatically with reduced cholesterol levels after plasma exchange. It may also reduce clinical events,[66] but data of regression on serial angiograms are inconsistent.[95] Evidence that a sustained decrease in plasma cholesterol concentration had a favorable effect on the atherosclerotic process was inconclusive.

Ultrasound Studies in Man

Doppler sonography is particularly useful for the detection of abnormal flow velocity patterns induced by stenosing plaques but will not detect secondary flow phenomena near the initial stage of plaque formation most likely to regress.[65,96] Ultrasound echotomography however, allows repeated imaging of the extent and size of small plaques and demonstrates early vessel wall alterations.[45,97-101] It pro-

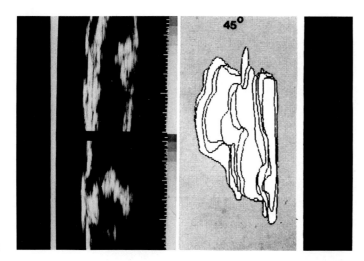

FIGURE 4.5. In vitro high-resolution 2D echotomograms (a) of a soft plaque at the posterior wall of the carotid bifurcation in the neck (upper row: longitudinal section, lower row: cross section) and its 3D reconstruction of the plaque surface from serial longitudinal sections (b).

a

b

vides a two-dimensional intraarterial contour and surface image of the adjacent structures, comparable in resolution to the macroscopic anatomy.[102] It is particularly useful for follow-up studies: in two recent preliminary studies regressive phases of carotid atheroma were demonstrated in 19% and 14%.[27,103]

Unfortunately, with "complication" and calcium deposition in the plaque, high-resolution echotomography becomes increasingly attenuated, producing reflections from surface tissues close to the ultrasound transducer, resulting in dense echo-shadows in more distant zones. Obstructive, advanced lesions (>80% stenosis) are more difficult to visualize and to quantify. Combined Doppler sonography and echotomography produces a simultaneous display provided by the recently introduced color-coded duplex sonographic technique (Fig. 4.4. See the color plate.).[99,104] In addition there are new techniques for three-dimensional analysis of carotid plaque using computer-assisted reconstructions of a series of two-dimensional sections taken from different angles of insonation[82] (Fig. 4.5). These are risk-free, cost-effective, and well tolerated.

Application of these high-quality methods is still restricted to a few segments of the vascular tree. Individual plaques must be followed separately, and investigations are restricted to local lesions rather than to atherogenesis in general. At present the cervical carotid artery is best for the application of these methods, rather than the coronary and visceral arteries and the aorta.[105]

We assessed 389 observations in the spontaneous history of 117 carotid plaques prospectively studied in 60 patients; follow-up was at 2 and 67 months (mean 37.7 months).[106] High-resolution ultrasound B-mode imaging, combined with a specially designed three-dimensional plaque contour and volume reconstruction analysis, and multigate pulsed Doppler intraarterial flow velocity examination, evaluated plaque morphology and local hemodynamics.[82] There was progression in 99 (25%), regression in 28 (7%) (Fig. 4.6), and no change in 262 examinations (68%). Regression was frequent in minor, flat homogeneous and ulcerated plaques, and progression occurred more often in soft, heterogeneous and irregularly surfaced ones. Secondary slow-flow zones and turbulence were significantly associated with irregular plaque surfaces and ulceration, but neither their incidence nor their extent correlated with the plaque size and volume.

A marked but statistically insignificant reduction in platelet and endothelial eicosanoid metabolites thromboxane (TXB_2) and prostacyclin (6-keto-PGF_1), as well as beta-thromboglobulin and platelet factor 4, was found at the repair versus progressive phases. Whether or not these metabolites and proteins therefore predict plaque progression in the presence of unstable morphologic and hemodynamic plaque conditions remains to be further evaluated.

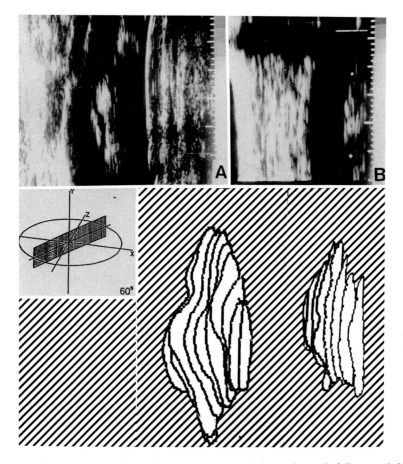

FIGURE 4.6. Longitudinal high-resolution echotomograms (A,B) and 3D displays (lower row) of a regressive soft plaque at the posterior wall of the common carotid artery during a 6-month follow-up (left: initial image, right: late image). (From Hennerici and Steinke, *Carotid Artery Plaques*. Basel: Karger. Reprinted by permission.)

Conclusion

1. The encouraging results of regression of atherosclerosis with hypocaloric diet or drug treatment that occur in animals are less convincing in man, where reduced progression rather than regression of established plaques may occur.
2. "Scarring" of atheroma occurs more frequently than "healing" in experimental models.
3. Qualitative rather than quantitative angiography was the only method available for the investigation of the blood vessels in man, but this provides no data on arterial wall changes. The risks of the procedure limit angiograms to patients with clinical indications. Noninvasive methods such as Doppler sonography and ultrasound echotomography or combinations of both may provide better results particularly with regard to carotid studies. Refined techniques such as color-coded duplex sonography are promising tools for the future to study the mechanisms involved in human plaque regression.[107]

References

1. Armstrong ML, Warner ED, Connor WE. Regression of coronary atheromatosis in rhesus monkeys. *Circ Res*. 1970;27:59–67.
2. Vesselinovitch D, Wissler RW, Hughes R, et al. Reversal of advanced atherosclerosis in rhesus monkeys. *Atherosclerosis*. 1976;23:155. 155–161.

3. Stary HC. Regression of atherosclerosis in primates. *Virchows Arch A Path Anat*. 1979;383:117–134.

4. Wagner WD, Saint-Clair RW, Clarkson TB. A study of atherosclerosis regression in macaca mulatta. *Exptl Molec Pathol*. 1980;32:162–174.

5. Wagner WD, St-Clair RW, Clarkson TB, Connor JR. A study of atherosclerosis regression in macaca mulatta. *Am J Pathol*. 1980;100:633–650.

6. Malinow MR. Atherosclerosis: progression, regression and resolution. *Am Heart J*. 1984;108:1523–1537.

7. Armstrong ML. Regression of atherosclerosis. *Atherosclerosis Reviews*. 1976;1:137–141.

8. Wissler RW, Vesselinovitch D. Regression of atherosclerosis in experimental animals and man. *Mod Concepts Cardiovasc Dis*. 1977;46:27–32.

9. Malinow MR. Regression of atherosclerosis in humans. A new frontier. *Postgrad Med*. 1983;73:232–235.

10. Brensike JF, Levy RI, Kelsy SF, et al. Effects of therapy with cholestyramine on progression of coronary arteriosclerosis: results of the NHLBI Tape II Coronary Intervention Study. *Circulation*. 1984;69:313–324.

11. Adams CWM, Morgan RS. Regression of atheroma in the rabbit. *Atherosclerosis*. 1977;28:399–404.

12. Okamoto R, Hatani M, Tsukitani M, et al. The effect of oxygen on the development of atherosclerosis in WHHL rabbits. *Atherosclerosis*. 1983;47:47–53.

13. Constantinides P. Overview of studies on regression of atherosclerosis. *Artery*. 1981;9:30–43.

14. Mathur KS, Kashyap SK, Kumar V. Correlation of the extent and severity of atherosclerosis in the coronary and cerebral arteries. *Circulation*. 1963;27:929–934.

15. Bullock BC, Moossy J. Cerebral infarction with atherosclerotic occlusion of the middle cerebral artery in a squirrel monkey (Saimiri sciureus) fed an atherogenic diet. *J Neuropathol Exp Neurol*. 1972;31:177–180.

16. Holme I, Enger SC, Helgeland A. Risk factors and raised atherosclerotic lesions in coronary and cerebral arteries. Statistical analysis from the Oslo study. *Arteriosclerosis*. 1981;1:250–256.

17. Weber G, Fabbrini P, Resi L, et al. Ultrastructural aspects of cynomologous atherosclerotic carotid artery lesions on cholestyramine "regression" treatment. *Appl Pathol*. 1986;45:225–232.

18. Brown MS, Ho YK, Goldstein JL. The cholesterol ester cycle in macrophage foam cells. *J Biol Chem*. 1980;255:9344–9352.

19. Brown MS, Kovanen PT, Goldstein JL. Regulation of plasma cholesterol by lipoprotein receptors. *Science*. 1981;212:628–635.

20. Kottke BA. Lipid markers for atherosclerosis. *Am J Cardiol*. 1986;57:11C–17C.

21. Henry PD. Atherosclerosis, calcium, and calcium antagonists. *Circulation*. 1985;72:456–459.

22. Parmley WW, Blumlein S, Sievers R. Modification of experimental atherosclerosis by calcium-channel blockers. *Am J Cardiol*. 1985;55:165B–171B.

23. Willis AL, Smith DL. Therapeutic impact of eicosanoids in atherosclerotic disease. *Eicosanoids*. 1989;2:69–72.

24. Schmitz-Hübner U, Thompson SG, Balleisen L, et al. Lack of association between haemostatic variables and the presence or extent of coronary atherosclerosis. *Br Heart J*. 1988;59:287–291.

25. Vesselinovitch D. Animal models and the study of atherosclerosis. *Arch Pathol Lab Med*. 1988;112:1011–1017.

26. Bond MG, Insull W, Glagov S, et al. Clinical Diagnosis of Atherosclerosis. New York, NY: Springer-Verlag; 1983.

27. Hennerici M, Rautenberg W, Trockel U, Kladetzky RG. Spontaneous progression and regression of small carotid atheroma. *Lancet*. 1985;1:1415–1419.

28. Anitschkow NN, Chalatow S. Über experimentelle Cholesterinsteatose. *Zentralbl Allg Path*. 1913;24:1–6.

29. Munro JM, van der Walt J, Munro CS, et al. An immunohistochemical analysis of human aortic fatty streaks. *Hum Pathol*. 1987;18:375–380.

30. Wissler RW, Vesselinovitch D, Komatsu A, et al. The arterial wall and atherosclerosis in youth. Proceedings of the 8th International Symposium on Atherosclerosis, 1988; Siena: 265.

31. Ross R. Atherosclerosis: a problem of the biology of arterial wall cells and their interaction with blood components. *Arteriosclerosis*. 1981;1:293–311.

32. del Zoppo GJ, Harker L. Blood/vessel interaction in coronary disease. *Hosp Practice*. 1984;163–165, 169–177, 181–182.

33. Sterne J. The present state of knowledge on the mode of action of the antidiabetic diguanides. *Metabolism*. 1964;13:791–796.

34. Horlick L, Katz LN. Retrogression of atherosclerotic lesions on cessation of cholesterol feeding in the chick. *J Lab Clin Med*. 1949;34:1427–1431.

35. Wagner WD, Clarkson TB. Effect of regression potential of atherosclerosis produced by intermittent continuous hypercholesterolemia. *Atherosclerosis*. 1977;27:369–381.

36. Jokinen MP, Clarkson TB, Prichard RW. Recent advances in molecular pathology. Animal models in atherosclerosis research. *Exp Mol Path*. 1985;42:1–28.

37. Daoud AS, Jarmolych J, Augustyn JM, et al. Sequential morphologic studies of regression of advanced atherosclerosis. *Arch Pathol Lab Med.* 1981;195:233–239.

38. Fisher M, Levine PH, Weiner BH. Omega-3 fatty acids and atherosclerosis. In: Hennerici M, Sitzer G, Weger H-D, eds. *Carotid Artery Plaques.* Basel: Karger; 1988:92–100.

39. Lee TH, Hoover RL, Williams JD, et al. Effects of dietary enrichment with eicosapentaenoic acid and docosahexaenoic acids on in-vitro neutrophil and monocyte leukotriene generation and neutrophil function. *N Engl J Med.* 1985;312:1217–1224.

40. Hartung HP, Kladetzky RG, Melnik G, et al. Stimulation of the scavenger receptor on monocytes-macrophages evokes release of arachidonic acid metabolites and reduced oxygen species. *Lab Invest.* 1986;55:209–216.

41. Fisher M, Upchurch KS, Levine PH, et al. Effects of dietary fish oil supplementation on polymorphonuclear leukocyte inflammatory potential. *Inflammation.* 1986;10:387–392.

42. Davis HR, Bridenstine RT, Vesselinovitch D, et al. Fish oil inhibits development of atherosclerosis in rhesus monkeys. *Arteriosclerosis.* 1987;7:441–449.

43. Hadjiisky P, Bourdillon MC, Grosgogeat Y. Histoire naturelle de la regression de l'atherosclerose: des modeles animaux a l'homme. *Arch Mal Coeur.* 1988;81:1411–1417.

44. Hollander W, Kirkpatrick B, Paddock J, et al. Studies on the progression and regression of coronary and peripheral atherosclerosis in the cynomologous monkey. *Exp Mol Pathol.* 1979;30:55–73.

45. Hennerici M, Bürrig KF, Daffertshofer M. Flow pattern and structural changes at carotid bifurcation in hypertensive cynomologous monkeys. *Hypertension.* 1989;13:315–329.

46. Saint-Clair RW. Atherosclerosis regression in animal models: current concepts of cellular and biochemical mechanisms. *Prog Cardiovasc. Dis.* 1983;26:109–112.

47. Malinow MR, Blaton VW. Regression of atherosclerotic lesions. Arteriosclerosis 1984;4:292–295.

48. Pick R, Glick G. Effects of propranolol, minoxidil and clofibrate in cholesterol-induced atherosclerosis in stumptail macaques (macaca arctoides). *Atherosclerosis.* 1977;27:71–77.

49. Vesselinovitch D, Wissler RW. Correlation of types of induced lesions with regression of coronary atherosclerosis in two species of macaques. In: Noseda G, Fragiacomo C, Fumagalli R, et al., eds. *Lipoproteins and Coronary Atherosclerosis.* Amsterdam: Elsevier Publishers; 1982:401.

50. Vartiainen I, Kanerva K. Arteriosclerosis and war time. *Ann Med Int Fenniae.* 1947;36:748.

51. Wanscher O, Clemmesen J, Nielson A. Negative correlation between atherosclerosis and carcinoma. *Br J Cancer.* 1951;5:172–177.

52. Strong JP, Solberg LA, Restrepo C. Atherosclerosis in persons with coronary heart disease. *Lab Invest.* 1968;18:527–531.

53. Malinow MR, Senner JW. Arterial pathology in cancer patients suggests atherosclerosis regression. *Med Hypotheses.* 1983;11:353–357.

54. Solberg LA, Strong JP. Risk factors and atherosclerotic lesions. *Arteriosclerosis.* 1983;3:187–198.

55. Solberg LA, McGarry PA, Moossy J, et al. Severity of atherosclerosis in cerebral arteries, coronary arteries, and aortas. *Ann NY Acad Sci.* 1968;149:956–962.

56. Weber G, Fabbrini P, Resi L, et al. An ultrastructural comparison of diet-induced atherosclerosis of arteries supplying the central nervous system in cynomologous and rhesus monkeys. *Appl Pathol.* 1983;1:121–138.

57. Malinow MR. Regression and resolution in atherosclerosis. In: *Recent Advances in Arterial Disease: Atherosclerosis, Hypertension and Vasospasm.* 1986:31–38.

58. Clarkson TB, Lehner ND, Wagner, WD, et al. A study of atherosclerosis regression in macaca mulatta. *Exp Mol Pathol.* 1979;30:360–385.

59. Clarkson TB, Bond MG, Bullock BC, et al. A study of atherosclerosis regression in macaca mulatta. *Exp Mol Pathol.* 1981;34:345–368.

60. Bond MG, Adams MR, Bullock BC. Complicating factors in evaluating coronary artery atherosclerosis. *Artery.* 1981;9:21–29.

61. Zarins CK, Weisenberg E, Kolettis G, et al. Differential enlargement of artery segments in response to enlarging atherosclerotic plaques. *J Vasc Surg.* 1988;7:386–394.

62. Stary HC, Eggen DA, Strong JP. The mechanisms of atherosclerosis regression. In: Schettler G, et al., eds. *Atherosclerosis IV.* New York, NY: Springer-Verlag; 1977. p 394.

63. Hennerici M, Rautenberg W, Mohr S. Stroke risk from symptomless extracranial disease. *Lancet.* 1982;2:1180–1183.

64. Chambers BR, Norris JW. Outcome in patients with asymptomatic neck bruits. *N Engl J Med.* 1986;315:860–865.

65. Hennerici M, Hülsbömer HB, Hefter H, et al. Natural history of asymptomatic extracranial arterial disease. Results of a long-term prospective study. *Brain.* 1987;110:777–791.

66. Thompson GR, Lowenthal R, Myant NB. Plasma exchange in the management of homozygous familial hypercholesterolaemia. *Lancet*. 1975;1: 1208–1211.

67. Eisenhauer T, Armstrong VW, Wieland H, et al. Selective removal of low density lipoproteins (LDL) by precipitation at low pH: first clinical application of the HELP system. *Klin Wschr*. 1987;65:161–168.

68. Stary HC. What is the nature of coronary atherosclerotic lesions that have been shown to regress in experiments with nonhuman primates and by angiography in man? *VASA*. 1984;13:298–304.

69. Hennerici M, Kleophas W, Gries FA. Regression of carotid plaques during HELP therapy. In preparation.

70. Daoud AS, Fritz KE, Jarmolych J, et al. Roles of macrophages in regression of atherosclerosis. *Ann NY Acad Sci*. 1985;454:101–114.

71. Yatsu FM. Atherosclerosis and stroke. In: Hennerici M, Sitzer G, Weger H-D, eds. *Carotid Artery Plaques*. Basel: Karger, 1988:p 10–25.

72. Watanabe T, Hirata M, Yoshikawa Y, et al. Role of macrophages in atherosclerosis. *Lab Invest*. 1985; 53:80–90.

73. Hartung HP, Hennerici M. Role of macrophages in atherosclerosis. In: Hennerici M, Sitzer G, Weger H-D, eds. *Carotid Artery Plaques*. Basel: Karger; 1988:p 47–63.

74. Yamamoto A, Hara H, Takaichi S, et al. Effect of probucol on macrophages, leading to regression of xanthomas and atheromatous vascular lesions. *Am J Cardiol*. 1988;62:31B–36B.

75. Armstrong ML, Heistad DD, Marcus ML, et al. Hemodynamic sequelae of regression of experimental atherosclerosis. *J Clin Invest*. 1983;71:104–113.

76. Williams JK, Armstrong ML, Heistad DD. Vasa vasorum in the atherosclerotic coronary arteries: responses to vasoactive stimuli and regression of atherosclerosis. *Circulation Res*. 1988;62:515–523.

77. Smith EB, Slater RS. Relationship between low density-lipoproteins in aortic intima and serum lipid levels. *Lancet*. 1972;1:463–469.

78. Hort W, Lichtli H, Kalbfleisch H, Kohler F, et al. The size of human coronary arteries depending on the physiological and pathological growth of the heart, the age, the size of the supplying areas and degree of coronary sclerosis: a post-mortem study. *Virchows Arch A*. 1982;397:37–59.

79. Glagov S, Weisenberg E, Zarins CK, et al. Compensatory enlargement of human atherosclerotic coronary arteries. *N Engl J Med*. 1987;316:1371–1375.

80. LoGerfo F. Discussion. *J Vasc Surg*. 1988;7:393–395.

81. Schmid-Schönbein H, Wurzinger LJ. Vortex transport phenomena of the carotid trifurcation: inter-

action between fluid dynamic transport phenomena and hemostatic reactions. In: Hennerici M, Sitzer G, Weger H-D, eds. *Carotid Artery Plaques*. Basel:Karger;1988:p 64–91.

82. Steinke W, Hennerici M. Three-dimensional ultrasound imaging of carotid artery plaques. *J Cardiovasc Tech*. 1989;8:15–17.

83. Detre KM, Kelsy SF, Passamani ER, et al. Reliability of assessing change with sequential coronary arteriography. *Am Heart J*. 1982;104:816–823.

84. Reiber JHC, Serruys PW, Kooijman CJ, et al. Assessment of short-, medium-, and long-term variations in arterial dimensions from computer-assisted quantitation of coronary cineangiograms. *Circulation*. 1985;71:280–288.

85. Waters D, Lespérance J. Regression of coronary atherosclerosis-angiographic perspective. *Drugs*. 1988;36 (suppl 3):37–42.

86. Blankenhorn DH, Nessim SA, Johnson RL, et al. Beneficial effects of combined colestipol-niacin therapy on coronary atherosclerosis and coronary venous bypass grafts. *JAMA*. 1987;257:3233–3240.

87. Clarkson TB, Bond MG, Bullock BC, et al. A study of atherosclerosis regression in Macaca mulatta. *Exp Mol Pathol*. 1984;41:96–118.

88. Glueck CJ. Role of risk factor management in progression and regression of coronary and femoral artery atherosclerosis. *Am J Cardiol*. 1986;57: 35G–41G.

89. Slater EE, MacDonald JS. Mechanism of action and biological profile of HMG CoA reductase inhibitors. *Drugs*. 1988;36 (suppl 3):72–82.

90. Waters D, Freedman D, Lesperance J, et al. Design features of a controlled clinical trial to assess the effect of a calcium entry blocker upon the progression of coronary artery disease. *Contr Clin Trials*. 1987;8:216–242.

91. Buchwald H, Moore RB, Varco RL. Surgical treatment of hyperlipidemia. *Circulation*. 1974;49 (suppl 1):122.

92. Buchwald H, Moore RB, Rucker RD, et al. Clinical angiographic regression of atherosclerosis after partial ileal bypass. *Atherosclerosis*. 1983;46:117–128.

93. Erikson U, Helmius G, Hemmingsson A, et al. Repeat femoral arteriography in hyperlipidemic patients. *Acta Radiol*. 1988;29:303–309.

94. Schoop W. Progression und Regression der peripheren arteriellen Verschlusskrankheit. *VASA*. 1987;20 (suppl):62–66.

95. Thompson GR, Myant NB, Kilpatrick D, et al. Assessment of long-term plasma exchange for familial hypercholesterolaemia. *Br Heart J*. 1980; 43:680–688.

96. Norris JW, Bornstein NM. Progression and regression of carotid stenosis. *Stroke*. 1986;17:755–757.

97. Hennerici M, Freund H-J. Evaluation of the efficacy of different ultrasound methods for the detection of extracranial arterial disease. *J Clin Ultrasound*. 1984;12:115–161.

98. Reneman RS, van Merode T, Hick P, et al. Flow velocity patterns in and distensibility of the carotid artery bulb in subjects of varying age. *Circulation*. 1985;71:500–509.

99. Steinke W, Kloetzsch C, Hennerici M. Carotid artery disease assessed by Doppler color flow imaging. *AJNR*. 259–266.

100. Baker DW, Daigle RJ. Noninvasive ultrasonic flowmetry. In: Hwang NHC, Norman NA, eds. Cardiovascular Flow Dynamics and Measurements. Baltimore, MD: University Park Press; 1977: p 151–159.

101. Pignoli T, Tremoli E, Poli A, et al. Intimal plus medial thickness of the arterial wall: a direct measurement with ultrasound imaging. *Circulation*. 1986;74:1399–1406.

102. Hennerici M, Reifschneider G, Trockel U, et al. Detection of early atherosclerotic lesions by duplex scanning of the carotid artery. *J Clin Ultrasound*. 1984;12:455–463.

103. Ehringer H, Bockelmann L, Konecny U, et al. Verschlusskrankheit der extrakraniellen A. carotis: "Spontanverlauf" und frühe Phase nach Thrombendarteriektomie im bildgebenden Ultraschall. *VASA*. 1987;20(suppl):71–76.

104. Merritt CRB. Doppler color flow imaging. *J Clin Ultrasound*. 1986;15:591–599.

105. Poli A, Paoletti R. Regression of the atherosclerotic lesion in man: the impact of non-invasive techniques. *Inter Angio*. 1987;6:327–329.

106. Hennerici M, Steinke W. Three-dimensional ultrasound imaging for the evaluation of progression and regression of carotid atherosclerosis. In: Hennerici M, Stear G, Weger H-D, eds. *Carotid Artery Plaques*. Basel: Karger; 1988:115–132.

107. Weber G, Bianciardi B, Toto P, et al. Some pathogenetic aspects of atherosclerotic lesions. *Int Angio*. 1987;6:37–43.

5

Drug Inhibition of Experimental Carotid Atherogenesis

Eberhard L. Betz

It is well known that a number of risk factors exists for atherogenesis and that reduction of these factors (cholesterol, smoking, hypertension, etc.) is recommended to prevent progression of this disease. Drugs that reduce hyperlipidemia or hypertension play a supporting role in the treatment of some forms of atherosclerosis. At the vessel wall level other factors are additionally involved (Table 5.1).

Producing Experimental Plaques

Because of the difficulty in documenting drug-induced inhibition of atherosclerotic changes in the human arterial wall directly, experimental models have been used. In the initial phase of atherosclerosis, disturbed permeability of the endothelial lining[1-14] and endothelial dysfunction occurs.[15-20] Then there is migration of leukocytes (mainly monocytes) from the vessel lumen through the endothelium and into the vessel wall,[21-34] and also of smooth muscle cells (SMC) from the media into the subendothelial space where they proliferate. The plaque (consisting of a mixture of blood-borne cells, SMC, and extracellular matrix synthesized by the newly migrated SMC) forms a stenosing intimal proliferation. If there is also hypercholesteremia, the proliferation contains increased amounts of intracellular lipids in macrophages, SMC and extracellular cholesterol. In thick, atheromatous plaques the endothelium sometimes ruptures or is denuded and platelets adhere to the underlying tissue. Thrombosis may now develop if antithrombotic components are not sufficient to prevent the for-mation of a thrombus. The resulting stenosis produces ischemia in the area supplied by the stenosed or occluded artery.

The carotid artery is particularly suitable to study the effects of drugs on experimentally induced atherosclerotic plaques because of its surgical accessibility. In some animals, e.g., the rabbit, the subendothelial space of the carotid arteries is only a cleft between the basal lamina of the endothelial cells and the internal elastic lamina. It is devoid of cells, and cells are found in the subendothelial space only if they have invaded this region. If the method to produce atheroma or a fibromuscular intimal plaque is standardized and restricted to the carotid artery, it is possible to quantify the effect of antiatherogenic drugs.

There are several techniques for experimental induction of stenosing arteriosclerosis in carotid arteries. These include sheathing the artery with a cuff[35-37] extensive local cooling with a precooled metal block,[38] mechanical injury of the endothelial lining and the subendothelial tissue by ballooning,[39,40] or repeated electrical transmural stimulation with weak electrical current.[41]

In normally fed animals these stimuli produce intimal accumulation and proliferation of SMC and an accumulation of leukocytes within the stimulated area. There are, however, some differences in the effects on the endothelial lining. In arteries mechanically injured by ballooning or local cooling, the endothelial lining is destroyed. However, in sheathing experiments, in arteries stimulated with weak impulses of direct current, or when proliferation is induced by hyperlipidemia, the endothelial lining is maintained, at least in the

TABLE 5.1. Typical changes in artery walls during athe-rogenesis.

Increase of endothelial permeability
Migration of leukocytes into the subendothelial space
Migration of smooth muscle cells from the media into the intima
Proliferation of smooth muscle cells in the intima
Modulation of proliferating smooth muscle cells
Endocytosis of lipids, foam cell formation
Necroses in the artery wall
Destruction of the endothelial lining
Adherence of platelets
Formation of thromboses, stenoses, and artery occlusion

initial stages. In arteries of rabbits stimulated with direct current (DC) impulses, intimal proliferation develops beneath the anode but not the cathode. The development of cell proliferation also depends on the intensity and duration of the stimuli. For instance, in sheathing experiments, the subendo-thelial proliferation is circular. Quantitation of the mechanical stimulus caused by a cuff is more diffi-cult than quantitation of an electrical current.

Drug Inhibition of Experimental Plaques

An accumulation of cells and extracellular material forming an intimal "cushion" is an essential com-ponent in the development of fibromuscular prolif-eration and atheroma. Suppression by drugs is the goal of secondary prevention of atherosclerosis.

The first experimental model used for induction of atherosclerosis has been described by Igna-towski,[42] who fed rabbits a diet enriched with egg yolk and fat. After some weeks, lipid-laden plaques developed in the aorta and coronary arteries and sometimes also in the carotid arteries. These experiments later formed the basis of the lipid the-ory of atherogenesis when it was realized that serum cholesterol is an essential component for the development of intimal atheromatous plaques. Numerous reviews and papers deal with the mech-anisms of lipid accumulation in the arterial walls in atherogenesis.[43-62]

Lowering serum cholesterol by reducing choles-terol intake, supplemented by drugs that lower the concentration of low-density lipoproteins (LDL), inhibits the development of this type of atheroscle-

rosis. It is difficult to predict the effect of this ther-apy on carotid atherosclerosis because the pattern of distribution of plaques induced by hyperlipide-mia is not uniform and differences exist in the response of arteries to this atherogenic stimulus. If the LDL level is increased and the high-density lipoprotein (HDL) level is low, antihyperlipidemic drugs are needed for primary as well as for second-ary prevention of carotid atherosclerosis.

The production of an intimal plaque by applica-tion of mechanical atherogenic stimuli gave rise to the "injury hypothesis" of atherogenesis. Based on the ballooning experiments of Baumgartner and Studer,[39] it was assumed by Ross and Glomset,[63] Ross et al.,[64-66] and Ross[67,68] that where the vessel is denuded of endothelial lining, platelets adhere and release growth factors, causing the under-lying SMC to migrate from the media into the intima and then proliferate. However, destruction of the endothelial lining is not a necessary pre-condition for the migration of SMC through the internal elastic lamina (IEL). For instance, ather-omatous plaque is produced by local, weak, trans-mural electrical stimuli[69,34] or by sheathing experi-ments in which cells migrate initially into the subendothelial space and then proliferate there without denudation of the endothelial lining. Elec-trical stimulation and intraluminal balloons are particularly suitable for testing antiatherogenic drug effects in carotid arteries.

Atheroma Induced by Repeated Electrical Stimulation

Rabbits are ideal experimental animals for the pro-duction of intimal proliferation in carotid arteries by local electrical stimulation. Graphite-covered gold electrodes mounted into a flexible cuff of sili-con or into a teflon cuff are attached to the adven-titia of an anesthetized rabbit in such a way that the electrodes are opposite to each other and the cur-rent passes transmurally through the carotid artery wall. Apfel[70,71] and Apfel et al.[72] studied in detail the amount of current that crosses the artery wall and the current that flows around the artery.

Leads from the electrodes are passed subcutane-ously to a socket made of plexiglass fixed with two fine screws in the skull, allowing the artery to be connected to a stimulator. The artery can be stim-ulated in the conscious unrestrained animal without

TABLE 5.2. Percent numbers of cells absorbing Ruthenium Red (= RR) in cross sections of carotid arteries.[a]

Treatment group	Number of examined arteries	Total % cells absorbing RR(mean)	Range	Sections counted	Cells counted
1. Unstimulated no Flunarizine	4	18[b]	11–29	4	278
2. Stimulated 30–60 min (beneath anode) no Flunarizine	5	100	–	5	450
3. Stimulated 60 min (beneath anode) no Flunarizine recovery 120 min	3	40	17–65	4	380
4. Unstimulated Flunarizine (0.1 mg/kg)	5	20	18–26	5	437
5. Stimulated 60 min (beneath anode) Flunarizine (examined immediately after stimulation)	6				
Animal 1		55	27–80	4	184
2		10	5–18	3	187
3		>90[c]	55–100	3	190
4		55	47–66	3	191
5		100	–	4	360
6		15	6–23	5	400
6. Chronic stimulation	3	33	8–56	6	400

[a]The differences in the numbers of cells counted per artery are caused by a variable number of electron microscopic pictures/artery that were suitable for evaluation.
[b]One animal in the unstimulated control group showed RR uptake in all cells of all sections examined.
[c]Two sections showed 100% RR uptake; the other, 59%.

causing pain. In order to standardize the procedure, DC impulses with an intensity of 0.1 mA, duration: 10 ms/impulse at a frequency of 10 Hz, are applied twice a day (30 minutes in the morning and 15 minutes in the afternoon). In this way, each stage of plaque development is controlled. In our laboratory, we studied the effect of single or repeated stimulation on functional and morphological reactions of the carotid artery wall and the sequence of events resulting in an atheromatous or fibromuscular intimal proliferation.

After a single stimulation period of 30 minutes, the endothelial luminal surface shows no change when examined by conventional scanning electron microscopy. Viele and Betz,[73] however, using Ruthenium Red in transmission electron microscopy, found that this substance (which in normal endothelial cells (EC) does not penetrate the membrane), was taken up by many EC. This indicates that the stimulation causes a disturbance in the glycocalyx of the endothelial lining. Table 5.2 shows the differences in Ruthenium Red staining of EC of rabbits in stimulated and nonstimulated carotid arteries. The glycocalyx dysfunction after one stimulation period is only transient and returns

to the normal state in 3 hours after termination of a stimulation period of 45 minutes. If the animal receives 0.1 mg Flunarizine/kg body weight 20 minutes prior to the stimulation, the uptake of Ruthenium Red is inhibited.

This is not the only effect of a single stimulation period. Apfel et al.[71] found that the electrical resistance between the electrodes increases transiently for some hours and then returns to normal. Transmission electron microscopy reveals a slightly increased content of fluid beneath the endothelial cells in the form of small blebs. Since these blebs remained in the subendothelial space for some hours, it was assumed that osmotically active material was trapped beneath the endothelial cells.

Endothelial Permeability in Carotid Arteriosclerosis

There is an increase of endothelial permeability to macromolecules in areas of arterial atherosclerosis.[3,5,11,12,74-79] Labeled albumin crosses the endothelial lining more easily in atherosclerotic than in normal arteries. Peroxidase of different molecular sizes has been used to study transport of macro-

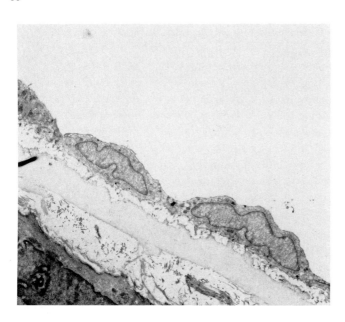

FIGURE 5.1. Endothelium of a normal carotid artery 6 minutes after an intravenous infusion of 10 000 units of peroxidase, molecular weight 40 000 d. Infusion time: 3 minutes. Magnification ×6300.

molecules through the walls of carotid arteries. Figure 5.1 shows the endothelial lining of a normal rabbit carotid artery 6 minutes after the intravenous infusion of 10 000 units of peroxidase (molecular weight 40 000 d). To stain the peroxidase reaction products, a modified technique of Karnovsky[80] and Forssmann[81] was used. The technique has been described in detail for measurements of permeability in atherosclerosis by Betz et al.[82]

In the experiment shown in Figure 5.2, the contralateral artery of the same animal shown in Figure 5.1 has been stimulated electrically with weak impulses (0.1 mA, 10 ms duration/impulse, 10 Hz) for 45 minutes. Three minutes before termination of the stimulation, the animal received an infusion of peroxidase, and 6 minutes later both arteries (the stimulated and nonstimulated artery) were dissected out and prepared for electron microscopy. Figure 5.2 shows that there is a massive accumulation of reaction products of peroxidase in the subendothelial space of the stimulated region. The transport of peroxidase was considerably higher beneath the anode than at the cathode. Higher magnification of the endothelial cells shows that the peroxidase crosses the endothelial lining through the interendothelial clefts (Fig. 5.3). Also, a number of intracellular vesicles are seen containing peroxidase reaction

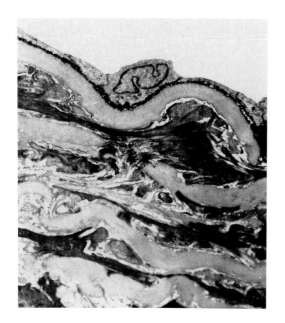

◄

FIGURE 5.2. Endothelium beneath the anode of an electrically stimulated carotid artery (0.1 mA, 10 ms/ impulse, 10 Hz) for 45 minutes, six minutes after an intravenous infusion of 10000 units of peroxidase (molecular weight 40000 d). The infusion (3 minutes) started at the end of the stimulation period. Massive uptake of peroxidase into the subendothelial space can be seen. Reaction products of peroxidase are black. Magnification ×6300.

FIGURE 5.3. Routes of transport of peroxidase through the endothelial lining are seen in this high magnification of the endothelium beneath the anode. With freeze-etching techniques it has been demonstrated that the tight junctions between the endothelial cells are patchy and remain present after one stimulation period. The interendothelial transport of peroxidase is therefore possible without destruction of the tight junctions. The interendothelial clefts are wider after stimulation in comparison to nonstimulated arteries (Figure 5.1). Magnification ×10 000.

▶

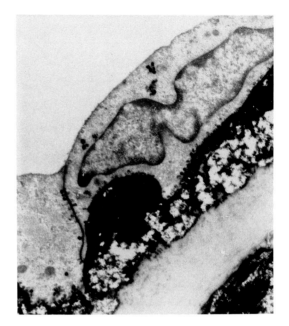

products. However, one cannot conclude that an increased transport rate exists just from the number of peroxidase-containing intracellular vesicles. Possibly, part of the peroxidase is transported transcellularly.

With densitometric techniques the subendothelial accumulation of peroxidase reaction products can be quantified. The optical density of ultrathin sections of the IEL in the immediate neighborhood of the subendothelial space in which peroxidase reaction products have accumulated is useful as a reference.[82] Electron micrographs with magnification of ×6300 were placed under a densitometer and 20 spots of the IEL beneath each endothelial cell were compared with the densities of 20 spots of the subendothelial space beneath the same cell. The density of the IEL was nearly homogenous and

was accordingly given the density 100% (= index 1). Measurements were conducted in several hundred ultrathin sections of normal and of stimulated arteries. Figure 5.4 shows that the increase of permeability after a single stimulation period is transient. It returns to normal values 1–5 hours after the stimulation has ended.

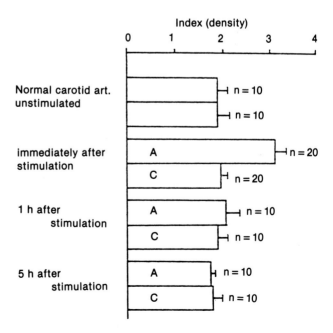

FIGURE 5.4. Densitometric measurement of the uptake of peroxidase into the subendothelial space beneath the anode (A) and the cathode (C) at different times after stimulation. Control: No stimulation. The increase of peroxidase transport through the endothelium after a stimulation period is transient and is considerably higher beneath the anode. A = beneath anode; C = beneath cathode.

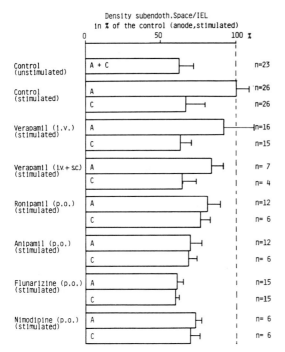

FIGURE 5.5. Densitometric measurements showing the inhibitory effects of various substances that inhibit the transendothelial transport of peroxidase. All columns show the densities immediately after the same stimulation time. All substances used in this experiment possess calcium-antagonistic properties. (However, pentoxifylline also inhibits transendothelial peroxidase transport and is not a calcium antagonist.) A = beneath anode, C = beneath cathode. p.o. = oral administration of the drug; i.v. = intravenous administration; s.c. = subcutaneous administration.

Various drugs inhibit the endothelial permeability of the carotid artery for macromolecules. Strohschneider et al.[83] found a concentration-dependent reduction of the permeability by pentoxifylline. Figure 5.5 shows the effects of various calcium antagonists. In the concentrations used, most of these drugs inhibit the permeation of peroxidase through the carotid endothelial lining after only one stimulation period. After injection of Flunarizine, the interendothelial transport, as well as the number of intracellular vesicles, was reduced. In arteries with fully developed atheromas that are still covered with an endothelium, the intercellular clefts are open for high-molecular-weight peroxidase. Figure 5.6 depicts the luminal part of an intimal proliferation in a rabbit carotid artery produced during 28

days; the last stimulation period was applied 24 hours prior to the peroxidase infusion (given 6 minutes prior to the excision of the artery). The peroxidase has filled the clefts between the endothelial cells and also the intercellular spaces between the cells forming the proliferate, consisting mainly of SMC. Some of these SMC take up small amounts of peroxidase in their cytoplasm. As demonstrated with densitometric techniques, pentoxifylline or Flunarizine partly reduce the inflow of macromolecules under these experimental conditions.

Intimal Cell Behavior in Carotid Arteriosclerosis

The response to atherogenic stimuli includes an accumulation of cells in the subendothelial space. The sequence of cellular reactions is best studied by using electrical stimuli for producing the intimal plaque. As shown by Kling et al.,[33,34] leukocytes appear in the subendothelial space (SES) after only two periods of stimulation. The cells adhere to the endothelium of the stimulated area and then migrate through the endothelial lining, mainly through the interendothelial clefts into the

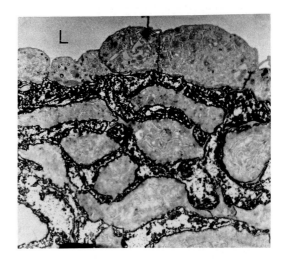

FIGURE 5.6. Typical atheromatous proliferate in a rabbit carotid artery after 28 days of electrical stimulation (30 minutes in the morning, 15 minutes in the afternoon). The proliferate developed beneath the anode. The rabbit was fed 1% cholesterol in its diet. The interendothelial spaces are filled with peroxidase reaction products (same staining procedure as in Figures 5.1, 5.2, and 5.3). L = lumen. Magnification ×6300

FIGURE 5.7. Intima of a rabbit carotid artery 1 day after the first stimulation period. The animal received normal food.

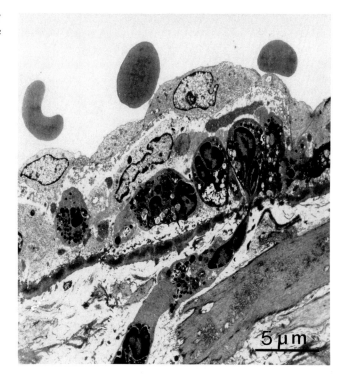

widened SES. Figure 5.7 depicts an area that was stimulated twice within 24 hours and produced an accumulation of leukocytes consisting mainly of granulocytes and mononuclear cells. If the animal had received 1% cholesterol in its food during the 3-day period prior to the stimulations, mononuclear cells would contain considerable lipid-laden vacuoles (foam cells). In other arteries foam cells are not found regularly in such a short period after the addition of 1% cholesterol to the chow.

Two days after stimulation, SMC appear in the SES, migrating through the preformed pores of the IEL. They arrange themselves longitudinally along the longer axis of the vessel and divide in the SES. Figure 5.8 shows a longitudinal section through an early plaque taken 14 days after onset of the stimula-

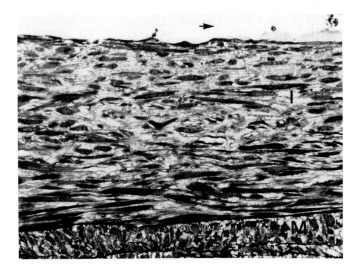

FIGURE 5.8. Longitudinal section through a fresh plaque induced by electrical stimulation, 3 weeks after the onset of the stimulation. The proliferated SMC arrange along the longer axis of the vessel. Arrow: direction of blood flow; I = intimal proliferate; M = media. Magnification ×2100.

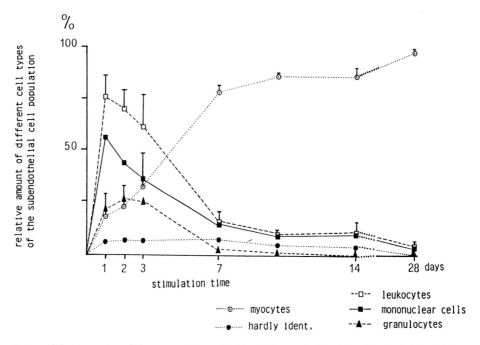

FIGURE 5.9. Dynamics of the composition of intimal plaques induced by electrical stimulation.

tion. Figure 5.9 shows the dynamics of cellular composition of the intima during development of a carotid artery plaque in rabbits fed a normal diet. The granulocytes disappear after a couple of days and the number of mononuclear cells also diminishes gradually during the development of the plaque, whereas the SMC proliferate and remain in the intima. In lipid-laden plaques the number of mononuclear cells is considerably higher than in lipid-free fibromuscular proliferates.

Figure 5.10 shows an SMC on its way from the media into the intima. Carotid artery plaques in animals stimulated for 7 days are depicted in Figure 5.11. Figure 5.11a shows the reaction of an animal fed 1% cholesterol in its chow, while 5.11b shows a proliferating plaque in an animal fed a normal diet. The rate of growth is high within the initial 14 days but diminishes with time. This is determined by counting the layer number of proliferating cells (Fig. 5.12) in serial sections. Plaque growth eventually ceases despite continual stimulations. If stimulation is stopped for 4 weeks

FIGURE 5.10. Migrating SMC (arrow) through the internal elastic lamina (E). The cell contains filaments that are typical for SMC. With immunological techniques it was demonstrated that the migrating cells contain smooth muscle myosin and α-actin, typical markers for SMC. Magnification ×10 000. (Obtained from D. Kling, Institute of Physiology I, Tuebingen.)

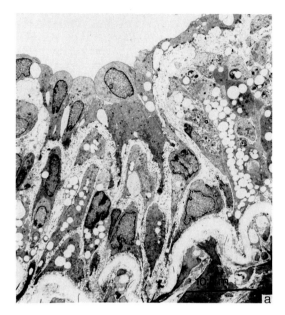
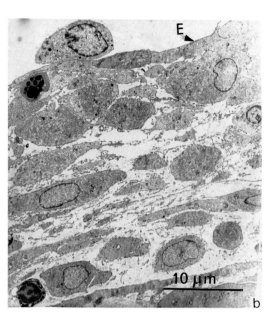

FIGURE 5.11. (a) Carotid artery proliferate 7 days after the start of the experiment. The rabbit received 1% cholesterol in its chow during the electrical stimulation. (b) Carotid artery proliferate 7 days after the start of the experiment. A monocyte adheres on the endothelium (E). The rabbit received normal food. (Obtained from D. Kling, Institute of Physiology I, Tübingen.)

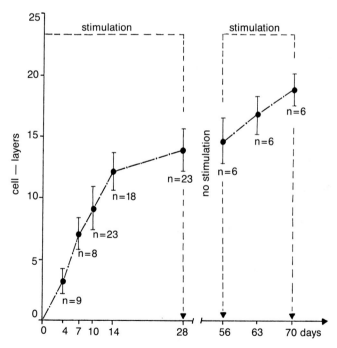

FIGURE 5.12. Time course of the growth of intimal plaques within two periods of proliferation-inducing stimulations in rabbits fed a normal diet. The first stimulation period lasted 28 days. The growth rate was initially higher than in the later phase of the first stimulation period. The second period, in which no stimuli were applied, lasted 4 weeks. During this period no further growth could be seen. In the third period of 14 days, the artery was stimulated with the same stimuli as in the first period. Within this third period the plaque grew again considerably.

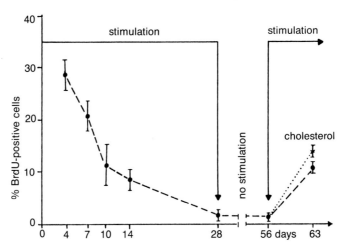

FIGURE 5.13. Measurements of the mitotic rates of cells within the plaque. The stimulation program was identical to that of Figure 5.11, and the same animals were used for labeling the S-phase of dividing cells with BrdU. One group of animals received in the third period 1% cholesterol in addition to the electrical stimuli. The response of this group was stronger. BrdU was given subcutaneously as a depot 18 hours prior to the excision of the artery and once more 8 hours before excision.

after a 28-day period of repeated daily stimuli and then the stimuli are reapplied as before, growth begins again (Fig. 5.12).

Measurement of the mitotic rate of the intimal cells is possible by labeling the dividing cells with bromo-desoxy-uridin (BrdU), staining them with an antibody that can be identified by fluorescence (see Refs. 84–86 for description of technique). With this method the mitotic rate of the SMC is found to be high in the initial phase of plaque development and then to decrease to nearly initial levels. The mitotic rate increases again during restimulation after an interval of 4 weeks in which no stimuli are applied. Figure 5.13 shows this effect and also that other atherogenic stimuli cause a rapidly reappearing mitotic response if the atheromatous plaque has already developed. This is similar to the well-known periodic growth of atheromas in humans in which "silent" plaques are suddenly activated without observ-

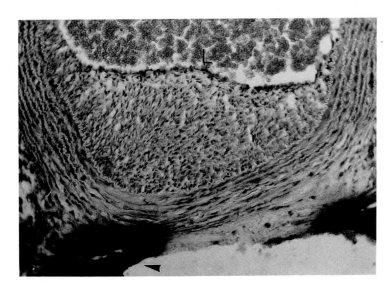

FIGURE 5.14. Atheroma beneath the anode, 28 days stimulation.

TABLE 5.3. Inhibition of carotid intimal proliferates in rabbits by oral (o) or subcutaneous (sc) administration of various drugs.[a]

Substance	Daily doses (mg/kg body weight)	% change of plaque growth in comparison with controls (number of cell layers)	% change of serum cholesterol in treated animals	% change of serum triglycerides in treated animals
Etofibrate	200 (o)	−25% (ns)	−15% (ns)	+80% (ns)
SP 54	25 (sc)	−55% (s)	−25% (ns)	+280% (s)
Flunarizine	30 (o)	−68% (s)	−35% (ns)	−30% (ns)
Verapamil	21.5 (o + sc)	−48% (s)	− 5% (ns)	+50% (ns)
Oktimibate	30 (o)	− 5% (ns)	−25% (ns)	+15% (ns)

[a]Controls = 100%. The third column shows the changes of total serum cholesterol, and the last column the changes of serum triglycerides. The numbers give the percentage of reduction (s = significant change, ns = nonsignificant; student test).

able changes in risk factors. Thus the artery walls may adapt to atherogenic stimuli, while in "silent," atheromatous plaques failure of adaptation may reactivate the plaque by the same atherogenic stimulus.

Growth of intimal plaque is inhibited not only by a reduction of risk factors but also by drugs. To study drug effects on atherogenesis, the following technique for plaque production was standardized. The carotid artery was stimulated with 0.1 mA, 10 ms/impulse, 10 Hz for 30 minutes in the morning and 15 minutes in the afternoon for 28 days in unrestrained animals. The control group of animals received no cholesterol in their food, while other groups received either 1% or 0.5% cholesterol. Figure 5.14 shows a fully developed plaque. The stimulation time was 28 days in a rabbit also given 1% cholesterol in its diet. To quantify the response, the plaque (beneath the 5-mm-long electrode) was cut in series for histological examination, and the maximal number of cell layers was counted. Some sectors were stained with hematoxylin-eosin and others with oil red (staining lipids).

Table 5.3 lists the effects of some antiatherogenic drugs and illustrates the lack of clear relationship between the cholesterol content of the blood and the thickness of the proliferation. The lipid content of the plaque is indexed, 0 being a plaque with no lipid, and 1, if one-third of the plaque (luminal portion) contained stainable lipid; 2, if the whole plaque contained lipids, and index 3 was given if both the proliferation and the underlying media contained lipid droplets. This method allows a gross classification of lipid content of the plaques. Only SP54 and Flunarizine moderately inhibited the uptake of lipids into the proliferate.

With some drugs a concentration-dependent antiproliferative response could be obtained. Figure 5.15 shows the response after oral application of varying doses of Flunarizine. The calcium antagonist Verapamil was effective only in hyperlipidemic animals, whereas in normolipidemic animals no inhibition of plaque growth was seen.

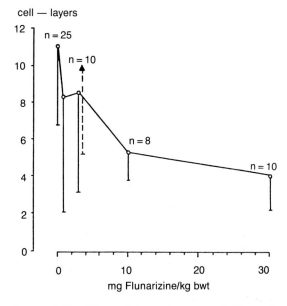

FIGURE 5.15. Effects of increasing concentrations of Flunarizine in the chow of rabbits on the development of electrically induced atheromas. All groups except one (arrow) received 1% cholesterol in their chow during the whole period of stimulation. It can be seen that the one group fed a normal diet plus Flunarizine (arrowhead) responded with almost the same reduction of proliferate growth as the cholesterol group with the same concentration of Flunarizine in the diet.

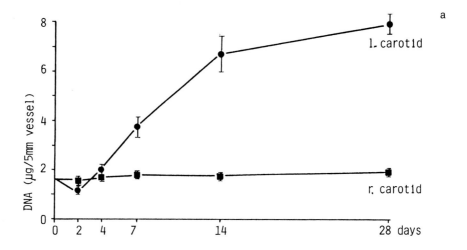

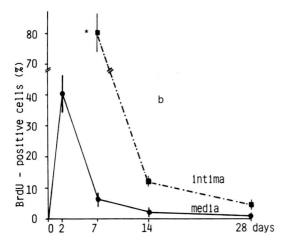

FIGURE 5.16. (a) Comparison of the DNA content of a group of four ballooned and four normal contralateral rat carotid arteries. (b) Comparison of mitotic rates of intimal and medial SMC measured by labeling ballooned carotid arteries of rats with BrdU. BrdU (30 mg/kg) was given as a depot subcutaneously 18 hours before excision. (By permission of Fotev et al., manuscript in preparation.)

Atheroma Induced by Intraluminal Balloon

In the following experiments balloons were inserted, in rats or rabbits, through an arterial branch into the carotid artery. It was then inflated and moved three times back and forth. The proliferative response started 2 or 3 days afterwards. The mitotic rate reaches its maximal value between the second and seventh days and then declines. The proliferative response of the intima of normally fed animals stimulated with electrical current was identical to those damaged by balloon, except that the endothelium remained intact in the electrostimulation model but was denuded in the ballooned model.

To quantify the proliferative response in ballooned carotid arteries, they were kept at their nor-

mal length during excision and then cut into 5-mm-long segments. The DNA content of one dissected artery segment was then determined using the method of Labarca and Paigen.[87] The second segment was used for histological analyses, and the contralateral nonstimulated carotid artery served as a control. Since the ballooned arteries proliferated circumferentially, cell counts were used for quantification from four sectors of the artery 90 degrees to each other. Figure 5.16a shows the DNA level of the stimulated and contralateral nonstimulated artery, and Figure 5.16b shows the mitotic rate in the proliferated area. There is a striking similarity between the responses of the electrostimulated carotid arteries and the ballooned arteries. Various drugs reduce plaque development (Table 5.4), and this may be close related (see Fig. 5.17).

TABLE 5.4. The effect on the proliferative response in ballooned carotid arteries of rats to subcutaneously injected (sc) 1. heparin, 2. low-molecular-weight heparin, 3. and 4. dextran sulfate.[a]

	Substance	Molecular weight (Dalton)	Doses per day/kg body weight	% sulfatation	Intimal DNA content (μ/5 mm vessel)	% inhibition of plaque growth	n
A.	Control (NaCl 0.9%)		1 ml (sc)	–	3.82 ± 0.32	–	7
	1. Sigma-heparin	15 000–18 000	3 mg (sc)	11.9	2.11 ± 0.08	45	4
	2. LMW-heparin	3900	3 mg (sc)	11.5	2.30 ± 0.39	40	4
	3. Dextran sulfate (I)	9245	3 mg (sc)	9.4	3.37 ± 0.72	12	4
	4. Dextran sulfate (II)	4210	3 mg (sc)	17.0	1.67 ± 0.32	56	4
B.	Control		–	–	4.07 ± 0.17	–	13
	5. Fendiline	351.9	20 mg (o)	–	2.30 ± 0.34	43	4

[a]The ballooned controls A received 3 ml 0.9% NaCl daily but no drug. In another series Fendiline (a calcium-calmodulin antagonist) was administered orally (o). The ballooned controls B received no further treatment. The arteries were excised 14 days after ballooning, and the DNA contents of the vessels were measured immediately after excision. Administration of the drugs started 2 days prior to ballooning and was continued until the day of artery excision.

Conclusion

Numerous drugs act by inhibiting the growth of intimal proliferation, and their effect on the invasion of granulocytes and monocytes into the wall of a carotid artery after a local atherogenic stimulation has been evaluated by various techniques. For instance, Kling (personal communication) found that Flunarizine did not significantly inhibit the early migration of leukocytes but did suppress SMC proliferation.

In vivo models provide little information about the mechanisms of drug actions because of frequent toxicity to proliferating cells. Similar limitations apply to the drug effects on the proliferation or migration of SMC. The drugs may affect other cell types, or the inhibitory action may be directly on the SMC or may be indirect, such as via endothelial cell mediators. Hence, in vivo experiments must be supplemented by investigating the effects of drugs on cultures of SMC, fibroblasts and EC. Table 5.5 gives an overview of the effects of drugs on SMC and fibroblast cultures. Some experiments utilize cells from human carotid arteries (h), others from human bypass veins or from animal aorta. Fibroblasts were not obtained from the adventitia but from subcutaneous tissue. Betz et al.[82] showed that cells stained with ethidiumbromide and fluoresceinacetate enable living cells to be distinguished from dead cells, thus indicating which concentration of drugs is cytotoxic.[88-90]

By treatment of mass cultures and clone cultures of different cells from the arterial wall with the same concentration of a drug, the differences in effect on growth inhibition can be tested. Some

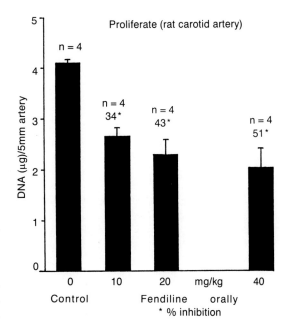

FIGURE 5.17. Effect of increasing concentrations of Fendiline (a calcium + calmodulin antagonist from Thie-mamn, Waltrop) on the development of a fibromuscular proliferate after ballooning. There is a dose-dependent inhibition of the proliferation. (By permission of Fotev, unpublished data.)

TABLE 5.5. Effects of various drugs on cultures of SMC of human arteries (h) or rabbit arteries and fibroblasts.[a]

Substance	Concentration ml/l	Inhibition of SMC proliferation after 4 days of culture. Controls = no inhibition ($=0\%$)	Inhibition of fibroblast proliferation after 4 days of culture. Controls = no inhibition ($=0\%$)
Etofibrate	$8 \cdot 10^{-5}$	95	98
SP 54	$1.2 \cdot 10^{-5}$	62	0
Flunarizine (h)	10^{-5}	37	42
Verapamil (h)	10^{-5}	17	10
Nimodipine	10^{-5}	98	120

[a]Inhibitions $> 100\%$ indicate toxicity of the applied concentration because the number of cells decreases below the number of cells initially seeded. Nimodipine (10^{-5} mol/l) has such an effect in vitro but no observable effect in vivo (see Table 5.3). This discrepancy is caused by a strong first-pass effect when the drug is applied via an oral route. The concentrations in the blood of rabbits are very low. This may be different in other animal species.

drugs, such as heparinoids or dextran sulfates, inhibit the growth of SMC but have no effect on EC or fibroblast growth. SP 54 (Bene-Chemie, Munich) is one such drug.[69] For studies of drug actions on the inhibition of stenosing plaques, in vivo studies can be combined with in vitro studies.[82,91-110]

Recently developed cell culture experiments (coculture systems) imitate the interplay among the media, endothelium, and macrophages of normal arteries.[111-112] In addition, these new techniques produce early atheroma in vitro and appear extremely promising as models for future drug research on the inhibition of atherogenesis.[113]

References

1. Friedman M, Byers S. Endothelial permeability in atherosclerosis. *Arch Pathol.* 1963;76:111–117.
2. Friedman RJ, More S, Singal DP. Repeated endothelial injury and induction of atherosclerosis in normolipidemic rabbits by human serum. *Lab Invest.* 1975;32:404.
3. Bell FP, Adamson JL, Schwartz CJ. Aortic endothelial permeability of albumin. Focal and regional patterns to uptake and transmural distribution of 131-J-albumin in the young pig. *Exp Mol Path.* 1974;20:57–61.
4. Constantinides P. The role of the endothelium in atherosclerosis. *Verh Dtsch Ges Inn Medizin.* 1975; 81:839–843.
5. Kurozumi T. Electron microscopic study on permeability of the aorta and basilar artery of the rabbit—with special reference to the changes of permeability by hypercholesteremia. *Exp Mol Path.* 1975;23:1–11.
6. Jellinek H, Elemer G. Die Transportstörungen der Arterienwand als Initialfaktor der zellulären Reaktion. *Atherogenese.* 1976;1:20.
7. Adams CWM, Bayliss OB, Morgan RS. Permeability in atherosclerosis: Fluorescence test in green light with trypan blue. *Atherosclerosis.* 1977;27: 353–359.
8. Bratzler RL, Chisholm GM, Colton CK, et al. The distribution of labelled albumin across the rabbit thoracic aorta in vivo. *Circulat Res.* 1977;40:182–190.
9. Constantinides P. The morphological basis for altered endothelial permeability in atherosclerosis. *Atherosclerosis.* 1977;82:969–974.
10. Schwartz SM. Role of endothelial integrity in atherosclerosis. *Artery.* 1980;8:305–314.
11. Caro CG, Lever MJ, Laver-Rudich Z, et al. Net albumin transport across the wall of the rabbit common carotid artery perfused in situ. *Atherosclerosis.* 1980;37:497–511.
12. Schmid G. Permeabilität der Arterienwand bei tierexperimenteller Arteriosklerose. In: Betz E, Fischer H, eds. *Das Gefässendothel.* Stuttgart: Wissenschaftliche Verlagsgesellschaft mbH; 1981: 96–109.
13. Pfeffer R, Ganatos P, Nir A, Weinbaum S. Diffusion of macromolecules across the arterial wall in the presence of multiple endothelial injuries. *J Biochmech Engn.* 1981;103:197–203.
14. Fujino M. Ultrastructural studies of the mouse aorta and its endothelial pinocytosis in diet-induced arteriosclerosis. *Acta Path Jpn.* 1983;33:1115–1130.
15. Veress B, Balint A, Kocze A, et al. Increasing aortic permeability by atherogenic diet. *Atherosclerosis.* 1970;11:369–370.
16. Holle G, Massmann J, Weidenbach H. Experimentally induced early changes in arteries. *Path Eur.* 1974;9:125–132.

17. Minick CR, Stemerman MB, Insull W. Role of endothelium and hypercholesterinaemia in intima thickening and lipid accumulation. *Am J Pathol.* 1979;95:131–158.
18. Copley AL. The physiological significance of the endothelial fibrin lining (EEFL) as the critical interface in the "vessel-blood organ" and the importance of in vivo "fibrinogen formation" in health and disease. *Thromb Res.* 1983;(suppl. 5):105–145.
19. Lindner V. Permeabilitätsänderungen der Arterienwand im Initialstadium experimenteller Atherosklerose. Diss. Tübingen 1984
20. Apfel H, Betz E, Strohschneider T. Änderungen der Permeabilität und der elektrischen Leitfähigkeit von Arterienwänden bei der experimentellen Atherogenese. *Funktionsanalyse biologischer Systeme.* 1986;15:27–33 (Stuttgart: Steiner Verlag).
21. Gerrity RG. The role of the monocyte in atherogenesis: I. Transition of blood-borne monocytes into foam cells in fatty lesions. *Am J Pathol.* 1981;103:181–190.
22. Gerrity RG. The role of the monocyte in atherogenesis: II. Migration of foam cells from atherosclerotic lesions. *Am J Pathol.* 1981;103:191–200.
23. Trillo AA. The cell population of aortic fatty streaks in African green monkeys with special reference to granulocytic cells: an ultrastructural study. *Atherosclerosis.* 1982;43:259–275.
24. Joris J, Zand T, Nunnari JJ, et al. Studies on the pathogenesis of atherosclerosis: I. Adhesion and emigration of mononuclear cells in the aorta of hypercholesterolemic rats. *Am J Pathol.* 1983;113:341–358.
25. Faggiotto A, Ross R, Harker E. Studies of hypercholesterolemia in the nonhuman primate: I. Changes that lead to fatty streak formation. *Arteriosclerosis.* 1984;4:323–346.
26. Faggiotto A, Ross R. Studies of hypercholesterolemia in the nonhuman primate: II. Fatty streaks conversion to fibrous plaques. *Arteriosclerosis.* 1984;4:341–356.
27. Rosenfeld ME, Faggiotto A, Ross R. The role of mononuclear phagocyte in primate and rabbit models of atherosclerosis. Proceedings of the Fourth Leiden Conference on Mononuclear Phagocytes. The Hague: Martinus Nijhoff; 1985.
28. Watanabe T, Hirata M, Yoshikawa Y, et al. Role of macrophages in atherosclerosis: Sequential observations of cholesterol-induced rabbit aortic lesion by the immunoperoxidase technique using monoclonal antimacrophage antibody. *Lab Invest.* 1985;53:80–90.
29. Schwartz CJ, Sprague EA, Kelley JL, et al. Aortic intimal monocyte recruitment in the normo and hypercholesterolemic baboon (Papio cynocephalus). An ultrastructural study: implications in atherogenesis. *Virchows Arch A Pathol Anat Histopath.* 1985;405:175–191.
30. Nilsson J. Growth factors and the pathogenesis of atherosclerosis. *Atherosclerosis.* 1986;62:185–199.
31. Jonasson L, Holm J, Skalli O, et al. Regional accumulations of T cells, macrophages, and smooth muscle cells in the human atherosclerotic plaque. *Arteriosclerosis.* 1986;6:131–138.
32. Schwartz CJ, Valente AJ, Sprague EA, et al. Monocyte-macrophage participation in atherogenesis: Inflammatory components of pathogenesis. *Seminars in Thrombosis and Hemostasis.* 1986;12:79–86.
33. Kling D, Holzschuh T, Strohschneider T, et al. Enhanced endothelial permeability and invasion of leukocytes into the artery wall as initial events in experimental arteriosclerosis. *Inter Angio.* 1987;6:21–28.
34. Kling D, Holzschuh T, Betz E. Temporal sequence of morphological alterations in artery walls during experimental atherogenesis. *Res Exp Med.* 1987;187:237–250.
35. Meessen H, Kojimahara M, Franken T, et al. Alteration of the rabbit aorta following feeding of cholesterol diet in combination with sheathing of aortic segments by polyethylene tubes. *Beitr Path.* 1975;154:218–232.
36. Booth RFG, Honey AC, Moncada S, et al. Enhancement of focal intimal proliferation in the rabbit carotid by cholesterol feeding. Proceedings of the Eighth International Symposium on Atherosclerosis; 1988;Rome:CI C Edizioni Internazionali Stampa Tekno Press; 1988:p 98. Abstract
37. Booth RFG, Martin JF, Honey AC, et al. Rapid development of atherosclerotic lesions in the rabbit carotid artery induced by perivascular manipulation. *Atherosclerosis.* 1989;76:257–268.
38. Seuter F, Sitt R, Busse WD. Experimentally induced thromboatherosclerosis in rats and rabbits. *Folia Angiol.* 1980;28:85–87.
39. Baumgartner HR, Studer A. Gezielte Überdehnung der Aorta abdominalis am normo- und hypercholesterinämischen Kaninchen. *Path Microbiol.* 1963;26:129–148.
40. Baumgartner HR, Studer A. Smooth muscle cell proliferation and migration after removal of arterial endothelium in rabbits. In: Schettler G, Stange E, Wissler RW, eds. *Atherosclerosis—is it reversible?* New York, NY: Springer-Verlag; 1978: pp 12–18.
41. Betz E, Schlote W. Responses of vessel walls to chronically applied electrical stimuli. *Basic Res Cardiol.* 1979;74:10–20.

42. Ignatowski AC. Influence of animal food on the organism of rabbits. *S Peterb Izviest Imp Voyenno-Med Akad.* 1908;16:154–173.

43. Kritchevsky D, Moyer AW, Tesar WC, et al. Effects of cholesterol vehicle in experimental atherosclerosis. *Am J Physiol.* 1954;178:30–32.

44. Schettler G, ed. *Arteriosklerose. Ätiologie, Pathologie, Klinik und Therapie.* Stuttgart: Georg Thieme Verlag; 1961.

45. Meyer WW. Die Arteriosklerose im Tierexperiment. In: Kaufmann E, Staemmler M, Erg Bd I, eds. *Lehrbuch der speziellen pathologischen Anatomie.* 1. Hälfte. Berlin: Walter de Gruyter; 1969:591–652.

46. Kritchevsky D. Role of cholesterol vehicle in experimental atherosclerosis. *Am J Clin Nutr.* 1970;23: 1105–1110.

47. Schettler G, Weizel A, ed. *Atherosclerosis III.* New York, NY: Springer-Verlag; 1974.

48. Ross R, Harker L. Hyperlipidemia and atherosclerosis. *Science.* 1976;193:1094–1100.

49. Schettler G, Goto Y, Hata Y, et al., eds. *Atherosclerosis IV.* New York, NY: Springer-Verlag; 1977.

50. Kritchevsky D, Davison LM, Kim HK, et al. Influence of semipurified diet on atherosclerosis in African green monkeys. Exp Mol *Pathol.* 1977; 26:28–51.

51. Wissler RW. Risk factors and regression. In: Schettler G, Stange E, Wissler RW, eds. *Atherosclerosis —is it reversible?* New York, NY: Springer-Verlag; 1978:93–101.

52. Goldstein JL, Anderson RGW, Brown MS. Coated pits, coated vesicles, and receptor-mediated endocytosis. *Nature.* 1979;279:679–685.

53. Gerrity RG, Naito HK, Richardson M, et al. Dietary induced atherogenesis in swine. *Am J Pathol.* 1979;95:775–785.

54. Vesselinovitch D, Fischer-Dzoga K. Techniques in pathology in atherosclerosis research. *Adv in Lipid Res.* 1981;18:1–63.

55. Wissler RW. Neuste Studien über die Pathogenese und Rückbildung der Atherosklerose. *Therapiewoche.* 1982;32:3735–3745.

56. Kritchevsky D. Experimental atherosclerosis. diet and drugs. In: Born GVR, Catapano AL, Paoletti R, eds. *Factors in Formation and Regression of the Atherosclerotic Plaque.* New York, NY: Plenum Publ Corp; 1982: pp 95–105.

57. Schettler G. Zur Pathogenese der Arteriosklerose. Hämostaseologie. 1982;2:3–6.

58. Assmann G. Zur Ätiologie der Atherosklerose. *Hämostaseologie.* 1982;2:162–168.

59. Assmann G. Lipidstoffwechsel und Atherosklerose. Stuttgart: Schattauer-Verlag, 1982.

60. Joris I, Billingham ME, Majno G. Human coronary arteries: an ultrastructural search for the early changes of atherosclerosis. *Fed Proc.* 1984;43:710.

61. Goldstein JL, Brown MS, Anderson GW, et al. Receptor-mediated endocytosis. Concepts emerging from the LDL receptor system. *Ann Rev Cell Biol.* 1985;1:1–39.

62. Haust MD. Recent concepts on the pathogenesis of atherosclerosis. *Can Med Assn J.* 1989;140:929.

63. Ross R, Glomset JA. The pathogenesis of atherosclerosis. *N Engl J Med.* 1976;295:420–425.

64. Ross R, Glomset J, Harker L. Response to injury and atherogenesis. *Am J Pathol.* 1977;86:675–684.

65. Ross R, Glomset J, Harker L. The response to injury and atherogenesis: The role of endothelium and smooth muscle. *Atherosclerosis Rev.* 1978;3: 69–75.

66. Ross R, Faggiotto A, Bowen-Pope D, et al. The role of endothelial injury and platelet and macrophage interactions in atherosclerosis. *Circulat.* 1984;70: III–77–III–82.

67. Ross R. Platelets—endothelial and smooth muscle proliferation. In: Dingle JT, Gordon JL, eds. *Cellular Interactions.* Elsevier, North-Holland: Biomed Press; 1981;6:177.

68. Ross R. Growth factors in the pathogenesis of atherosclerosis. *Acta Med Scand.* 1987;221(Suppl. 715):33–38.

69. Betz E, Hämmerle H. Arterienwandproliferate und Zellkulturen als Indikatoren für Hemmstoffe der Atherogenese. *Funkt Biol Med.* 1984;3:46–55.

70. Apfel H. Ein zwei-Elektroden-Messverfahren zur in vivo-Bestimmung der elektrischen Impedanz arterieller Blutgefässe im Frequenzbereich von 1 kHz bis 100 kHz. *Biomed Technik.* 1988;33(Erg. Bd 2):309–310.

71. Apfel H. Electrical impedance of the carotid artery in response to various types of stress. In: Liepsch D, ed. *Proceedings of the second International Symposium on Biofluid Mechanics and Biorheology* Munich Institut für Biotechnik, 1989; pp 267–276.

72. Apfel H, Kaufmann J, Betz E. Electrical conductivity of the vessel wall in normal and arteriosclerotic carotid arteries. *Pflügers Arch.* 1988; 412(suppl. 1):R88.

73. Viele D, Betz E. Effect of the calcium entry blocker, Flunarizine, on ruthenium red uptake by endothelial cells following acute electrical stimulation of rabbit carotid arteries. *Basic Res Cardiol.* 1985;80:58–65.

74. Jellinek H. Stofftransport in der Gefässwand bei Frühveränderungen der Arteriosklerose. *Z Ges Inn Med.* 1978;33:599–601.

75. Heinle H, Lindner V. The binding of Evans blue to collagen and elastin in elastic tissue. *Arch Int Physiol Biochem*. 1984;92:13–17.

76. Strohschneider T, Betz E. Hemmwirkungen von Calciumeintrittsblockern auf den transendothelialen Transport von Peroxidase. *Angio Archiv*. 1985; 7:100–103.

77. Jellinek H, Füzesi S, Solti F, et al. Ultrastructural study of canine aortic damage caused by disturbance of transmural transport. *Exp Mol Path*. 1986;44:67–75.

78. Strohschneider T, Betz E. Densitometric measurement of increased endothelial permeability in arteriosclerotic plaques and inhibition of permeability under the influence of two calcium antagonists. *Atherosclerosis*. 1989;75:135–144.

79. Strohschneider T, Betz E. Die Wirkung von Pentoxifyllin auf die Arterienwandpermeabilität. *Perfusion*. 1988;2/88:50–55.

80. Karnovsky MJ. The ultrastructural basis of capillary permeability studied with peroxidase as a tracer. *J Cell Biol*. 1967;35:213–236.

81. Forssmann WG. A method for in vivo diffusion tracer studies combining perfusion fixation with intravenous tracer injection. *Histochemie*. 1969; 20:277–286.

82. Betz E, Hämmerle H, Strohschneider T. Inhibition of smooth muscle cell proliferation and endothelial permeability with Flunarizine in vitro and in experimental atheromas. *Res Exp Med*. 1985;185:325–340.

83. Strohschneider T, Kling D, Betz E. The effect of pentoxifylline on endothelial permeability of rabbit carotid artery wall. *Europ J Pharmacol*. 1988;150: 287–293.

84. Gratzner HG. Monoclonal antibody to 5-Bromo- and 5-Jododeoxy-uridine: a new reagent for detection of DNA replication. *Science*. 1982;218:474–475.

85. Morstyn G, Hsu SM, Kinsella T, et al. Bromodeoxyuridine in tumors and chromosomes detected with a monoclonal antibody. *J Clin Invest*. 1983; 72:1844–1850.

86. Fingerle J, Kraft T. The induction of smooth muscle cell proliferation in vitro using an organ culture system. *Inter Angio*. 1987;6:65–72.

87. Labarca C, Paigen K. A simple, rapid and sensitive DNA assay procedure. *Ann Biochem*. 1980;102: 344–352.

88. Rotman B, Papermaster BW. Membrane properties of living mammalian cells as studied by enzymatic hydrolysis of fluorogenic esters. *Proc Natl Acad Sci USA*. 1966;55:134–141.

89. Netuschil L, Schmalz G. Lebendbestimmung kariogener Bakterien mittels Fluoresceindiacetat. *Kariesprophylaxe*. 1981;3:75–79.

90. Netuschil L: Vitalfärbung von Plaque-Mikroorganismen mit Fluorescein-diacetat und Ethidiumbromid. *Dtsch zahnärztl Z*. 1983;38:914–917.

91. Lippman MM, Mathews, MB: Heparins. Varying effects on cell proliferation in vitro and lack of correlation with anticoagulant activity. *Fed Proc*. 1977;36:55–59.

92. Guyton JR, Rosenberg RD, Clowes AW, et al. Inhibition of rat arterial smooth muscle cell proliferation by heparin. In vivo studies with anticoagulant and nonanticoagulant heparin. *Circulat Res*. 1980; 46:625–634.

93. Hoover RL, Rosenberg R, Haering W, et al. Inhibition of rat arterial smooth muscle cell proliferation by heparin. *Circulat Res*. 1980;47:578–583.

94. Nakao J, Ito H, Ooyama T, et al. Calcium dependency of aortic smooth muscle cell migration induced by 12-L-hydroxy-5,8,10,14-eicosatetraenoic acid. Effects of A23187, Nicardipine and Trifluoperazine. *Atherosclerosis*. 1983;46:309–319.

95. Blaes N, Boisell JP. Growth-stimulating effect of catecholamines on rat aortic smooth muscle cells in culture. *J Cell Physiol*. 1983;116:167–172.

96. Majack RA, Clowes AW. Inhibition of vascular smooth muscle cell migration by heparin-like glycosaminoglycans. *J Cell Physiol*. 1984;118:253–256.

97. Engelberg H: Heparin and the atherosclerotic process. *Pharmacol Rev*. 1984;36:91–110.

98. Castellot JJ, Rosenberg RD, Karnovsky MJ. Endothelium, heparin, and the regulation of vascular smooth muscle cell growth. In: Jaffee EA, ed. *Biology of Endothelial Cells*. Boston: Martinus Nijhoff; 1984: pp 118–128.

99. Thilo-Körner DGS, Bödeker RH. Human smooth muscle cells of the aorta and vena cava: Different sensitivity to the inhibition of proliferation by heparin in vitro. *Klin Wsch*. 1985;63:702–705.

100. Betz E, Hämmerle H. Effects of Etofibrate and its metabolites on atheromas of rabbits and on smooth muscle cell cultures. *Arzneim-Forsch/Drug Res*. 1986;36:92–98.

101. Betz E, Hämmerle H, Kling D, et al. The actions of Verapamil on the model of arteriosclerosis. In: Rosenthal J, ed. *Calcium antagonists and Hypertension: Current Status*. Amsterdam: Exc Med; 1986:83–96.

102. Reilly CF, Fritze LMS, Rosenberg RD. Inhibition of smooth muscle cell proliferation by heparin-like molecules. *Med J Australia*. 1986;144:HS10–HS15.

103. Castellot JJ, Choay J, Lormeau JC, et al. Structural determinants of the capacity of heparin to inhibit the proliferation of vascular smooth muscle cells: II. Evidence for a pentasaccharide sequence that contains a 3-0-sulfate group. *J Cell Biol*. 1986; 102:1979–1984.

104. Orekhov AN, Tertov VV, Kudryashov SA, et al. Primary culture of human aortic intima cells as a model for testing antiatherosclerotic drugs. Effects of cyclic AMP, prostaglandins, calcium antagonists, antioxidants, and lipid-lowering agents. *Atherosclerosis*. 1986;60:101–110.

105. Orekhov AN, Tertov VV, Khashimov KA, et al. Evidence of antiatherosclerotic action of Verapamil from direct effects on arterial cells. *Am J Cardiol*. 1987;59:495–496.

106. Thyberg J, Palmberg L. The calcium antagonist nisoldipine and the calmodulin antagonist W-7 synergistically inhibit initiation of DNA synthesis in cultured arterial smooth muscle cells. *Biol o t Cell*. 1987;60:125–132.

107. Orekhov AN, Ruda MY, Baldenkov GN, et al. Atherogenic effects of beta blocker on cells cultured from normal and atherosclerotic aorta. *Am J Cardiol*. 1988;61:1116–1117.

108. Nomoto A, Mutho S, Hagihara H, et al. Smooth muscle cell migration induced by inflammatory ceil products and its inhibition by a potent calcium antagonist, nilvadipine. *Atherosclerosis*. 1988;72:213–219.

109. Herbert JM, Maffrand JP. Heparin interactions with cultured human vascular endothelial and smooth muscle cells: incidence on vascular smooth muscle cell proliferation. *J Cell Physiol*. 1989; 138:424–432.

110. Roth D, Dartsch PC, Betz E. Wirkung von Flunarizin auf die Proliferation von Gefäßwandzellen des Menschen. In: Betz E, ed. *Die Anwendung aktueller Methoden in der Arteriosklerose-Forschung*. Tübingen: Selbstverlag Dtsch Ges Arterioskleroseforschung e.V.; 1989: pp 276–279.

111. Fallier P, Hämmerle H, Betz E. Transfilterkulturen als Modelle für Untersuchungen von Frühveränderungen bei der Atherogenese. In: Betz E, ed. Frühveränderungen bei der Atherogenese. Munich: Zuckerschwendt Verlag; 1987: pp 112–116.

112. Fallier-Becker P, Wolburg-Buchholz K, Betz E. Co-cultures of smooth muscle and endothelial cells from the arterial wall. *Pflügers Arch*. 1988;412 (suppl 1):R 84.

113. Fallier-Becker P, Wolburg-Buchholz K, Baur R, et al. Einflüsse von Adventita und Endothel in Explantatkulturen. In: Betz E, ed. *Die Anwendung aktueller Methoden in der Arteriosklerose-Forschung*. Tübingen: Selbstverlag der Dtsch Ges Arterioskleroseforschung 1989: pp 332–339.

6
Stroke Risk Factors

Mark L. Dyken

The ideal treatment for stroke, is of course, prevention. This book is dedicated to that premise. To prevent stroke one must be able to identify that portion of the population that is at high risk and to identify factors that contribute to this risk. The remarkable decline in stroke mortality must be related to either a decreased risk for stroke or better treatment. The data suggest that both may be true to some degree. Nevertheless, although better treatment of stroke may have something to do with this decline, the evidence is compelling that recognition, treatment, and altering risk factors to prevent stroke are major reasons. If the purposes of this book are to be accomplished, it is imperative to identify potential risk factors, establish the relative degree of risk, and to remove or treat them appropriately.

Despite the decline in death rate, stroke is still the third leading cause of death in the United States, following heart disease and cancer, and is the most common reason for major disability.[1-3] Around a half million new strokes and 150 000 deaths occur each year. It is estimated that the annual cost for health care in 1989 will be $13.5 billion. Thus, if stroke could be greatly prevented, in addition to the incalculable decrease in human suffering, the economic benefits would be major.

The true prevalence of the types of cerebrovascular disease has not been definitely established. Estimates vary widely depending upon whether the data are from hospital records or from epidemiological population surveys. Each has defects, but since prevention of stroke depends upon risk factors being identified in the general population, for this presentation, whenever possible, population studies will be used. These indicate that atherothrombotic ischemic infarction is the most common type, accounting for nearly two thirds of all stroke.[4,5] Cerebral embolization from a cardiac source is reported to occur in 5% to 14% of all strokes, but as hospital-based diagnoses become more sophisticated, an increased percentage of infarctions previously diagnosed as atherothrombotic are now being attributed to embolus. Hemorrhage, including intraparenchymal and subarachnoid, is present in about 14% to 20%.

To prevent stroke it is necessary to identify and correct the predisposing factors in persons at high risk. The frequency and relative impact of these factors have been and are being identified in free-living populations through means of epidemiological studies, such as those performed in Framingham, Massachusetts,[4] and in Rochester, Minnesota.[5] It is likely that these concerted efforts to better identify, reduce, and eliminate risk factors will continue to decrease the incidence of stroke.

Although epidemiological studies have firmly established a number of factors that may be altered, ongoing studies are continuing to identify and verify others. In the 5 years since the last review of risk factors in stroke by a panel of the Stroke Council of the American Heart Association (AHA),[6] many factors that were then suspected have now been established, and others are in the process of study and evaluation. Since this report was a consensus statement and no controversial or isolated viewpoint was given without qualification, it will be referred to in all debatable areas.

Since the purpose of this book is stroke prevention, risk factors will be considered first by the

TABLE 6.1. Stroke risk factors.

I. Treatment specifically effective
  A. Established factors
    1. Hypertension!
    2. Cardiac disease
    3. Transient ischemic attacks
    4. Cigarette smoking
    5. Alcohol consumption
    6. Other drug abuse
  B. Factors not well established
    1. Abnormal lipids
    2. Diet
    3. Oral contraceptives
    4. Sedentary activity
    5. Obesity
    6. Hyperuricemia
    7. Infection
    8. Homocysteinemia
II. Treatment of associated factors effective
  A. Established factors
    1. Age
    2. Gender
    3. Heredo-familial
    4. Race
    5. Diabetes mellitus
    6. Prior stroke
    7. Increasing hematocrit
    8. Elevated fibrinogen
    9. Sickle cell disease
    10. Lupus anticoagulant
    11. Asymptomatic structural lesions (bruits)
  B. Factors not well established
    1. Migraine and migraine equivalents
III. Treatment not possible
  A. Factor not well established
    1. Geographic location
    2. Season and climate
    3. Socioeconomic factors
    4. Personality type
IV. Treatment of factors in combination

effectiveness of preventing them or altering them by treatment, and then by the firmness of their relationship to stroke. A number of factors that are not now well documented is associated with other factors that do have a relationship to stroke and may be treated. Thus, in many cases, the general health could be improved if each factor was recognized and treated. Therefore, factors will be considered individually and in combination. Although some are major risks for stroke by themselves, others become more important when in combination, and some are important only when in combination with others. Table 6.1 outlines the approach that will be followed.

Treatment Specifically Effective

Established Factors

Hypertension

Hypertension is the most important of all the risk factors for stroke. In addition to being strongly related to both atherothrombotic brain infarction and intraparenchymal hemorrhage, it is also very common.[7,8] In the Framingham study, the risk of stroke was directly related to the elevation of blood pressure.[9] Women with hypertension were at as great a risk for stroke as men, and the risk persisted in the elderly, in whom most strokes occur. Systolic pressure was most closely linked to stroke. In the Multiple Risk Factor Intervention Trial[10] the risk for stroke was also most strongly related to systolic hypertension. In a Japanese population, a single blood pressure measurement was not sufficient to predict risk.[11] An accumulated value or average over time was required. Also, an increase in blood pressure with time was a particular risk factor for cerebral hemorrhage. In that population, cerebral hemorrhage was more strongly related to diastolic than to systolic blood pressure, while cerebral infarction appeared to be more strongly related to systolic than to diastolic blood pressure. A hospital study in Cincinnati indicated that if a more inclusive definition of hypertension including history, electrocardiography, and chest radiography was used, relative risk increased from 3.9 to 5.4.[12] The Framingham study also suggests that antecedent blood pressure elevation is a significant risk factor for subarachnoid hemorrhage.[13]

The Framingham study indicated a declining incidence of stroke only for women who had more intensive treatment and effective control of blood pressure than men.[14,15] Effective treatment of hypertension cannot be accepted unequivocally as the only reason for the overall decline in stroke because stroke mortality was already declining before effective antihypertensive therapy became available. Nevertheless, all evidence in balance overwhelmingly supports the conclusion that efforts to control hypertension have been a major contribution to the recent decline in death rate from stroke. Clinical studies continue to show a reduction in stroke incidence and mortality when hypertension is treated.[16-29] These reductions are reported in a number of countries, for mild as well as severe hypertension, and in young and old people. In the United States from 1972 to 1977, age-adjusted death rates for hypertension-related cardiovascular disease declined 20%; whereas for hypertension-unrelated cardiovascular disease, the decline was only 9%.

Cardiac Disease

In the Framingham study, independent of blood pressure, persons with cardiac impairment of any sort, whether symptomatic or not, had more than twice the risk of stroke than persons with normal cardiac function. This is true whether cardiac impairment was determined by the presence of overt diseases such as coronary heart disease and congestive heart failure or by evidence of left ventricular hypertrophy by ECG and X-ray readings, or arrhythmias.[4] Coronary heart disease is also the major cause of death among stroke survivors, as well as for patients with transient ischemic attacks or carotid bruits.[30] The Honolulu Heart Program[31] followed 7560 men for 12 years. Those with baseline electrocardiographic abnormalities, including major ST depression, left ventricular strain, left ventricular hypertrophy, major T wave inversion, and overall major abnormalities, had considerably higher incidence rates for both thromboembolic and hemorrhagic stroke than those with normal baseline studies.

In the Framingham study atrial fibrillation, whatever the cause, was strongly correlated with embolic stroke.[14,32] Even after adjustment for increased age and blood pressure, patients with chronic nonrheumatic atrial fibrillation develop strokes more than five times as often as those without fibrillation, suggesting a direct association.[33] Atrial fibrillation with rheumatic heart disease had a 17-fold increase. Stroke occurrence increased as the duration of the atrial fibrillation increased, with no evidence of a particularly vulnerable period. However, recent reports from other studies suggest that much of this risk may be due to other associated factors. In Rochester, Minnesota,[34] a prospective study of 1804 residents followed for 13 years reported that individual relative risk for age was 1.6, 2.0 for males, 4.0 for definite hypertension, 3.9 for transient ischemic attacks, 2.2 for hypertensive heart disease, 2.2 for coronary heart disease, 1.7 for congestive heart failure,

and 1.7 for diabetes mellitus. Yet atrial fibrillation was not a significant risk factor. In addition, lone atrial fibrillation was associated with a very low risk of stroke in patients who were under the age of 60 at diagnosis and were followed for 14.8 years.[35] Other studies recently have reported that the increased stroke rate in atrial fibrillation may be accounted for by other factors.[36,37]

Mitral valve prolapse has been demonstrated to have an association with stroke in young people,[38] but the incidence is so low that even if there was an established prophylactic treatment, it would not be indicated unless it was absolutely innocuous.

Transient Ischemic Attacks

Transient ischemic attacks (TIAs) are generally considered to be episodes of focal ischemic neurological deficit in the distribution of an arterial vessel to the brain that last <24 hours. The 24-hour limit is probably far too high since attacks average only 8 to 14 minutes[39]; and, when they last over an hour, they are less likely to reverse.[40] When they last several hours, subclinical infarctions are frequently visualized with magnetic resonance imaging.[41,42] Whether TIAs are risk factors or are strokes can be debated; but, since they leave no clinical deficits, the opportunity exists to identify a high-risk patient and initiate a program with the potential to prevent permanent deficits. Although TIAs are associated with a high risk for stroke,[43] in the Framingham study[4] patients with TIAs also had many other significant risk factors, (hypertension and cardiac disease, coronary heart disease, left ventricular hypertrophy by ECG examination, and congestive heart failure) than those of the same age and sex. Therefore, TIA is not a totally independent risk factor for stroke, and this suggests that the risk might be greatly reduced by treating associated conditions. Although it is clear that TIAs are strong predictors for stroke, only about 10% of all strokes are preceded by them.[44-47] In addition, it is estimated that atherothrombotic disease of the large extracranial arteries, including the carotid arteries, is associated with no more than one third of all strokes, and a surgically accessible lesion accounts for no more than 15%.

Nevertheless, we now have means to decrease appreciably the risk for stroke in individuals who have TIAs. Established current therapy includes platelet antiaggregating medications. To date, eight prospective, double-blinded studies have been reported for aspirin (five with TIAs and three with TIAs and mild stroke). In seven studies, the end points were TIAs, stroke, and death,[48-55] and in one, only ischemic events.[56] Although each of these studies might have had defects, they are minimal when compared to those of anecdotal case reports. When one combines all groups receiving aspirin and all receiving placebo in these studies, a 15% to 35% decrease in stroke and death is noted. The probability of this occurring by chance is extremely small.[57] None of the studies of patients with TIAs only demonstrated an independent effect for women, but two of the three studies of patients with TIA or mild stroke did.[48,54] Recently, two very large, prospective, double-blind studies compared ticlopidine and aspirin in stroke prevention. One was of patients with TIA[58] and the other of patients who had stroke.[59] Both showed a statistical decrease in all strokes and for stroke and death combined in those receiving ticlopidine. These differences were present in all patients and for women as a subgroup.

Cigarette Smoking

Five years ago when the AHA published a consensus Statement for Physicians[6] on risk factors in stroke, the evidence was not strong enough to establish cigarette smoking as a definite risk for stroke. Although it was a recognized risk factor for cardiopulmonary and peripheral vascular disease, its relationship to atherothrombotic brain infarction was not clear. At that time the Framingham study suggested that smoking was an apparent risk factor for atherothrombotic brain infarction only in men below age 65.[4] The Elkhart study suggested that smoking was a risk for men.[60] Paffenbarger and Williams[61] found smoking to be one of the major risk factors in college students who later developed fatal occlusive stroke at twice the rate of nonsmokers. Since then, a number of studies have established cigarette smoking not only as a risk factor for stroke, but a substantial one. After a 26-year follow-up, the Framingham study[62] established that cigarette smoking was a significant risk factor for stroke independent of age, hypertension, and pertinent cardiovascular disease risk factors. The risk increased with the number of cigarettes. The possible effectiveness of treatment was sup-

ported by a significant decrease in risk two years after cessation, reverting to that of nonsmokers at five years. Other large epidemiological studies have reported similar results, including a study of young and middle-aged women,[63] middle-aged men,[64] residents of Copenhagen,[65] and males of Japanese ancestry,[66] among others. A meta-analysis of 32 separate studies reported in March of 1989 concluded that the evidence was strong that cigarette smokers had an excess risk for stroke.[67]

Alcohol Consumption

Studies in the last five years have better clarified the relationship of alcoholic consumption to various types of stroke. The earlier reported positive association of hemorrhagic stroke with alcohol intake observed in the Honolulu heart study and the Hisayama study in Japan[68,69] have been reinforced.[70-72] In more recent reports, alcohol intake was associated with two to three times the risk for hemorrhagic stroke, particularly subarachnoid hemorrhage, but was not related independently to ischemic stroke.[71] Studies in Scandinavia have implicated alcohol intoxication as a precipitating factor, both for infarction and subarachnoid hemorrhage.[73-74] The Framingham study suggested an association between alcohol intake and the incidence of stroke in general, as well as brain infarction in men.[4] Recent reports have offered possible explanations for the different results from the various studies. Gill et al.[75] reported that low levels of alcoholic intake were associated with a decreased risk for stroke and moderate-to-heavy drinking with an increased risk. Also, Gorelick et al.[76] reported that apparent effects of acute alcohol consumption were not independent of smoking. Alcohol consumption and cigarette smoking have been shown to increase blood viscosity,[77] and cigarette smoking is more frequent among heavy drinkers, as is hemoconcentration with increased hematocrit. Rebound thrombocytosis during abstinence from alcohol has been suggested as a mechanism predisposing to stroke. Cardiac rhythm disorders also have been associated with acute alcohol intoxication.[78]

Other Drugs

In addition to alcohol and cigarettes, other drug abuse has become an increasing problem in the United States and in other countries.[79] Common drugs known to be associated with stroke include opiates (heroin), amphetamines and related drugs, cocaine, and phencyclidine. Stroke may be produced by either the direct effect of the drug or by complications of its method of administration, e.g., infection or emboli from intravenous injection. Heroin may be associated with either ischemic or hemorrhagic stroke. Amphetamines, amphetamine-related drugs (phenylpropanolamine), cocaine, and phencyclidine are more likely to be associated with hemorrhage because of elevated blood pressure and/or vasculitis. Recent studies suggest that stroke related to cocaine use is increasing, occurs primarily in the young, follows any route of administration, is frequently associated with intracranial aneurysms and malformations, and that hemorrhage is more common than infarction.[80]

Factors Not Well Established

Abnormal Lipids

Although evidence is quite convincing that elevated blood cholesterol and lipids, particularly low-density lipoproteins, are risks for cardiac disease, the evidence for stroke is not convincing.[81-84] Although reports of types of familial hyperlipidemia indicate a very high incidence of stroke,[85] for those that do not belong to these families, the evidence is not conclusive. In the Framingham study an increased risk appeared to be present for those under age 50.[83] In Gothenburg, Sweden,[86] a 12-year population study of 1462 women, aged 38 to 60, revealed that patients with high serum triglyceride values had a higher incidence of stroke after adjusting for other risk factors, but serum cholesterol did not predict any end points when adjusted for other risk factors.

Diet

Despite the evidence that control of salt and fat intake in the diet has a favorable effect on decreasing heart disease, no convincing data exist establishing a favorable effect on stroke. From the review of lipids as risk factors, this is not unexpected. In a study of men of Japanese ancestry living in Oahu,[87] by univariate analysis there was an inverse relation between dietary fat intake and thromboembolic and total stroke incidence. In addition, an inverse relation was also shown between protein intake and total stroke incidence.

Neither relationship was significant by multivariate analysis. In a 12-year prospective study of an upper-middle-class white community in California, by multivariate analyses a high intake of potassium from food sources was associated with a 40% reduction in the risk of stroke-associated mortality.[88] The effect was independent of other dietary variables and was apparently independent of other known cardiovascular risk factors. Further studies are needed to confirm this.

Oral Contraceptives

A 4- to 13-fold increase in the relative risk for cerebral infarction has been associated with oral contraceptive use in retrospective case control studies.[89-91] The risk of stroke appears to be enhanced by coexistent hypertension, a history of migraine, age exceeding 35 years, oral contraceptives rich in estrogen, prolonged use of oral contraceptives, presence of diabetes or hyperlipidemia, and, in particular, cigarette smoking.[90] When smoking was controlled as a risk factor, Petitti et al.[92] found no independent effect related to the use of birth control pills except for subarachnoid hemorrhage. This will be discussed further in the section on multiple risk factors.

A number of reviews suggest that the evidence for an association of oral contraceptives with stroke is inconclusive.[93-95] A recent, very large prospective study of past use of oral contraceptive agents,[96] regardless of length of previous use, did not raise the risk of subsequent cardiovascular disease. In the United States the incidence of stroke in the 15-to-45-year age group is equal in men and women; further, no substantial increase in stroke mortality has been noted in these age groups since oral contraceptives became available.[97] However, in Denmark there was an increase in this age group in women but not in men.[98] Five years ago the Subcommittee on Risk Factors of the Stroke Council of the AHA[6] did not reach agreement concerning the risk of oral contraceptive use and advised readers to review the referenced studies to draw an independent conclusion.

The data concerning estrogen use in postmenopausal women are conflicting. The Framingham study[99] reported estrogen users had a significant increase in cerebrovascular disease, and when they smoked it was more than twofold. Another prospective study reported a significant decrease in stroke death in users,[100] and a third one noted a decrease in coronary heart disease.[101]

Sedentary Activity

Studies of the incidence of stroke in a variety of occupations have shown no significant differences in the incidence of stroke between sedentary and physically active occupations.[102-106] In a study of longshoremen,[105] men with sedentary jobs had coronary death rates one third higher than cargo handlers, but the rates for stroke were similar in both groups. A prospective study of men of Japanese ancestry in the Honolulu Heart Program[106] indicated after 18 years of follow-up that carpenters, compared to other occupations, had a lower rate of definite coronary heart disease but no differences in stroke.

Obesity

In most studies, obesity is not a separate risk factor for stroke independent of hypertension and diabetes.[4,107] Studies of men born in 1913 in Gothenburg, Sweden,[108] indicated by both univariate and multivariate analyses that larger waist circumference and higher waist/hip ratio were significant risk factors for stroke. Regardless, obesity can be related to hypertension, and an increase in weight is often associated with an increase in severity of hypertension. Obesity also contributes to impaired glucose tolerance. Therefore, although obesity may or may not be a direct risk factor for stroke, it is a very potent risk factor for other factors, such as hypertension and glucose intolerance, which definitely are risk factors for stroke. For this reason, treatment might be effective in reducing the risk for stroke.

Hyperuricemia

Although it is stated that hyperuricemia is associated with stroke, no good evidence supports this. A recent study of women in Gothenburg, Sweden, correlated serum uric acid concentration to 12-year overall mortality but showed no relationship to stroke or heart disease.[109]

Infection

Associated preceding infection has been reported by one group to be an important risk factor for infarction in young and middle-aged patients.[110-111]

This was based on small series of patients with cerebral infarction compared to matched, randomly selected, community controls and will require further confirmation.

Homocysteinemia

Premature arteriosclerosis and thromboembolic events are known complications of homozygous homocysteinuria due to cystathionine synthase deficiency. Recently it has been suggested that heterozygous hemocysteinuria is also a risk factor for stroke.[112] A study of 25 patients with occlusive cerebrovascular disease, 25 with peripheral arterial disease and 25 with myocardial infarction, revealed that seven patients in each of the first two groups and none in the last were heterozygous for homocysteinuria. This was determined by methionine loading and cystathionine synthase deficiency in skin fibroblast cultures. Because of these results and also because the frequency of heterozygosity in the general population is < 1 in 70, the authors assumed a relationship. If further studies establish this to be a cause-and-effect relationship, treatment with folic acid or pyridoxine might be effective.[113,114]

Treatment of Associated Factors Effective

Many factors are not at first glance specifically treatable, but they may identify individuals who are at high risk and can be singled out for focused treatment on associated factors that can be altered by treatment.

Established Factors

Age

Age is the single most important risk factor for stroke, and as the population ages, those at high risk are increasing disproportionately. For each successive 10 years after 55 years of age, the stroke rate more than doubles.[115] Since age is not treatable, the recognition of other factors and their treatment are even more critical as the numbers of elderly persons increase. It must be noted, however, that despite the strong relationship between stroke and increasing age, in the National Survey of Stroke[44] 29.6% of strokes occurred before 65 years of age. Therefore, youth does not necessarily prevent stroke.

Gender

If one were to look casually at the overall statistics for the United States, it would appear that women are at greater risk for stroke than men. In any given year many more women die from a stroke—for example, in 1984, 92 630 women compared to 61 697 men.[116] Nevertheless, men are at greater risk for stroke than women. Age is the most important risk factor for stroke, and women tend to live much longer. The ratio of women to men before age 65 is about 1:1, but after 65 is about 1.5:1, and this difference increases as age increases. Thus when one adjusts the stroke mortality statistics for age, the rates reverse. In 1984 it was 31.1 per 100 000 for women and 36.4 for men (a 17% increase). The National Survey of Stroke[115] reported that in short-term general hospitals for each 10-year period between 35 and 65 years of age, the average annual initial stroke incidence rate was always higher for men than women.

It has been suggested that administration of female sex hormones will retard the formation of atherosclerosis and reduce the mortality from coronary and cerebrovascular disease,[117-120] but long-term studies comparing estrogens to placebo have failed to demonstrate any beneficial effect on men with cerebral infarction.[121] Not only did estrogens fail to reduce the incidence of cerebral infarction, transient ischemia, or death; they were associated with an overall higher death rate, largely due to cancer and various other diseases.

Heredo-Familial

A marked excess of stroke deaths among the parents and male and female relatives of patients with cerebrovascular disease has been reported.[61,108,122,123] In these studies, all of the excess could not be accounted for by an increase in other familial diseases such as hypertension and diabetes mellitus. Nevertheless, the evidence is becoming more convincing that the risk may be primarily related to the inheritance of other risk factors, some of which are treatable. A controlled study of siblings of stroke patients revealed an excess of combinations of hypertension, heart disease, and stroke in siblings over other controls.[124]

Race

A number of recent reports report that much of the risk for stroke that appears to be related to race is related to either environmental risk factors or the inheritance of other risk factors that in turn increases the risk for stroke. Risk factors that have excess prevalence in blacks are hypertension and cigarette smoking in men.[125] In the Lehigh Valley study,[126] the relative frequencies of hypertension, myocardial infarction, other heart diseases, and diabetes were higher for blacks. Consistently, blacks in the United States have higher death rates from stroke than whites,[127] but this may be altered. In the Minnesota Heart Survey a 58% decrease in stroke mortality was observed between 1968–73 and 1979–84.[128] This was associated with significant decreases in mean systolic blood pressure in both sexes and diastolic blood pressure in men. The proportion of men and women hypertensives on medication and under control increased. Although the overall prevalence of cigarette smoking changed very little, the proportion of heavy smokers decreased significantly.

Studies conducted in Japan and Hawaii strongly suggest that racial variation is environmentally and not genetically determined. In Japan the incidence and mortality rates for stroke have been very high for most of this century and exceed those for heart disease.[103,129-131] In Hawaii stroke incidence rates for Japanese residents appear similar to those of Caucasian Americans.[69,87,132] Thus, if the death rates truly reflect stroke incidence in Japan, then environmental factors would be the most likely explanation for the difference. Some evidence suggested that high sodium diet is related to the higher incidence of hypertension and that this might be a potent environmental factor,[133,134] but studies of dietary and other stroke risk factors in Hawaiian Japanese men do not demonstrate any relation between salt intake and the incidence of stroke.[87] In this cohort of Japanese ancestry, the risk factors were remarkably consistent with other American studies. For thromboembolic infarction, the independent risk factors included elevated blood pressure, glucose intolerance, age, electrocardiographic evidence of left ventricular hypertrophy or strain, cigarette smoking, and proteinuria. For intracranial hemorrhage they included age, elevated blood pressure, cigarette smoking, serum uric acid, and, inversely, serum cholesterol level.

Electrocardiographic evidence of left ventricular hypertrophy or strain significantly increased the risk of cerebral hemorrhage but was not associated with subarachnoid hemorrhage. Other Japanese studies support these observations.[135-138] Pathological studies do show that Japanese in Japan have more intracranial than extracranial occlusive disease compared to Occidentals or Hawaiian Japanese.[139-141]

Diabetes Mellitus

Diabetes mellitus is a major risk factor for stroke, along with hypertension and heart disease. Although diabetes is commonly associated with other risk factors, most importantly hypertension,[4,43] it does have a separate and significant independent impact. Although diabetes should be treated, to date there is no evidence that this treatment will reduce the risk for stroke.[142,143] The Honolulu Heart Program[144] examined the 12-year risk of stroke in 690 diabetic and 6908 nondiabetic men of Japanese ancestry. Not only was diabetes an independent risk factor for stroke, but among those without diabetes the relative risk for those at the 80th percentile of serum glucose level compared with those at the 20th percentile was 1.4. In those with glucosuria, the relative risk was 2.7.

Previous Stroke

Once a stroke has occurred, the risk of recurrent stroke increases 10 to 20 times.[115,145] Although it might at first appear to be too late, the knowledge of this increased risk offers the opportunity to institute vigorous therapy for associated diseases and other risk factors that might decrease the likelihood of a repeat insult and more severe dysfunction or death. In addition, several studies have shown that aspirin or ticlopidine in patients who have experienced a mild stroke will decrease subsequent recurrent stroke and death.[48,54,59]

Increasing Hematocrit

Although several studies have established a relationship between high hematocrit and the incidence of cerebral infarction, this factor was placed in this section with some trepidation because of the controversy concerning the effectiveness of treatment. The Framingham study[146] established a relationship between high hemoglobin (or high hematocrit) and increased incidence of cerebral infarction. Within the normal range the risk was directly proportional to the hemoglobin concentration. This was true for both sexes. However, when the study results were adjusted for blood pressure and smoking, the hemoglobin level, as a separate risk factor, was not statistically significant. Nevertheless, a Japanese autopsy study[103] and several clinical and radiologic studies of patients with stroke[147,148] support these observations. In patients with elevated hematocrit values, the associated decreased cerebral blood flow was increased by 50% following venesection.[149] Harrison et al.[150] found a direct correlation between hemoglobin levels and the size of brain infarcts and suggested that this was caused by decreased collateral flow secondary to increased viscosity. The Lehigh Valley Stroke Register, comparing the relationship between hematocrit and stroke subtype, indicated that hematocrit was higher in patients with lacunes but was significant only when systolic blood pressure was elevated.[151] Two studies of the relationship of hematocrit to clinical outcome in acute cerebral infarction reported quite different results.[152,153] One showed that cases with more intense admission deficit had lower admission hematocrit and that cases with poorer outcome had lower hematocrit levels on the second and fourth day, but hematocrit was not independently related to outcome.[152] The other indicated an increased mortality at the extremes.[153] Experience with venesection in acute polycythemia can reverse stroke. However, two multicenter controlled hemodilution studies showed no benefit.[154,155]

Fibrinogen

Two prospective long-term studies indicated that increased blood fibrinogen level was an independent risk factor for stroke. The results of the two studies, one performed in Sweden[156] and the other part of the Framingham study,[157] were similar. Although fibrinogen levels were related to other risk factors, such as blood pressure, serum cholesterol, and cigarette smoking, fibrinogen still made an independent contribution to risk. The Framingham data were updated in 1987.[158] It was concluded that risk of stroke increased progressively with fibrinogen level in men but not in women. No studies have established that treatment of fibrinogen is directly effective, but it is associated with other risk factors that are. Although cause-and-effect cannot be assumed, if there is such a relationship, a number of therapeutic interventions may be possible since the theoretical adverse effects of increased fibrinogen might be at several different levels.

Sickle Cell Disease

The occurrence of stroke associated with homozygous sickle cell anemia varies from as low as 2.4% to as high as 17%. When the diagnoses have been substantiated by hemoglobin electrophoresis, hemiplegia has been reported in 13% to 17%.[159] Other neurological signs are much more common. Treatment of the neurologic complications once they occur does not have a beneficial effect. The effectiveness of prophylactic therapy in preventing stroke has not been established.

Lupus Anticoagulant and Anticardiolipin Antibodies

A number of reports have noted an association between lupus anticoagulant or abnormal anticardiolipin antibodies and an increased risk for stroke in patients with no overt evidence of collagen-vascular disease.[160-165] To date, no studies have shown any treatment to be effective in decreasing this risk.

Asymptomatic Carotid Arterial Lesions (Bruits)

Technology has evolved to the point that now lesions are increasingly being identified in the asymptomatic population. Since it is assumed that lesions of the arteries and of the brain are precursors of symptomatic stroke, the opportunity may exist to initiate preventive therapy. Although this concept is enticing, in addition to establishing the degree of risk for any stroke, it must also be determined if there is a close cause-and-effect relationship of the stroke to the asymptomatic lesion. The success of any interventional therapy depends upon this knowledge. Information concerning these asymptomatic carotid lesions comes primarily from either the physical examination or from imaging techniques. Cervical bruits have long been thought to identify carotid arteries with a high likelihood of atherosclerotic disease, and now, using ultrasound, radiology, and nuclear magnetic resonance, the identification of the supposed lesions is possible with minimal risk. Unfortunately, it has not yet been determined whether the benefit of current methods of therapy for the lesion outweighs the risk or even if there is any benefit. To put this in perspective, some of the available evidence needs to be reviewed.

First, prospective epidemiological studies have established that individuals with asymptomatic neck bruits have a much greater risk for stroke than those without.[166,167] Unfortunately, these studies indicate that this risk is not for ischemic stroke in the distribution of the artery with the bruit but for stroke in general. In the Framingham study,[167] 21 (12%) of 171 patients prospectively followed with neck bruit developed permanent stroke during up to 8 years of follow-up. Although the stroke rate was 2.6 times that of those without bruits, in only 6 was there an atherothrombotic infarction in the arterial distribution of the artery exhibiting the bruit. Of the 43 that died, the cause of death was cardiovascular in 34. The Evans County, Georgia, study was of a different population[166] than that of the Framingham study, a northern middle-class white community. Although Evans County is in the South and more than 40% black, the results were similar. Of 72 patients with bruits, 10 (13.9%) of 72 individuals with neck bruits developed a stroke compared to 52 (3.4%), of the 1548 without bruits. Of those with bruits, only 3 of the 10 had a spontaneous stroke on the same side as the bruit. Although each study concluded that an asymptomatic cervical bruit was a major risk factor for stroke, because the stroke occurred so infrequently in the distribution of the appropriate carotid artery, it is unlikely that removal of cause of the bruit in the artery would have affected the outcome. In the Hospital Frequency Study of Transient Ischemic Attacks, neither carotid bruit nor the degree of stenosis added any additional risk for stroke or death over the TIA alone.[168]

Bruits do not always indicate underlying atherosclerosis, and severe stenosis from atherosclerosis frequently occurs without associated bruit. Stenosis and atherosclerosis of an artery supplying the brain indicates an increased risk for stroke, but no study to date has shown an independent cause-and-effect relationship of stenosis to stroke. For a number of theoretical reasons, the removal of an atherosclerotic lesion is enticing. First they tend to progress.[169,170] Simplistically, one might reason that if the lesion were removed, progression would cease and this might be beneficial. A large number of studies of patients receiving noninvasive techniques after endarterectomy indicates that stenosis continues despite surgery.[169,170] In a few years up to 58% of the operated arteries become stenotic, and in 7% to 36% of them the stenosis is >50%. Several studies have compared operated carotid arteries to unoperated arteries with stenosis on the opposite side and have shown no differences or more progression on the operated side.

Although a number of studies indicate that as stenosis becomes more severe, the stroke rate increases, none has conclusively established an increased risk in the artery involved. A recent study reported the results of 640 patients with bruits who had ocular pneumoplethysmography (OPG).[171] Those with abnormal OPG had 2.3 times the risk for stroke of those with normal OPG, and 4.8 times that of the general population. Yet, of the strokes that occurred, 48% were not in the distribution of the abnormal artery. In the Hospital Frequency Study of Transient Ischemic Attacks,[168] the degree of stenosis had no relationship to infarction. Also, during the 8 years of follow-up, of those that had infarction, 51% had at least one infarction out of the distribution of the symptomatic artery. In addition, when endarterectomy was performed, subsequent infarction occurred most frequently in the distribution of the operated artery. Using positron emission tomography (PET), Powers and his colleagues[172] have established that hemodynamically significant stenosis has a very poor correlation with stroke. Studies of patients with dynamically significant carotid artery stenosis had no effect on the hemodynamic status of the cerebral circulation. They then followed a group of 30 medically treated patients with >75% stenosis of the intracranial carotid arterial system with PET evaluation of the hemodynamic status of the cerebral circulation.[173] During 1 year of follow-up, 1 of the 9 with normal hemodynamics and none of the 21 with abnormal hemodynamics developed an ipsilateral ischemic stroke. In another study of 44 patients who had PET evidence of hemodynamic compromise,[174] they compared 21 who had successful extracranial-intracranial arterial bypass without stroke with 23 who did not have surgery. During 1 year, 3 of the 21 who were operated had a stroke, and none of those who were not operated had a stroke. These data indicate that correction of hemodynamically significant stenosis is unlikely to greatly benefit the usual patient. The evidence indicates that asymptomatic lesions are potent risk factors for stroke or death but does not yet support the value of surgical intervention. Still, it is very important to identify the patient. Then an aggressive approach can identify other risk factors that may be treated.

Factors Not Well Established

Migraine and Migraine Equivalents

A relationship between migraine headaches and stroke is commonly reported. Persistence of ischemic deficit following an attack is defined as "complicated migraine" and appears to be one of the recognized causes of stroke, particularly in young people.[175-177] Although a number of reports suggests that those with migraine cephalgia are at increased risk for stroke, they are also associated with a number of other factors that are established risks for stroke.[179-181] In a thorough review, Henrich concluded that the contribution of migraine to other known risk factors for thromboembolic stroke needs to be examined further by controlled studies.[182]

Treatment Not Possible

The factors described in this section have an implied relationship to stroke, but treatment is not practicable.

Geographic Location

Cerebrovascular disease is more common in some parts of the world than in others. For example, in the United States stroke incidence is higher in the southeast than in the northern Midwest.[183-185] Despite this, no well-documented environmental factors have been established to contribute to the occurrence of stroke.

Season and Climate

Several studies report a general relationship between stroke deaths and extremes in temperature.[186-189] Recently a study in the Negev desert of Israel reported that the average daily incidence of stroke on relatively warm days was about twice as great as that on relatively cold ones.[190] In this study, it was hypothesized that increases in thromboembolic mechanisms were secondary to physiologic changes in response to heat. Another study in Iowa reviewed the seasonal occurrence of stroke in 2960 patients.[191] There was a significant increase in the rate of referral for cerebral infarction during the warmer months and less intracranial hemorrhage. Time of onset of ischemic stroke in 1167 patients was reported to occur more frequently in awake patients between 10:00 A.M. and noon than during any other 2-hour interval.[192]

Socioeconomic Factors

In England, a weak but direct correlation between cerebrovascular disease and high socioeconomic status was reported,[193] but in the United States, men who died because of strokes have been observed to be poorer than those in a control group.[194]

Personality Type

Type A behavior has been assumed to be an increased risk factor for heart disease and stroke. Prospective studies have shown no association.[195-197]

Treatment of Multiple Factors in Combination

Although some factors are of insignificant to moderate risk by themselves, in combination with other factors they become more important. These combinations, in addition to increasing the number of treatable factors, offer the opportunity to identify a subgroup of the population that can be singled out for intensive diagnostic and treatment programs. Most studies now analyze for unifactorial and multifactorial risks. Some of these combinations follow.

Systolic Blood Pressure, Serum Cholesterol, Glucose Intolerance, Cigarette Smoking, and Abnormal ECG

From the Framingham study, Kannel and Wolf reported that this combination would identify 10% of the population that would have at least one third of the strokes.[198]

Cigarette Smoking, Systolic Blood Pressure, and Low Ponderal Index

Paffenbarger and Williams[61] reported this combination to be associated with an increasing stroke mortality rate. When all three factors were present, risk was increased eightfold.

Body Height, a Parent Dead, and Not a Varsity Athlete

In addition, Paffenbarger and Williams noted that this combination resulted in a fourfold increase in the mortality rate secondary to stroke. The most important single factor in both groups was elevated blood pressure.

Women of Childbearing Age, Oral Contraceptives, Cigarette Smoking, and Older Than 35 Years

Longstreth and Swanson[199] in an in-depth review noted that much of the controversy concerning the relationship between oral contraceptives and stroke might be because most studies were of young populations with a lower incidence of stroke. Because of this a multiple-factor effect might be lost, particularly if an important component was older age. From their analysis they observed that most women who had strokes and were on oral contraceptives had other risk factors such as hypertension. They concluded that this combination of oral contraception, cigarette smoking, and age >35 years is particularly potent.

Increasing Blood Pressure, Abdominal Obesity, Increased Plasma Fibrinogen Level, and Maternal Death from Stroke

In Gothenburg, Sweden, these factors in combination were significant for stroke risk.[108]

Transient Ischemic Attacks, Myocardial Infarction, and Other Heart Disease

In the Lehigh Valley study, which used a logistic regression model for the odds ratio to study the relative contribution of several factors, these three constituted a significantly greater risk than other combinations studied.[200]

Summary

In this chapter those factors that are considered to be risk for strokes have been identified, with specific attention to treatment. For some of these, treatment of the factor has been established to decrease stroke significantly. Most important in this group are hypertension, cardiac disease, transient ischemic attacks, cigarette smoking, and alcohol consumption. Treatment of these conditions will reduce the incidence of stroke morbidity and mortality.

Factors that have not been well established but are treatable include abnormal lipids, diet, oral contraceptives, sedentary activity, obesity, hyperuricemia, and homocysteinemia.

Established factors that are not treatable but identify individuals with other treatable risk factors include age, sex, heredo-familial, race, diabetes mellitus, prior stroke, and asymptomatic structural lesions.

A number of factors of very low or no risk at all by themselves may be important in combination with others. These combinations also make risk-factor identification and treatment more practical. Although one cannot assume a cause-and-effect relationship for each of these multiple factors, it is quite important to identify them. When each is treated, the probability greatly increases that at least one will be effective in reducing stroke incidence and mortality.[201]

References

1. Mortality trends—United States, 1986–1988. *MMWR*. 1989;38:117–118.
2. American Heart Association. *Stroke Facts*. 1989: p 1.
3. Adelman SM. The National Survey of Stroke: economic impact. *Stroke*. 1981;12(suppl I):169–178.
4. Wolf PA, Kannel WB, Verter J. Current status of risk factors for stroke. In: Barnett HJM, ed. *Neurologic Clinics*. vol 1. no 1. Philadelphia: W.B. Saunders Company; 1983: pp 317–343.
5. Garraway WM, Whisnant JP, Furlan AJ, et al. The declining incidence of stroke. *N Engl J Med*. 1979; 300:449–452.
6. Dyken ML, Wolf PA, Barnett HJM, et al. Risk factors in stroke: a statement for physicians by the subcommittee on risk factors and stroke of the stroke council. *Stroke*. 1984;15:1105–1111.
7. Kannel WB, Wolf PA, McGee DL, et al. Systolic blood pressure, arterial rigidity, and risk of stroke; the Framingham study. *JAMA*. 1981;245:1225–1229.
8. Wolf PA. Hypertension as a risk factor for stroke. In: Whisnant JP, Sandok B, eds. *Cerebral Vascular Diseases*. New York, NY: Grune & Stratton; 1975: p 105.
9. Kannel WB, Wolf PA, Verter J, McNamara PM. Epidemiologic assessment of the role of blood pressure in stroke: the Framingham study. *JAMA*. 1970;214:301–310.
10. Rutan GH, Kuller LH, Neaton JD, et al. Mortality associated with diastolic hypertension and isolated systolic hypertension among men screened for the Multiple Risk Factor Intervention Trial. *Circulation*. 1988;77:504–514.
11. Shimizu Y, Kato H, Lin CH, et al. Relationship between longitudinal changes in blood pressure and stroke incidence. *Stroke*. 1984;15:839–846.
12. Brott T, Thalinger K, Hertzberg F. Hypertension as a risk factor for spontaneous intracerebral hemorrhage. *Stroke*. 1986;17:1078–1083.
13. Sacco RL, Wolf PA, Bharucha NE, et al. Subarachnoid and intracerebral hemorrhage: natural history, prognosis, and precursive factors in the Framingham study. *Neurology*. 1984;34:847–854.
14. Sacco RL, Wolf PA, Kannel WB, et al. Survival and recurrence following stroke: the Framingham study. *Stroke*. 1982;13:290–295.
15. Kannel WB, Thom TJ. Implications of the recent decline in cardiovascular mortality. *Cardiovasc Med*. 1979;4:983–997.
16. Carter AB. Hypotensive therapy in stroke survivors. *Lancet*. 1970;1:185.
17. Hypertension Detection and Follow-up Program Cooperative Group. Five year findings of the hypertension detection and follow-up program: III. Reduction in stroke incidence among persons with high blood pressure. *JAMA*. 1982;247:633–638.
18. Taguchi J, Freis ED. Partial reduction of blood pressure and prevention of complications in hypertension. *N Engl J Med*. 1978;291:329–331.

19. Veterans Administration Cooperative Study Group on Antihypertensive Agents. Effects of treatment on morbidity in hypertension: I. Results in patients with diastolic blood pressures averaging 115 through 129 mm Hg. *JAMA.* 1967;202:1028–1034.

20. Veterans Administration Cooperative Study Group on Antihypertensive Agents. Effects of treatment on morbidity in hypertension: II. Results in patients with diastolic blood pressures averaging 90 through 114 mm Hg. *JAMA.* 1970;213:1143–1152.

21. Ueda K, Omae T, Hasuo Y, et al. Prevalence and long-term prognosis of mild hypertensives and hypertensives in a Japanese community, Hisayama. *J Hypertens.* 1988;6:981–989.

22. Cox JP, O'Brien ET, O'Malley K. Treatment of elderly hypertensives: results and implications of recent trials. *J Cardiovasc Pharmacol.* 1987;10 (Suppl 2):S65–70.

23. Samuelsson OG, Wilhelmsen LW, Svardsudd KF, et al. Mortality and morbidity in relation to systolic blood pressure in two populations with different management of hypertension: the study of men born in 1913 and the multifactorial primary prevention trial. *J Hypertens.* 1987;5:57–66.

24. Davidson RA, Caranason GJ. Should the elderly hypertensive be treated? Evidence from clinical trials. *Arch Intern Med.* 1987;147:1932–1937.

25. MacMahon S, Cutler JA, Stamler J. Antihypertensive drug treatment. Potential, expected and observed effects on stroke and on coronary heart disease. *Hypertension.* 1989;13:145–150.

26. Peart S. Results of MRC (UK) trial of drug therapy for mild hypertension. *Clin Invest Med.* 1987;10:616–620.

27. Doyle AE. The Australian therapeutic trial in mild hypertension. *Nephron.* 1987;47(Suppl 1):115–119.

28. Tuomilehto J, Piha T, Nissinen A, et al. Trends in stroke mortality and in antihypertensive treatment in Finland from 1972 to 1984 with special reference to North Karelia. *J Hum Hypertens.* 1987;1:201–208.

29. Fieschi C, Carolei A, Salvetti M, etal. Systemic hypertension as a treatable risk factor for cerebrovascular disease. *Am J Cardiol.* 1989;63:19C–21C.

30. Toole JF, Janeway R, Choi K, et al. Transient ischemic attacks due to atherosclerosis: a prospective study of 160 patients. *Arch Neurol.* 1975;32:5–12.

31. Knutsen R, Knutsen SF, Curb JD, et al. Predictive value of resting electrocardiograms for 12-year incidence of stroke in the Honolulu Heart Program. *Stroke.* 1988;19:555–559.

32. Kannel WB, Abbott RD, Savage DD, et al. Epidemiologic features of chronic atrial fibrillation: the Framingham study. *N Engl J Med.* 1982;306:1018–1022.

33. Wolf PA, Dawber TR, Thomas HE Jr, et al. Epidemiologic assessment of chronic atrial fibrillation and risk of stroke, the Framingham study. *Neurology.* 1978;28:973–977.

34. Davis PH, Dambrosia JM, Schoenberg BS, et al. Risk factors for ischemic stroke: a prospective study in Rochester, Minnesota. *Ann Neurol.* 1987;22:319–327.

35. Kopecky SL, Gersh BJ, McGoon MD, et al. The natural history of lone atrial fibrillation: a population-based study over three decades. *N Engl J Med.* 1987;317:669–674.

36. Petersen P, Godtfredsen J. Risk factors for stroke in chronic atrial fibrillation. *Eur Heart J.* 1988;9:291–294.

37. Petersen P, Hansen JM. Stroke in thyrotoxicosis with atrial fibrillation. *Stroke.* 1988;19:15–18.

38. Asinger RW, Dyken ML, Fisher M, et al. Cardiogenic brain embolism. The second report of the Cerebral Embolism Task Force. *Arch Neurol.* 1989;46:727–743.

39. Dyken ML, Conneally M, Haerer AF, et al. Cooperative study of hospital frequency and character of transient ischemic attacks: I. Background, organization, and clinical surgery. *JAMA.* 1977;237:882–886.

40. Levy DE. How transient are transient ischemic attacks? *Neurology.* 1988;38:674–677.

41. Kinkel PR, Kinkel WR, Jacobs L. Nuclear magnetic resonance imaging in patients with stroke. *Semin Neurol.* 1986;6:43–52.

42. Salgado ED, Weinstein M, Furlan AJ, et al. Proton magnetic resonance imaging in ischemic cerebrovascular disease. *Ann Neurol.* 1986;20:502–507.

43. Schoenberg BS, Schoenberg DG, Pritchard DA, et al. Differential risk factors for complete stroke and transient ischemic attacks (TIA): study of vascular diseases (hypertension, cardiac disease, peripheral vascular disease) and diabetes mellitus. In: Duvoisin RC, ed. *Transactions of the American Neurological Association.* vol 105. New York, NY: Springer Publishing Company; 1980: p 165.

44. Weinfeld FD, ed. The National Survey of Stroke. National Institute of Neurological and Communicative Disorders and Stroke. *Stroke.* 1981;12 (suppl):I-1.

45. Mohr JP, Caplan LR, Melski JW, et al. The Harvard cooperative stroke registry. *Neurology.* 1978;28:754–762.

46. Whisnant JP. The role of the neurologist in the decline of stroke. *Ann Neurol.* 1983;14:1–7.

47. Whisnant JP. Epidemilogy of stroke: emphasis on transient cerebral ischemia attacks and hypertension. *Stroke.* 1974;5:68–70.

48. Bousser MG, Eschwege E, Haguenau M, et al. "AICLA" controlled trial of aspirin and dipyridamole in the secondary prevention of atherothrombotic cerebral ischemia. *Stroke.* 1983;14:5–14.

49. Canadian Cooperative Stroke Study Group. A randomized trial of aspirin and sulfinpyrazone in threatened stroke. *N Engl J Med.* 1978;299:53–59.

50. Fields WS, Lemak NA, Frankowski RF, Hardy RJ. Controlled trial of aspirin in cerebral ischemia. *Stroke.* 1977;8:301–316.

51. Fields WS, Lemak NA, Frankowski RF, Hardy RJ. Controlled trial of aspirin in cerebral ischemia. Part II: Surgical group. *Stroke.* 1978;9:309–318.

52. Sorenson PS, Pedersen H, Marquardsen J, et al. Acetylsalicylic acid in the prevention of stroke in patients with reversible cerebral ischemic attacks. A Danish cooperative study. *Stroke.* 1983;14: 15–22.

53. Swedish Cooperative Study. High-dose acetylsalicylic acid after cerebral infarction. *Stroke.* 1987; 18:325–334.

54. The ESPS Group. The European stroke prevention study (ESPS): principal end-points. *Lancet.* 1987; 2:1351–1354.

55. UK-TIA Study Group. United Kingdom transient ischaemic attack (UK-TIA) aspirin trial: interim results. *Br Med J (Clin Res).* 1988;296:316–320.

56. Ruether R, Dorndorf W. Aspirin in patients with cerebral ischemia and normal angiograms or nonsurgical lesions: the results of a double-blind trial. In: Breddin K, Dorndorf W, Lowe D, et al., eds. *Acetylsalicylic Acid in Cerebral Ischemia and Coronary Heart Disease.* Stuttgart: Schattauer; 1978: pp 97–106.

57. Dyken ML. Anticoagulant and platelet-antiaggregating therapy in stroke and threatened stroke. In: Barnett HJM, ed. *Neurologic Clinics.* vol 1. no 1. Philadelphia, PA: W.B. Saunders Company; 1983: pp 223–242.

58. Hass WK, Easton JD, Adams HP Jr, et al. A randomized trial comparing ticlopidine hydrochloride with aspirin for the prevention of stroke in high-risk patients. *N Engl J Med.* 1989;1321:501–507.

59. Gent M, Blakely JA, Easton JD, et al., the CATS Group. The Canadian American Ticlopidine study (CATS) in thromboembolic stroke. *Lancet.* 1989; 1:1215–1220.

60. Dyken ML. Precipitating factors, prognosis, and demography of cerebrovascular disease in an Indiana Community: a review of all patients hospitalized from 1963–1965 with neurologic examination of survivors. *Stroke.* 1970;1:261–269.

61. Paffenbarger RS Jr, Williams JL. Chronic disease in former college students: V. Early precursors of fatal stroke. *Am J Public Health.* 1967;57:1290–1299.

62. Wolf PA, D'Agostino RB, Kannel WB, et al. Cigarette smoking as a risk factor for stroke: the Framingham study. *JAMA.* 1988;259:1025–1029.

63. Colditz GA, Bonita R, Stampfer MJ, et al. Cigarette smoking and risk of stroke in middle-aged women. *N Engl J Med.* 1988;318:937–941.

64. Menotti A, Mariotti S, Seccareccia S, et al. The 25 year estimated probability of death from some specific causes as a function of twelve risk factors in middle aged men. *Eur J Epidemiol.* 1988;4: 60–67.

65. Boysen G, Nyboe J, Appleyard M, et al. Stroke incidence and risk factors for stroke in Copenhagen, Denmark. *Stroke.* 1988;19:1345–1353.

66. Abbott RD, Yin Y, Reed DM, et al. Risk of stroke in male cigarette smokers. *N Engl J Med.* 1986; 315:717–720.

67. Shinton R, Beevers G. Meta-analysis of relation between ciagarette smoking and stroke. *Br Med J.* 1989;298:789–794.

68. Kagan A, Harris BR, Winkelstein W Jr, et al. Epidemiologic studies of coronary heart disease and stroke in Japanese men living in Japan, Hawaii and California: demographic, physical, dietary and biochemical characteristics. *J Chronic Dis.* 1974; 27:345–364.

69. Kagan A, Popper JS, Rhoads GG, et al. Epidemiologic studies of coronary heart disease and stroke in Japanese men living in Japan, Hawaii and California: prevalence in stroke. In: Scheinberg P, ed. *Cerebrovascular Diseases.* New York, NY: Raven Press; 1976: p 267.

70. Klatsky AL, Armstrong MA, Friedman GD. Alcohol use and subsequent cerebrovascular disease hospitalizations. *Stroke.* 1989;20:741–746.

71. Donahue RF, Abbott RD, Reed DM, et al. Alcohol and hemorrhagic stroke. The Honolulu Heart Program. *JAMA.* 1986;255:2311–2314.

72. Stampfer MJ, Colditz GA, Willett WC, et al. A prospective study of moderate alcohol consumption and the risk of coronary disease and stroke in women. *N Engl J Med.* 1988;319:267–273.

73. Hillbom M, Kaste M. Alcohol intoxication: a risk factor for primary subarachnoid hemorrhage. *Neurology.* 1982;32:706–711.

74. Lee K. Alcoholism and cerebrovascular thrombosis in the young. *Acta Neurol Scand.* 1979; 59:270.

75. Gill JS, Shipley MJ, Hornby RH, et al. A community case-control study of alcohol consumption in stroke. *Int J Epidemio.* 1988;17:542–547.

76. Gorelick PB, Rodin MB, Langenberg P, et al. Is acute alcohol ingestion a risk factor for ischemic stroke? Results of a controlled study in middle-aged and elderly stroke patients at three urban medical centers. *Stroke.* 1987;18:359–364.

77. Dintenfass L. Elevation of blood viscosity, aggregation of red cells, haematocrit values and fibrinogen levels with cigarette smokers. *Med J Aust.* 1975;1:617–620.

78. Ettinger PO, Wu CF, De La Cruz C Jr, et al. Arrhythmias and the "Holiday Heart": Alcohol-associated cardiac rhythm disorders. *Am Heart J.* 1978;95:555–562.

79. Brust JCM. Stroke and substance abuse. In: Barnett HJM, Mohr JP, Stein BM, et al., eds. *Stroke Pathophysiology, Diagnosis and Management.* vol 2. New York, NY: Churchill Livingstone; 1986: pp 903–917.

80. Klonoff DC, Andrews BT, Obana WG. Stroke associated with cocaine use. *Arch Neurol.* 1989; 46:989–993.

81. Dyer AR, Stamler J, Paul O, et al. Serum cholesterol and risk of death from cancer and other causes in three Chicago epidemiological studies. *J Chronic Dis.* 1981;34:249–260.

82. Farid NR, Anderson J. Cerebrovascular disease and hyperlipoproteinemia. *Lancet.* 1972;1:1398–1399.

83. Kannel WB. Epidemiology of cerebrovascular disease. In: Russell RWR, ed. *Cerebral Arterial Disease.* Edinburgh: Churchill Livingstone; 1976: pp 1–23.

84. Mathew NT, Davis D, Meyer JS, et al. Hyperlipoproteinemia in occlusive cerebrovascular disease. *JAMA.* 1975;232:262–266.

85. Kaste M, Koivisto P. Risk of brain infarction in familial hypercholesterolemia. *Stroke.* 1988;19: 1097–1100.

86. Lapidus L, Bengtsson C, Lindquist O, et al. 1988 Triglycerides – main lipid risk factor for cardiovascular disease in women? *Acta Med Scan.* 1985; 217:481–489.

87. Kagan A. Popper JS, Rhoads GG, et al. Dietary and other risk factors for stroke in Hawaiian Japanese men. *Stroke.* 1985;16:390–396.

88. Khaw KT, Barrett-Connor E. Dietary potassium and stroke-associated mortality–a 12 years prospective population study. *N Engl J Med.* 1987;316: 235–240.

89. Collaborative Group for the Study of Stroke in Young Women. Oral contraception and increased risk of cerebral ischemia or thrombosis. *N Engl J Med.* 1973;288:871–878.

90. Handin RI. Thromboembolic complications of pregnancy and oral contraceptives. *Prog Cardiovasc Dis.* 1974;16:395–405.

91. Layde PM, Beral V, Kay CR. Further analyses of mortality in oral contraceptive users. (Royal College of General Practitioners' Oral Contraception Study). *Lancet.* 1981;1:541.

92. Petitti DB, Wingerd J, Pellegrin F, et al. Risk of vascular disease in women: smoking, oral contraceptives, noncontraceptive estrogens, and other factors. *JAMA.* 1979;242:1150–1154.

93. Comer TP, Tuerck DG, Bilas RA, et al. Comparison of strokes in women of childbearing age in Rochester, Minnesota and Bakersfield, California. *Angiology.* 1975;26:351–355.

94. Schoenberg BS, Whisnant JP, Taylor WF, et al. Strokes in women of childbearing age: a population study. *Neurology.* 1970;20:181–189.

95. Shearman RP. Oral contraceptives: where are the excess deaths? *Med J Aust.* 1981;1:698.

96. Stampfer MJ, Willett WC, Colditz GA, et al. A prospective study of past use of oral contraceptive agents and risk of cardiovascular diseases. *N Engl J Med.* 1988;319:1313–1317.

97. Wiseman RA, MacRae KD. Oral contraceptives and the decline in mortality from circulatory disease. *Fertil Steril.* 1981;35:277–283.

98. Lidegaard O. Cerebrovascular deaths before and after the appearance of oral contraceptives. *Acta Neurol Scand.* 1988;75:427–433.

99. Wilson PWF, Garrison RJ, Castelli WP. Postmenopausal estrogen use, cigarette smoking and cardiovascular morbidity in women over 50. *N Engl J Med.* 1985;313:1038–1043.

100. Paganini-Hill A, Ross RI, Henderson BE. Postmenopausal estrogen treatment and stroke: a prospective study. *Br Med J (Clin Res).* 1988;297:519–522.

101. Stampfer MJ, Willett WC, Colditz GA, et al. A prospective study of postmenopausal estrogen therapy and coronary heart disease. *N Engl J Med.* 1985;313:1044–1049.

102. Johnson KG, Yano K, Kato H. Cerebral vascular disease in Hiroshima, Japan. *Jpn J Chronic Dis.* 1967;20:545.

103. Katsuki S, Omae T, Hirota Y. Epidemiological and clinicopathological studies on cerebrovascular disease. *Kyushi J Med Sci.* 1964;15:127.

104. Marquardsen J. The natural history of acute cerebrovascular disease: a retrospective study of 769 patients. *Acta Neurol Scand.* 1969;45(suppl 38):11.

105. Paffenbarger RS Jr, Laughlin ME, Gima AS, et al. Work activity of longshoremen as related to death from coronary heart disease and stroke. *N Engl J Med.* 1970;282:1109–1114.

106. Miller FD, Reed DM, MacLean CJ. A prospective study of mortality and morbidity among carpenters in the Honolulu Heart Program Cohort. *J Occup Med.* 1988;30:879–882.

107. Kannel WB. Health and obesity: an overview. In: Conn HL Jr, DeFelice EA, Kuo P, eds. *Health and Obesity.* New York, NY: Raven Press; 1983: p 1.

108. Welin L, Svardsudd K, Wilhelmsen L, et al. Analysis of risk factors for stroke in a cohort of men born in 1913. *N Engl J Med.* 1987;317:521–526.

109. Bengtsson C, Lapidus L, Stendahl C, et al. Hyperuricaemia and risk of cardiovascular disease and overall death: a 12-year follow-up of population study of women in Gothenburg, Sweden. *Acta Med Scan.* 1988;224:549–555.

110. Syrjanen J, Valtonen VV, Iivanainen M, et al. Preceding infection as an important risk factor for ischaemic brain infarction in young and middle aged patients. *Br Med J Clin Res.* 1988;196:1156–1160.

111. Syrjanen J, Peltola J, Valtonen V, et al. Dental infections in association with cerebral infarction in young and middle-aged men. *J Intern Med.* 1989; 225:179–184.

112. Boers GH, Smals AG, Trijbels FJ, et al. Heterozygosity for homocystinuria in premature peripheral and cerebral occlusive arterial disease. *N Engl J Med.* 1985;313:709–715.

113. Mudd SH. Vascular disease and homocysteine metabolism. Editorial. *N Engl J Med.* 1985;313: 751–753.

114. Brattstrom LE, Israelsson B, Jeppsson JO, et al. Folic acid – an innocuous means to reduce plasma homocysteine. *Scand J Clin Lab Invest.* 1988;48: 215–221.

115. Robins M, Baum HM. The National Survey of Stroke. Incidence. *Stroke.* 1981;12(suppl):I45–I55.

116. Monthly Vital Statistics Report – Final Data From the National Center for Health Statistics. U.S. Department of Health and Human Services. vol. 35, no. 6. September 26, 1986.

117. London WT, Rosenberg SE, Draper JF, et al. The effect of estrogens on atherosclerosis: a postmortem study. *Ann Int Med.* 1961;55:63.

118. Marmorston J. Effect of estrogen treatment in cerebrovascular disease. In: *Cerebral Vascular Diseases.* New York, NY: Grune & Stratton, 1965: p 214.

119. Rivin AU, Dimitroff SP. The incidence and severity of atherosclerosis in estrogen-treated males, and in females with hypoestrogenic or a hyperestrogenic state. *Circulation.* 1954;9:533–539.

120. Stamler J, Pick R, Katz LN, et al. Effectiveness of estrogens for therapy of myocardial infarction in middle-aged men. *JAMA.* 1963;183:632–638.

121. Veterans Administration Cooperative Study Group. Estrogenic therapy in men with ischemic cerebrovascular disease: effect on recurrent cerebral infarction and survival. Final report of the Veterans Administration Cooperative Study of Atherosclerosis, Neurology Section. *Stroke.* 1972; 3:427–433.

122. Heyden S, Heyman A, Camplong L. Mortality patterns among parents of patients with atherosclerotic cerebrovascular disease. *J Chronic Dis.* 1969; 22:105–110.

123. Khaw KT, Barrett-Connor E. Family history of stroke as an independent predictor of ischemic heart disease in men and stroke in women. *Am J Epidemiol.* 1986;123:59–66.

124. Diaz JF, Hachinski VC, Federson LL, et al. Aggregation of multiple risk factors for stroke in siblings of patients with brain infarction and transient ischemic attacks. *Stroke.* 1986;17:1239–1242.

125. Sprafka JM, Folsom AR, Burke GL, et al. Prevalence of cardiovascular disease risk factors in blacks and whites: the Minnesota Heart Survey. *Am J Public Health.* 1988;78:1546–1549.

126. Friday G, Lai SM, Alter M, et al. Stroke in the Lehigh valley: racial/ethnic differences. *Neurology.* 1989;39:1165–1168.

127. Gillum RF. Stroke in blacks. *Stroke.* 1988;19:1–9.

128. Folsom AR, Gomez-Marin O, Sprafka JM, et al. Trends in cardiovascular risk factors in an urban black population, 1973–74 to 1985: the Minnesota heart survey. *Am Heart J.* 1987;114:1199–1205.

129. Katsuki S, Hirota Y, Akazome T, et al. Epidemiological studies on cerebrovascular diseases in Hisayama, Kyushu Island, Japan: Part I. With particular reference to cardiovascular status. *Jpn Heart J.* 1964;5:12–36.

130. Tanaka H, Ueda Y, Hayashi M, et al. Risk factors for cerebral hemorrhage and cerebral infarction in a Japanese rural community. *Stroke.* 1982;13:62–73.

131. Ueda K, Omae T, Hirota Y, et al. Decreasing trend in incidence and mortality from stroke in Hisayama residents, Japan. *Stroke.* 1981;12:154–60.

132. Worth RM, Kato H, Rhoads GG, et al. Epidemiologic studies of coronary heart disease and stroke in Japanese men living in Japan, Hawaii and California: mortality. *Am J Epidemiol.* 1975;102:481–490.

133. Sasaki N. The salt factor in apoplexy and hypertension: epidemiological studies in Japan. In: Yamori Y, Lovinberg W, Freis E, eds. *Perspectives in Cardiovascular Research.* New York, NY: Raven Press; 1979: pp 467–474.

134. Takahashi E, Sasaki N, Takeda J, et al. The geographic distribution of cerebral hemorrhage and hypertension in Japan. *Human Biol.* 1957;29:139–165.

135. Benfante R, Reed D, Brody J. Biological and social predictors of health in an aging cohort. *J Chronic Dis.* 1985;38:385–395.

136. Shimamoto T, Komachi Y, Inada H, et al. Trends for coronary heart disease and stroke and their risk factors in Japan. *Circulation.* 1989;79:503–515.

137. Tanaka H, Hayashi M, Date C, et al. Epidemiologic studies of stroke in Shibata, a Japanese provincial city: preliminary report on risk factors for cerebral infarction. *Stroke.* 1985;16:773–780.

138. Lin CH, Shimizu Y, Kato H, et al. Cerebrovascular diseases in a fixed population of Hiroshima and Nagasaki, with special reference to relationship between type and risk factors. *Stroke.* 1984;15:653–660.

139. Mitsuyama Y, Thompson LR, Hayashi T, et al. Autopsy study of cerebrovascular disease in Japanese men who lived in Hiroshima, Japan and Honolulu, Hawaii. *Stroke.* 1979;10:389–395.

140. Resch JA, Okabe N, Loewenson RB, et al. Pattern of vessel involvement in cerebral atherosclerosis: a comparative study between a Japanese and Minnesota population. *J Atheroscler Res.* 1969;9719.

141. Takeya Y, Popper JS, Shimizu Y, et al. Epidemiologic studies of coronary heart disease and stroke in Japanese living in Japan, Hawaii and California: incidence of stroke in Japan and Hawaii. *Stroke.* 1984;15:15–23.

142. Olivares L, Castaneda E, Grife A, et al. Risk factors in stroke: a clinical study in Mexican patients. *Stroke.* 1973;4:773–781.

143. Paffenbarger RS Jr, Wing AL. Chronic disease in former college students. XI. early precursors of nonfatal stroke. *Am J Epidemiol.* 1971;94:524–530.

144. Abbott RD, Donahue RP, MacMahon SW, et al. Diabetes and the risk of stroke: the Honolulu heart program. *JAMA.* 1987;257:949–952.

145. Viitanen M, Eriksson S, Asplund K. Risk of recurrent stroke, myocardial infarction and epilepsy. *Eur Neurol.* 1988;28:227–231.

146. Kannel WB, Gordon T, Wolf PA, et al. Hemoglobin and the risk of cerebral infarction: the Framingham study. *Stroke.* 1972;3:409–420.

147. Pearson TC, Thomas DJ. Physiological and pharmacological factors influencing blood viscosity and cerebral blood flow. In: Tognoni G, Garattini S, eds. *Drug Treatment and Prevention in Cerebrovascular Disorders.* Amsterdam: Elsevier North Holland; 1979: p 33.

148. Tohgi J, Yamanouchi H, Murakami M, et al. Importance of the hematocrit as a risk factor in cerebral infarction. *Stroke.* 1978;9:369–374.

149. Thomas DJ, Marshall J, Russell RWR, et al. Effect of haematocrit on cerebral blood-flow in man. *Lancet.* 1977;2:941–943.

150. Harrison MJG, Pollock S, Kendall BE, et al. Effect of haematocrit on carotid stenosis and cerebral infarction. *Lancet.* 1981;2:114.

151. LaRue L, Alter M, Lai SM, et al. Acute stroke, hematocrit, and blood pressure. *Stroke.* 1987;18:565–569.

152. Ozaita G, Calandre L, Peinado E, et al. Hematocrit and clinical outcome in acute cerebral infarction. *Stroke.* 1987;18:1166–1168.

153. Lowe GDO, Jaap JL, Forbes CD. Relation of atrial fibrillation to acute stroke. *Lancet.* 1983;I:784–786.

154. Scandinavian Stroke Study Group. Multicentre trial of hemodilution in acute ischemic stroke: I. Results in the total patient population. *Stroke.* 1987;18:691–699.

155. Italian Acute Stroke Study Group. Haemodilution in acute stroke: results of the Italian Haemodilution Trial. *Lancet.* 1988;I:318–321.

156. Wilhelmsen L, Svardsudd K, Korsan-Bengtsen K, et al. Fibrinogen as a risk factor for stroke and myocardial infarction. *N Engl J Med.* 1984;311:501–505.

157. Wolf PA, Kannel WB, Meeks SL, et al. Fibrinogen as a risk factor for stroke, the Framingham study. *Stroke.* 1985;16:139.

158. Kannel WB, Wolf PA, Castelli WP, et al. Fibrinogen and risk of cardiovascular disease. The Framingham study. *JAMA.* 1987;258:1183–1186.

159. Portnoy BA, Herion JC. Neurological manifestations in sickle-cell disease: with a review of the literature and emphasis on the prevalence of hemiplegia. *Ann Intern Med.* 1972;76:643–652.

160. Kushner M, Simonian N. Lupus anticoagulants, anticardiolipin antibodies, and cerebral ischemia. *Stroke.* 1989;20:225–229.

161. Levine SR, Welch KM. Cerebrovascular ischemia associated with lupus anticoagulant. *Stroke.* 1987;18:257–263.

162. Young SM, Fisher M, Sigsbee A, et al. Cardiogenic brain embolism and lupus anticoagulant. *Ann Neurol.* 1989;26:390–392.

163. Coull BM, Bourdette DN, Goodnight SH, et al. Multiple cerebral infarctions and dementia associated with anticardiolipin antibodies. *Stroke.* 1987;18:1107–1112.

164. Levine SR, Kim S, Deegan MJ, et al. Ischemic stroke associated with anticardiolipin antibodies. *Stroke.* 1987;18:1101–1106.

165. Hart RG, Miller VT, Coull BM, et al. Cerebral infarction associated with lupus anticoagulants — preliminary report. *Stroke.* 1984;15:114–118.

166. Heyman A, Wilkinson WE, Heyden S, et al. Risk of stroke in asymptomatic persons with cervical arterial bruits: a population study in Evans County, Georgia. *N Engl J Med.* 1980;302:838–841.

167. Wolf PA, Kannel WB, Sorlie P, et al. Asymptomatic carotid bruit and risk of stroke. The Framingham study. *JAMA*. 1981;245:1442–1445.

168. Conneally PM, Dyken ML, Futty DE, et al. Cooperative study of hospital frequency and character of transient ischemic attacks: VIII. Risk factors. *JAMA*. 1978;240:742–746.

169. Dyken ML. Should the efficacy of carotid endarterectomy in symptomatic patients be examined in a controlled clinical trial? A study is needed. In: Raichle ME, Powers WJ, eds. *Cerebrovascular Diseases*. New York, NY: Raven Press; 1987.

170. Dyken ML. Carotid endarterectomy studies: a glimmering of science. *Stroke*. 1986;17:355–358.

171. Meissner I, Wiebers DO, Whisnant JP, et al. The natural history of asymptomatic carotid artery occlusive lesions. *Ann Neurol*. 1986;20:122.

172. Powers WM, Press GW, Grubb RL Jr, et al. The effect of hemodynamically significant carotid artery disease on the hemodynamic status of the cerebral circulation. *Ann Intern Med*. 1987;106: 27–35.

173. Powers WJ, Tempel LW, Grubb RL. Influence of cerebral hemodynamics on stroke risk: one-year follow-up of 30 medically treated patients. *Ann Neurol*. 1989;25:325–330.

174. Powers WJ, Grubb RL Jr, Raichle ME. Clinical results of extracranial-intracranial bypass surgery in patients with hemodynamic cerebrovascular disease. *J Neurosurg*. 1989;70:61–67.

175. Bogousslavsky J, Regli F, VanMelle G, et al. Migraine stroke. *Neurology*. 1988;38:223–227.

176. Bogousslavsky J, Regli F. Ischemic stroke in adults younger than 30 years of age: cause and prognosis. *Arch Neurol*. 1987;44:479–482.

177. Rothrock JF, Walicke P, Swenson MR, et al. Migrainous stroke. *Arch Neurol*. 1988;45:63–67.

178. Hilton-Jones D, Warlow CP. The causes of stroke in the young. *J Neurol*. 1985;232:137–143.

179. Chen TC, Leviton A, Edelstein S, et al. Migraine and other diseases in women of reproductive age: The influence of smoking on observed associations. *Arch Neurol*. 1987;44:1024–1028.

180. Pfaffenrath V, Pollmann W, Autenrieth G, et al. Mitral valve prolapse and platelet aggregation in patients with hemiplegic and nonhemiplegic migraine. *Acta Neurol Scand*. 1987;75:253–257.

181. Hogan MJ, Brunet DG, Ford PM, et al. Lupus anticoagulant, antiphospholipid antibodies and migraine. *Can J Neurol Sci*. 1988;15:420–425.

182. Henrich JB. The association between migraine and cerebral vascular events: an analytical review. *J Chronic Dis*. 1987;40:329–335.

183. Kuller L, Anderson H, Peterson D, et al. Nationwide cerebrovascular disease morbidity study. *Stroke*. 1970;1:86–99.

184. Nefzger MD, Acheson RM, Heyman A. Mortality from stroke among U.S. veterans in Georgia and five western states: I. Study plan and death rates. *J Chronic Dis*. 1973;26:393–404.

185. The WHO MONICA Project. Geographical variation in the major risk factors of coronary heart disease in men and women aged 35-64 years. *World Health Stat Q*. 1988;41:115–140.

186. Bull GM. Meteorological correlates with myocardial and cerebral infarction and respiratory disease. *Br J Prev Soc Med*. 1973;27:108–113.

187. Haberman S, Capildeo R, Rose FC. The seasonal variation in mortality from cerebrovascular disease. *J Neuro Sci*. 1981;52:25.

188. Knox EG. Meteorological associations of cerebrovascular disease mortality in England and Wales. *J Epidemiol Community Health*. 1981;35: 220–223.

189. Rogot E, Padgett SJ. Associations of coronary and stroke mortality with temperature and snowfall in selected areas of the United States, 1962–1966. *Am J Epidemiol*. 1976;103:565–575.

190. Berginer VM, Goldsmith J, Vardi H, et al. Clustering of strokes in association with meteorologic factors in the Negev desert of Israel. 1981–1983. *Stroke*. 1989;20:65–9.

191. Biller J, Jones MP, Bruno A, et al. Seasonal variation of stroke–does it exist? *Neuroepidemiology*. 1988;7:89–98.

192. Marler JR, Price TR, Clark GL, et al. Morning increase in onset of ischemic stroke. *Stroke*. 1989; 20:473–476.

193. Acheson RM, Fairbairn AS. Record linkage in studies of cerebrovascular disease in Oxford, England. *Stroke*. 1971;2:48–57.

194. Acheson RM, Heyman A, Nefzger MD. Mortality from stroke among U.S. veterans in Georgia and five western states: III. Hypertension and demographic characteristics. *J Chronic Dis*. 1973;26: 417–429.

195. Mann AH, Brennan PJ. Type A behavior score and the incidence of cardiovascular disease: a failure to replicate the claimed associations. *J Psychosom Res*. 1987;31:685–692.

196. Ragland DR, Brand RJ. Type A behavior and mortality from coronary heart disease. *N Engl J Med*. 1988;318:65–69.

197. Eaker ED, Castelli WP. Type A behavior and mortality from coronary disease in the Framingham study. *N Engl J Med*. 1988;319:1480–1481.

198. Kannel WB, Wolf PA. Epidemiology of cerebrovascular disease. In: Ross Russell RW, ed. *Vascular Disease of the Central Nervous System*. 2nd ed. London: Churchill Livingston; 1983.

199. Longstreth WT Jr, Swanson PD. Oral contraceptives and stroke. *Stroke*. 1984;15:747–750.

200. Sobel E, Alter M, Davanipour Z, et al. Stroke in the Lehigh valley: combined risk factors for recurrent ischemic stroke. *Neurology.* 1989;39:669–672.

201. Miettinen TA, Huttunen JK, Naukkarinen V, et al. Multifactorial primary prevention of cardiovascular diseases in middle-aged men: risk factor changes, incidence, and mortality. *JAMA*. 1985; 254:2097–2102.

7
Head and Neck Bruits in Stroke Prevention

John W. Norris

> Where observation is concerned, chance favours only the prepared mind.
>
> *Louis Pasteur, 1822–1895*

Pathogenesis of Bruits

Vascular bruits result from loss of laminar flow in blood vessels. Increased blood velocity or vessel tortuosity cause turbulence, which produces vibration of the vessel wall. If laminar flow is maintained, even with increased blood velocity, no bruit will result (Fig. 7.1). Neck bruits conducted from cardiac murmurs, e.g., aortic stenosis, similarly represent carotid wall vibration secondary to turbulence distal to the abnormal heart valve.

As the stenosis progresses, arterial bruits become louder, until the stenosis reaches about 50%, when volumetric blood flow falls and the bruit becomes fainter and finally inaudible as stenosis becomes occlusion (Fig. 7.2).[1] The frequency of the bruit increases with the degree of stenosis, but intraobserver error is wide, and, because of this subjectivity, this sign is not reliable.[2] The duration of the bruit also increases with the stenosis; in severe stenoses the bruit may be continuous with a clearly audible diastolic component. This should not be confused with the to and fro "machinery" murmur heard in arteriovenous malformations. Therefore, severe arterial stenoses are characterized by high-pitched, continuous, but often faint, bruits.

However, bruits may vary from day to day in the same patient, may change in character with posture (sitting or supine) and with the degree of activity or anxiety preceding auscultation. This wide margin of observer error may explain the frequent discovery of apparently new neck bruits at the consultant's ward round, previously missed by the resident at the patient's admission.

Clinical Significance of Cephalic Bruits

Although most published reviews of neck and head bruits commend auscultation of the head and neck,[3,4] this is far from routine in medical practice. In fact, in 1928 Bailey and Cushing stated: "By a strange human frailty, auscultation of the skull seems to be the one thing to be neglected in a routine neurological examination."[5] However, the value of this examination dates back to at least 1809, when an English physician, Dr. Travers, felt a pulsatile thrill over the acutely protuberant eye of a young lady who suddenly heard a "whooshing" sound in her head. He diagnosed an "aneurism" and successfully tied off the ipsilateral carotid artery, so curing her symptoms and signs. He is probably therefore the first physician to prevent stroke by being alerted by a cephalic bruit.[6]

When 50 family physicians in Toronto were questioned about their practice of auscultating the neck in routine physical examinations, 62% replied "nearly always," 30% "sometimes," and 8% "never."

Despite rapidly expanding noninvasive technology of imaging the carotid arteries, neck auscultation remains the simplest, most effective, and cheapest method for detecting carotid artery disease; in about half of neck bruits there is an underlying carotid stenosis of >35%, though only 10% have stenoses >75%.[2]

Ocular Bruits

Bruits around or over the eye usually indicate carotid siphon stenosis, but other causes include:

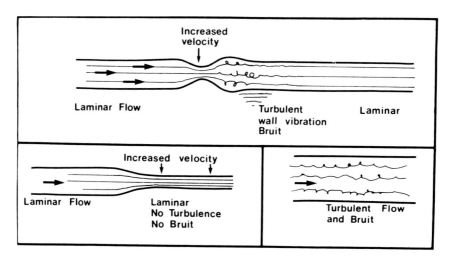

FIGURE 7.1. Relationship between laminar flow and turbulence. (Reprinted with permission from Martinus Nijhoff, Publishers, Ref. 1.)

1. Periorbital lesions – angiomas of the scalp and orbit, severe Paget's disease.
2. Intracranial lesions – cerebral angiomas and arteriovenous malformations, cortico-cavernous fistulas, large saccular aneurysms, vascular tumors – e.g., meningiomas, carotid arteritis, and dissection.
3. Systemic illnesses – hyperdynamic circulatory states that increase blood velocity, including anemia, thyrotoxicosis, and fever.

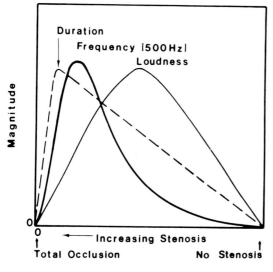

FIGURE 7.2. Change in duration, loudness, and pitch of vascular bruits with increasing stenosis. (Reprinted with permission from Martinus Nijhoff, Publishers, Ref. 1.)

4. In children orbital bruits may be physiological and of no pathological significance, disappearing as the child grows older.[7]

Ocular bruits are best heard using the stethoscope bell over the eye, asking the patient then to open his eyes to diminish blinking artifact.[8] Confirmation of the carotid origin of the ocular bruit (in one or both eyes) is readily obtained by abolishing it (or them) by digital compression of the carotid artery. In patients with cerebrovascular disease, ocular bruits are distinctly uncommon. They accounted for only about 2% of bruits heard in our Doppler laboratory, which corresponds to the 1 in 150 incidence previously documented in consecutive cases of cerebrovascular disease.[9]

C. Miller Fisher suggested that ocular bruits occur contralateral to carotid occlusion.[8] Pessin et al. also noted that 10 of 13 ocular bruits related to carotid occlusion, and 9 of these were contralateral to the occluded artery. None had intracranial carotid lesions.[9] However, Hu and colleagues studied 50 patients with 72 ocular bruits, confirming carotid occlusion by Doppler and, in 28 cases, by angiography. They found that ocular bruits due to contralateral carotid augmented flow occurred in one third of cases and that the most common cause was ipsilateral siphon stenosis.[5] Orientals tend to have more intracranial disease. This may not necessarily be true of other racial groups.[10]

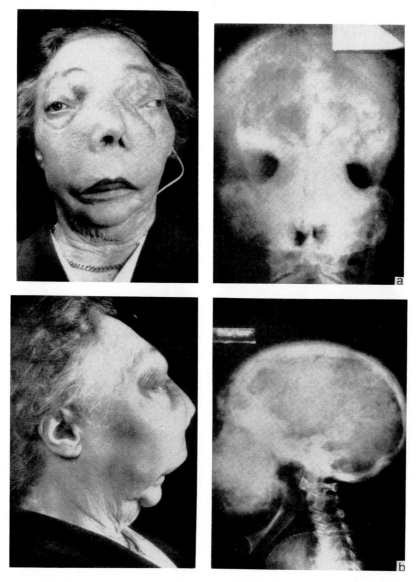

FIGURE 7.3. Patient with severe Paget's disease and loud, generalized head bruits. (Reprinted with permission from *Brain*, Ref. 11.)

Intracranial Bruits in Health and Disease

Wadia and Monckton[11] examined >700 otherwise normal individuals, auscultating six pre-determined regions in each person's head. There were 228 adults examined in the hospital out-patient department, and 513 normal school children. Only 3 adults (1%) had bruits in the head, one "ascribed to arteriosclerosis," and two without explanation. In the pediatric group, there were 98 cases (19%) with head bruits, but none was thought to be pathological.

The authors recommend routine cranial auscultation in all cases of suspected intracranial disease, from epilepsy to stroke. However, their figure of 1% of intracranial bruits in hospital outpatients must be far greater than that experienced by most physicians.

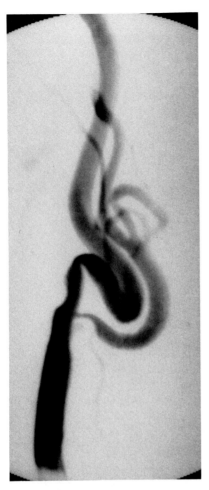

FIGURE 7.4. Coiled carotid artery producing loud, unilateral neck bruit with normal Doppler.

After reviewing the topic, they suggested that intracranial angiomas were the commonest cause of intracranial bruit, probably occurring in 80% of cases, depending on how carefully the patient is examined. They also illustrate their case history by a striking case of Paget's disease with a temporal bruit due to arteriovenous shunting in the thickened skull (Fig. 7.3).

Neck Bruits

Venous Neck Bruits

Bruits heard over veins are termed "hums" because of their soft to-and-fro character. They are inappropriately termed "bruits du diable" since they are always benign. They are almost always confined to children or young adults, are heard in the supraclavicular fossa, appear when the patient sits up, and become louder when the head is turned away from the auscultated side.[11] They occur predominantly on the right side.[12] They are produced by venous return to the heart, and so are abolished by breath holding.

They are of no pathological significance and, with a modicum of clinical experience, are easily differentiated from arterial bruits.

Arterial Neck Bruits

Clinical correlation of neck bruits with carotid Doppler examination indicates that about 40% are harmless or, at least, noncarotid in origin.[2] Neck bruits with normal Doppler evaluation are frequently seen in Doppler laboratories,[2,13] because of arterial kinks and coils or physiological arterial anomalies such as aberrant uptake of the superior thyroid artery, and are best differentiated by angiography (Fig. 7.4).

Increased velocity in the carotid artery due to hyperdynamic circulatory conditions, such as anemia, thyrotoxicosis, or fever, produces generalized arterial bruits that disappear when the systemic condition resolves, e.g., blood transfusion.[3,14]

Ziegler et al., correlating angiographic data and neck auscultation in 199 patients, commented that neck bruits were "highly fallible" indices of carotid arterial disease.[15] They found 73% false negatives (stenosis without bruit) and 10% false positives (bruit without stenosis). However, in a similar study comparing auscultation to carotid Doppler, Hennerici and colleagues found 23% false positives and 16% false negatives. This discrepancy may be based on the prior exclusion of certain bruits that are not associated with an arterial lesion (e.g., cardiac) by the Hennerici group.[13]

Bruits conducted from the heart are always due to aortic valve stenosis or, occasionally, incompetence, presumably representing turbulence of the cardiac ejection conducted upstream. The bruit is traditionally alleged to diminish as the auscultation is continued up the neck. However, our experience in the carotid Doppler laboratory is that only ultrasound can differentiate for certain between conducted murmurs and in situ bruits, and that clinical differentiation is unreliable.

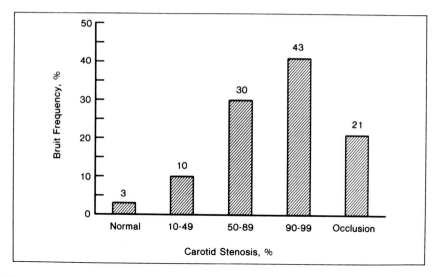

FIGURE 7.5. Percentage of carotid bruits associated with carotid stenosis. (Reprinted with permission from Ref. 16.)

Frequency of Neck Bruits in Patients with Carotid Stenosis

There have been numerous attempts to evaluate the importance of neck bruits in localizing carotid disease. These range from angiographic surveys to more recent series correlating Duplex ultrasound data. The result depends largely upon whether the investigations start with carotid imaging and correlate the bruits or start with the neck bruits and correlate the imaging. Each method brings its own bias depending on the referral base. Several excellent comprehensive reviews exist.[16,17]

In general, underlying carotid stenosis is usually "silent"; only about one in three patients with moderate to severe stenosis will have neck bruits.[15,16] In patients with unilateral neck bruits, two of three will have underlying carotid stenosis ipsilateral to the bruit, and 30% will have contralateral stenosis in the "silent" artery.[2]

Most published series correlating neck bruits have estimated the incidence of bruits in patients undergoing carotid angiography. The overall frequency is therefore irrelevant, since it depends upon the reason for angiography and will vary from center to center. Restricting the evaluation only to patients with 50% to 100% stenosis produces a more consistent picture. Ziegler et al.[15] found that 29% of patients with carotid stenosis >50% had neck bruits, while David et al.[18] found bruits in 88% in a similar group. This discrepancy may relate to how "blindly" the results were interpreted, since no mention is made in early series whether the examiners had a preview of the angiographic results.

In the Mayo Clinic study,[16] there were 196 neck bruits in 1004 patients, but the frequency depended on the severity of stenosis; this was never >43%, even in >90% stenotic lesions (Fig. 7.5).

Restricting the carotid lesions to those with lumens <2 mm (about 80% to 90% stenosis), Pessin et al. found localized bifurcation bruits in 34 (87%) of 37 severely stenosed arteries.[9] The lack of bruits in very stenosed or occluded arteries was attributed to slow flow where turbulence no longer occurred.

Frequency of Carotid Stenosis in Patients with Neck Bruits

Localization of the neck bruit is important, and bruits in the upper neck have a much greater correlation with underlying carotid stenosis than those in the lower neck (Figs. 7.6 and 7.7).[2]

About 4% of "normal" adults have neck bruits,[19,20] and this figure rises to 8% to 12% in asympto-

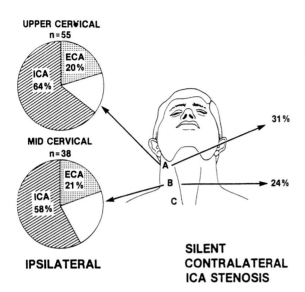

FIGURE 7.6. Frequency of carotid stenosis in 93 patients with unilateral neck bruits. (Reprinted with permission from *Neurology*, Ref. 2.)

matic patients over 70.[21] Prospective evaluations of asymptomatic patients with neck bruits also indicate that only 17% of carotid lesions have stenoses >75%[22]; so the frequency of significant carotid disease in the normal population, even in the elderly, is only 1% to 2%.

Howard et al.[17] evaluated 1107 patients with carotid disease referred to their Doppler laboratory by phonoangiography and B-mode ultrasonography (17). There were 917 without neck bruits, 119 with unilateral neck bruits, and 71 with bilateral neck bruits. Some had ischemic cerebral

SCREENING FOR ICA STENOSIS (one or both sides)

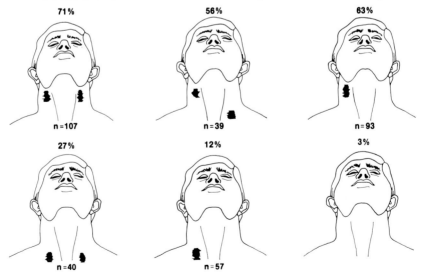

FIGURE 7.7. Prevalence of carotid artery stenosis in 336 patients with various locations of neck bruits. N = number of patients. Number above each figure represents percentage incidence of carotid stenosis. (Reprinted with permission from *Neurology*, Ref. 2.)

or cardiac disease, and some were asymptomatic. They concluded that although neck bruits were associated with an increased risk of carotid atherosclerosis, the bruit did not indicate which side was involved. The risk appeared to be random.

Data from other studies indicate a slight predilection for more severe carotid stenosis on the side of the bruit. For instance, in the Toronto study of asymptomatic neck bruits, a unilateral neck bruit had greater predictive value for ipsilateral carotid stenosis.[2] Similarly, Ingall et al., evaluating neck bruits by angiography, found a significantly higher incidence of carotid stenosis in 196 patients with neck bruits compared to 808 without bruits, but again, without much localizing value.[16]

However, all prospective studies of neck bruits utilizing carotid imaging lead to similar conclusions; bruits indicate underlying carotid disease, whether or not they have lateralizing value, and are associated with a significantly increased (though low) risk of stroke compared with the general population.[22,23] Earlier population studies[18,19] indicated that subsequent strokes in patients with neck bruits occur at random and irrespective of the bruit side, but they did not have the benefit of carotid imaging.

We compared the incidence and severity of carotid stenosis in three groups of patients: carotid strokes, carotid transient ischemic attacks (TIAs), and those with asymptomatic neck bruits.[24] There was a striking effect on the incidence and severity of carotid stenosis in the presence of neck bruits in the symptomatic groups, 23% in the TIA patients without bruits, compared with 70% in those with bruits, and 31% in the stroke group without bruits compared with 86% in those with bruits (Figs. 7.8 and 7.9). There was a hierarchy of degree of carotid artery stenosis from asymptomatic patients to those with stroke. Stroke patients had more severe carotid disease than the TIA group, who in turn had more severe carotid stenosis than the asymptomatic patients (Fig. 7.10).

Sex Differences in Neck Bruits

Men outnumber women in the incidence of symptomatic cerebrovascular disease in all prospective studies of TIAs and stroke.[25] However, population studies of patients with asymptomatic neck bruits indicate that detectable carotid stenosis is more common in men than in women (Fig. 7.11).

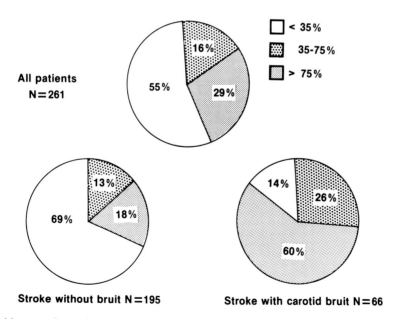

FIGURE 7.8. Incidence and severity of carotid artery stenosis in 261 consecutive patients with carotid ischemic stroke in the Toronto Stroke Unit.

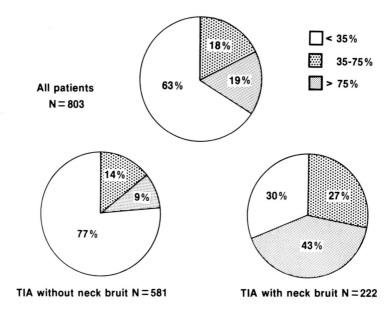

FIGURE 7.9. Incidence and severity of carotid artery stenosis in 803 consecutive patients with carotid TIAs admitted to the Toronto Stroke Unit.

Women are predisposed to carotid bruits in the absence of carotid stenosis. This is not related to caliber of vessels, hematocrit, presence of heart murmurs, differences in pulse rate, or body habitus.[26] It may represent referral bias, assuming that men are more likely to be symptomatic before being referred to a physician.

Conclusion

Most head and neck bruits do not represent underlying cerebrovascular disease, especially in children and young adults. Nevertheless, they are valuable indicators of intracranial or extracranial vascular lesions in a large minority of patients, and

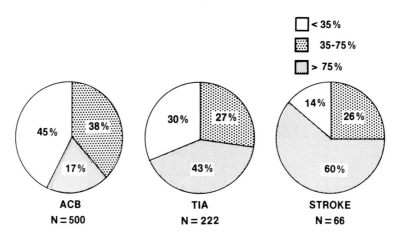

FIGURE 7.10. Incidence and severity of carotid stenosis in symptomatic and asymptomatic patients with neck bruits. (Reprinted with permission from *Stroke*, Ref. 24.)

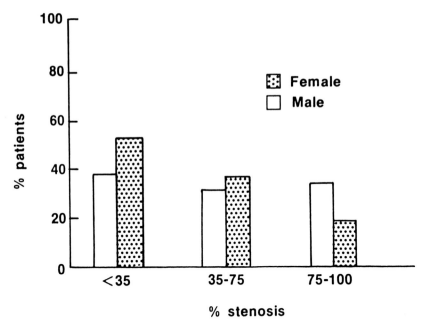

FIGURE 7.11. Differences in severity of carotid stenosis (%) between men and women presenting with asymptomatic neck bruits. (Data from the Toronto Asymptomatic Bruit Study.)

their significance becomes more sinister the older the patient.

Head bruits may indicate intracranial vascular tumors or arterial stenoses, while neck bruits more likely indicate carotid or subclavian atherosclerosis. In both symptomatic and asymptomatic patients, neck bruits indicate an increased risk of stroke. However, they do not localize the artery at risk, since severe carotid stenosis often has no associated neck bruits, while otherwise normal arteries may produce bruits due to increased flow and turbulence from contralateral carotid disease.

Head and neck auscultation is an inexpensive and effective method of screening for patients vulnerable to stroke and therefore should be an integral part of the routine physical examination.

References

1. Spencer M. Vascular murmurs. In: Spencer MP, Reid JMR. eds. *Cerebrovascular Evaluation with Doppler Ultrasound*. The Hague: Martinus Nijhoff; 1981: pp 89–96.
2. Chambers BR, Norris JW. Clinical significance of asymptomatic neck bruits. *Neurology.* 1985;35: 742–745.
3. Mackenzie I. The intracranial bruit. *Brain.* 1955; 78:350–368.
4. Hu HH, Liao KK, Wong WJ, et al. Ocular bruits in ischemic cerebrovascular disease. *Stroke.* 1988;19: 1229–1233.
5. Cushing H, Bailey P. *Tumours Arising from the Blood Vessels of the Brain.* London: 1928.
6. Travers B. A case of aneurism by anastomosis in the orbit, cured by ligature of the common carotid artery. *Med-Chir Trans.* 1813;2:1
7. Fowler NO, Marshall WJ. The supraclavicular arterial bruit. Am Heart J. 1965;69:410–418.
8. Fisher CM. Cranial bruit associated with occlusion of the internal carotid artery. *Neurology.* 1957;7: 299–306.
9. Pessin MS, Panis W, Prager RJ, et al. Auscultation of cervical and ocular bruits in extracranial carotid occlusive disease: A clinical and angiographic study. *Stroke.* 1983;14:246–251.
10. Inzitari D, Hachinski VC, Taylor DW, Barnett HJM. Racial differences in the anterior circulation of cerebrovascular disease: how much can be explained by risk factors. *Arch Neurol.* In press.
11. Wadia NH, Monckton G. Intracranial bruits in health and disease. *Brain.* 1957;80:492–509.
12. Fowler, NO, Gause R. The cervical venous hum. *Am Heart J*. 1964;67:135–136.

13. Hennerici M, Aulich A, Sandmann W, et al. Incidence of asymptomatic extracranial arterial disease. *Stroke*. 1981;12:750–755.
14. Allen N, Mustian V. Origin and significance of vascular murmurs of the head and neck. *Medicine*. 1962;41:227–247.
15. Ziegler DK, Zileli T, Dick A, et al. Correlation of bruits over the carotid artery with angiographically demonstrated lesions. *Neurology*. 1971;21:860–865.
16. Ingall TJ, Homer D, Whisnant JP, et al. Predictive value of carotid bruit for carotid atherosclerosis. *Arch Neurol*. 1989;46:418–422.
17. Howard VJ, Howard G, Harpold GJ, et al. Correlation of carotid bruits and carotid atherosclerosis detected by B-mode real-time ultrasonography. *Stroke*. 1989;20:1331–1335.
18. David TE, Humphries AW, Young JR, et al. A correlation of neck bruits and arteriosclerotic carotid arteries. *Arch Surg*. 1973;107:729–731.
19. Heyman A, Wilkinson WE, Heyden S, et al. Risk of stroke in asymptomatic persons with cervical arterial bruits. *N Engl J Med*. 1980;302:838–841.
20. Wolf PA, Kannel WB, Sorlie P, et al. Asymptomatic carotid bruit and risk of stroke. The Framingham study. *JAMA*. 1981;245:1442–1445.
21. Cutler JL. Cerebrovascular disease in an elderly population. *Circulation*. 1967;36:394–399.
22. Roederer GO, Langlois YE, Jager KA, et al. The natural history of carotid arterial disease in asymptomatic patients with cervical bruits. *Stroke*. 1984;15:605–613.
23. Hennerici M, Aulich A, Freund H-J. Carotid system syndromes. In: Vinken PJ, Bruyn GW, Klawans HL, eds. *Handbook of Clinical Neurology*. Amsterdam: Elsevier Science Publishers; 1989: pp 291–337.
24. Zhu CZ, Norris JW. Role of carotid stenosis in ischemic stroke. *Stroke*. 1990;21:1131–1134.
25. Wolf PA, Kannel WB, Verter J. Current status of risk factors for stroke. In: Barnett HJM, ed. *Neurologic Clinics, Symposium on Cerebrovascular Disease*. W.B. Saunders; 1981:317–320.
26. Ford CS, Howard VJ, Howard G, et al. The sex difference in manifestations of carotid bifurcation disease. *Stroke*. 1986;17:877–880.

8
Hypertension and Stroke Prevention

J.D. Spence

The management of hypertension is now more effective than ever before, but even today there is a problem with recognition of the goal of therapy. Since hypertension is asymptomatic, its treatment cannot improve a person's wellbeing; in fact, it may detract from it through the adverse effects of therapy. The goal of treatment is to prevent hypertensive vascular complications[1,2]; so it is necessary to understand the pathophysiologic mechanisms of these complications and their responses to treatment. Some effects of hypertension respond to lowering of blood pressure, while others are less responsive,[3-11] and both responses give insight into the way that vascular complications occur.

We have studied this problem at Victoria Hospital in London, Ontario, since the initiation of a hypertension detection and treatment program by the University of Western Ontario Department of Family Medicine in 1978.[12] Our initial data (since the advent of computerized tomographic (CT) scanning routinely performed in all patients) indicated that about half the strokes were associated with hypertension; of these, approximately 75% were hypertensive intracerebral hemorrhages, and 25% were due to lacunar infarction.

In the Family Medicine project, 34 physicians followed 32 124 patients for five years, with nursing assistants assigned to half the practices to improve detection and treatment of hypertension. By 1983, 94% of hypertensive patients in the London area were detected, and 92% were on treatment; 72% were considered well controlled.[13] By 1984, despite an increase in the population by nearly one third and a rising elderly population, the number of stroke patients admitted annually to our hospital decreased from 500 to 250. There was also a striking change in the type of the strokes. Fewer than 10% could be attributed to hypertension, and the proportion of strokes associated with cerebral atherosclerosis (mainly extracranial carotid disease) increased from 35% to 70%. There was no reduction in the number of atherosclerotic strokes, despite a dramatic decline in the number of strokes due to hypertensive disease.

Pickering, commenting on the relationship of blood pressure to arteriolar events, and later Russell, indicated that strokes due to high blood pressure were either hypertensive hemorrhages or lacunar infarctions, so that treatment to reduce blood pressure could prevent only these types of stroke.[1,14] These observations highlight the need for a clearer understanding of how hypertension causes vascular change, and so improve the use of antihypertensive drugs in the prevention of the atherosclerotic complications of hypertension.

Hypertensive Arteriolar Disease

Hypertensive Encephalopathy

Giese[15] noted that during severe hypertensive crises, vasospasm is the normal response to markedly increased pressure. Skinhoj, Strandgaard, and others confirmed[16,17] that the areas of vasodilation are the "injured" part of the arteriole, while the spastic segments are "normal." Hypertensive encephalopathy is, therefore, a forced vasodilation due to breakthrough of cerebral auto-regulation. There is increased cerebral blood flow, vascular congestion associated with cerebral edema, and areas of

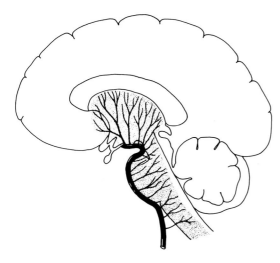

FIGURE 8.1. The vascular centrencephalon, showing the arterial system arising from the basal arterial trunks. (From Ref 22, with permission.)

cerebral ischemia due to fibrinoid necrosis and occlusion of some small vessels. The occipital cortex is particularly susceptible to edema, perhaps accounting for the cortical blindness and visual hallucinations seen in patients with eclampsia. Hypertensive encephalopathy is not confined to patients with very high blood pressure, but often occurs in those with moderate elevations. The pressure at which cerebral autoregulation "breaks through" is determined by the blood pressure to which the arterioles have recently been exposed. Patients with low normal premorbid levels will experience breakthrough at moderately elevated pressures, whereas those with long-standing severe hypertension will tolerate much higher pressures, presumably because of structural adaptation of the arterioles to high pressure.[18]

Individual tolerance to blood pressure is often surprisingly high and underlines the need for target pressures for treatment in the acute management of hypertensive emergencies. For most patients, a target blood pressure of approximately 120 mm Hg Mean Arterial Pressure (MAP) is desirable, and those with long-standing severe hypertension will not tolerate reduction of blood pressure to normal levels.

Effects of Antihypertensive Drugs

Certain drugs should be avoided in the treatment of hypertension. For instance, sublingual nifedipine (a popular treatment in many emergency rooms)

and intramuscular hydralazine produce uncontrollable blood pressure changes, and severe hypotension may cause cerebral infarction. The term *sublingual* is a misnomer for nifedipine, since absorption from the buccal mucosa is very slow; the rapid action results from swallowing nifedipine administered sublingually on the mistaken assumption that its rapid action is related to rapid absorption from the mouth.[19]

Blood pressure decreases more dramatically when it is initially very high, resulting in adverse effects such as myocardial infarction.[20] The management of severe hypertension in patients with hypertensive encephalopathy or acute stroke should ensure that sudden decreases in blood pressure are avoided, especially below the threshold for cerebral autoregulation. Small, repeated intravenous doses (or infusions) of potent intravenous drugs such as diazoxide, sodium nitroprusside, or intravenous beta-blockers in combination with vasodilators, under careful observation, are preferable.[21]

Hypertensive Strokes

Cerebral Hemorrhage

Rupture of arteriolar microaneurysms produces intracerebral hemorrhage in the basal ganglia, thalamus, pons, or cerebellum. The location of these events is perhaps best explained by the concept of the vascular centrencephalon,[22] where the arteries are short, straight vessels with few branches (Fig. 8.1). They are functional end arteries, supplying the mesial and basal portions of the brain and brain stem from the ventral surface, penetrating in the dorsal direction. Since the arteries arise from large basal trunks, the gradation between arterial and capillary pressure occurs over a relatively short distance, requiring the arterioles to withstand high pressures. In contrast, pressures are dissipated in the long, branching, penetrating vessels that perfuse the newer parts of the brain.

The detection and treatment of hypertension has resulted in a marked reduction in hypertensive intracerebral hemorrhage, and now the commonest cause is amyloid angiopathy, seen usually in the elderly and sometimes associated with Alzheimer's disease.[23] Characteristically, the location of hemorrhages in amyloid angiopathy is at the junction of cortex and white matter, often in the posterior parietal lobe.[24]

Lacunar Infarction

These are small white-matter infarctions in the same distribution as hypertensive intracerebral hemorrhages,[25] due to occlusion of arterioles and small arteries of the centrencephalon, from fibrinoid necrosis. They should not be confused with small infarctions from embolism of atheromatous debris from the carotid bifurcation. Since the advent of CT scanning, it has become popular to describe any visualized small white-matter infarct as a lacune. This is one of the commonest diagnostic errors in the management of stroke.

Hachinski et al.[26] have recently described a condition that they termed leukoaraiosis. This may relate to episodes of hypotension in patients with reduced cerebral vascular reserve due to hypertensive thickening of small vessels. This idea is similar to that described by Floras, consisting of nocturnal hypotension below the autoregulatory threshold for myocardial perfusion.[27] This concept has been implicated in the "J-shaped curve" of survival in treatment of hypertension.[28]

Effects of Antihypertensive Drugs

Consistent lowering of blood pressure prevents hypertensive arteriolar strokes but does not play a large part in the prevention of atherothrombotic strokes. Therefore, as hypertensive arteriolar strokes decrease in frequency as a result of effective detection and treatment of hypertension, the proportion of strokes due to atherosclerosis is increasing.

Pathogenesis of Atherosclerosis

The relationship between hypertension and atherosclerosis is indirect and complex. Focal atherosclerotic lesions occur at areas predisposed to disturbances of flow patterns and reflect the influence of local hemodynamic factors.[29] Recently, Glagov et al. suggested that arteries remodel themselves as required to maintain a constant shear rate at the interface between the endothelium and blood stream.[30] If low shear stress develops at the near side of an arterial loop or bifurcation, the area will fill in, while if high shear stress develops at the far wall, the artery will tend to enlarge away from the high shear rate.[31-33]

Injury to the endothelium, in part due to arterial flow disturbances, leads to interaction between the arterial wall and platelets, with release of platelet growth factors that result in proliferation of smooth muscle cells in the endothelium.[33] Since the vascular endothelium is exposed to the kinetic energy associated with disturbed flow patterns, the effects of antihypertensive drugs on these flow patterns and their effects on pressure[11] are both important.

The initiation of atherosclerosis, the progression of atherosclerotic plaques, and the complications of atherosclerotic lesions include embolization of platelet thrombus or atheromatous debris, and intraplaque hemorrhage or dissection. They are all related more to arterial flow disturbances than to blood pressure.[34-48]

Turbulence and Laminar Flow

Normal blood flow is laminar, with the fastest flow in the central (axial) part of the stream and the slowest along the wall. Most of the total fluid energy in the blood is in the form of pressure energy,[48] and the endothelium is spared from exposure to high-velocity gradients (high shear rates) along the wall. Normally, the endothelium is not exposed to appreciable amounts of kinetic energy; so no endothelial damage occurs when flow patterns become disturbed. Conversion of pressure into kinetic energy occurs, and the energy that has been stored in the blood in the form of pressure now may injure the vessel lining.

Two factors may expose the endothelium to kinetic energy. First, arterial loops or bifurcations may bring the fast-moving axial stream into contact with the wall (sites of high shear). Second, at areas where the fast-moving stream tends to pull away from the wall, abnormal low-shear rates may develop; these are potentially important in the pathogenesis of atherosclerosis.[36,37] The anatomy of the vessels may cause disturbed flow patterns where flow would normally remain laminar. For steady flow in straight tubes, the factors that cause turbulence are the diameter of the vessel and the velocity and density of the fluid. The major factor reducing turbulence is viscosity.[38,40]

Turbulence is mainly a product of heart rate and blood velocity. For any bifurcation, the critical Reynolds number decreases as the angle of bifurcation widens (i.e., the blood has to go more slowly to remain laminar as the angle widens), and for pulsatile flow, blood must move more slowly to remain laminar.[41] Yellin[42] introduced the concept of diastolic damping time; as heart rate increases, there is a greater tendency for transitory flow disturbances at peak systole to become propagated from one cycle to the next, and so to extend downstream. This concept of diastolic damping time is important in coronary and cerebral arteries, where most flow occurs during diastole.[43]

Hence, slower heart rates contribute to smoother patterns of blood flow, and increased heart rates contribute to disturbed flow patterns. Increasing the heart rate increases the frequency and speed with which the blood accelerates and decelerates, magnifying oscillations in shear along the wall during the transition from forward flow during systole to reverse flow during diastole.[36]

The heart rate is an independent predictor of coronary risk in man[44] and the magnitude of heart rate increase in response to threat also predicts progression of coronary artery disease in a monkey model of stress-induced atherosclerosis.[45]

The Role of Shear Stress in Atherogenesis

Whether atherosclerosis develops from high or low shear stress is controversial. In high shear stress, injury to the vascular endothelium by high fluid shear stresses is the focus for the development of atherosclerosis as a repair process at the site of injury.[35] In low shear sites, exposure of the endothelium to low fluid shear produces atherosclerosis by adversely affecting the mass transfer of lipids across the arterial wall.[36] Friedman proposed that both high-shear and low-shear sites are important[46,47] and that atherosclerosis develops more quickly but to a limited extent at high-shear areas and more slowly but to a greater extent at low-shear areas. This, together with the work of Glagov et al.,[30] suggests that atherosclerosis is a remodeling process, the shape of the artery adapting to the flow pattern.

Effects of Antihypertensive Drugs on Lipoproteins

It is necessary to examine the effects of antihypertensive agents on lipoprotein profiles, blood velocity, heart rate, and arterial flow patterns to select drugs that may prevent atherosclerosis.

Since 1980, there is increasing evidence that antihypertensive drugs adversely affect lipoproteins. Nonselective beta-blockers, probably all kaliuretic diuretics, and most sympatholytic drugs, such as methyldopa, tend to increase triglyceride levels and lower high-density lipoprotein (HDL) cholesterol levels, with the result that the cholesterol/HDL ratio is adversely affected by about 15%.[1] A perspective on the significance of this change can be gained from the Lipid Clinics Coronary Prevention Trial, in which there was a 20% reduction in coronary mortality following a 9% reduction of cholesterol levels using diet and cholestyramine.[49] Thus, a 15% adverse effect on lipids is thought to completely offset the benefit of treating mild hypertension.[33] Relatively cardioselective beta-blockers and those with weak intrinsic sympathomimetic activity (ISA) may have neutral effects on lipids. Alpha-blockers, beta-blockers with strong ISA, and in patients on diuretics, potassium-and-magnesium-sparing diuretics and angiotensin-converting-enzyme inhibitors, all have beneficial effects on lipoproteins,[11] but there is no evidence yet that these effects change the risk.

Effects of Antihypertensive Drugs on Flow Patterns

Antihypertensive drugs have different effects on blood velocity in the carotid arteries of rhesus monkeys[50] and in the aorta of hypertensive man.[51] Carotid Doppler data indicate that hydralazine aggravates and propranolol diminishes high-velocity flow patterns associated with turbulence and vortex formation in patients with carotid stenosis.[52] Also, our data in hypertensive cholesterol-fed rabbits,[53] supported by experimental data of Scanapieco et al.[54] and Kaplan et al.,[55] indicate that beta-blockers significantly reduce the development of atherosclerosis.

The treatment of high blood pressure may not prevent atherosclerotic complications. Several studies showed that treating hypertension prevented progression to malignant hypertension and reduced the risk of stroke and death.[4,5,7] However, strokes prevented by treating high blood pressure are those due to small vessel occlusion (lacunar infarcts) and rupture (hypertensive intracerebral hemorrhages).[14] This may be because hypertension is a disorder resulting from increased fluid energy.[11] Pressure energy leads to arteriolar complications such as lacunar infarction, cerebral hemorrhage and nephropathy, heart failure, and medial necrosis. However, kinetic energy results in the endothelial damage causing atherosclerosis, progressive enlargement of berry aneurysms, and embolization of plaque fragments from ulcerated lesions.

Accelerated heart rate also produces arterial flow disturbances, and in the Framingham study, increased heart rate was an independent risk factor.[44] Kaplan et al.[55] showed experimentally that increased heart rate is associated with sympathetic activation and increased lipid levels, as well as worsening of stress-induced atherosclerosis. They emphasized the antiatherosclerotic effects of beta-adrenergic blockers, and their protection from sympathetic arousal due to stress. In addition, beta-blockers have a beneficial effect on platelet agglutination.[56]

Calcium channel antagonists[57] and angiotensin-converting-enzyme inhibitors[58] also have anti-atherosclerotic effects in animal models.

Summary

1. Hypertension is asymptomatic, and treatment does not increase the feeling of well-being. The goal of antihypertensive treatment is to prevent vascular complications.
2. Hypertensive strokes are due to occlusion of arterioles by fibrinoid necrosis (lacunar infarction), or rupture of arteriolar microaneurysms (intracerebral hemorrhage), rather than the result of atherosclerosis.
3. Hypertensive encephalopathy is due to breakthrough of cerebral autoregulation with engorgement of the brain following vasodilation, producing cerebral edema and multifocal ischemia as the result of arteriolar injury.
4. These arteriolar complications are best prevented by lowering the blood pressure, and the main criterion in selecting antihypertensive drugs is to avoid those that cannot be controlled and so lead to severe hypotension with attendant cerebral and myocardial ischemia.
5. Atherosclerosis is only indirectly related to high pressure. Some antihypertensive drugs have adverse effects on lipoproteins, which may offset the benefits of lowering pressure, and certain antihypertensive drugs have beneficial effects on flow disturbances, which may prevent some of the embolic complications of atherosclerosis. To date, the best evidence available in man supports the antiatherosclerotic effects of beta-blockers; further work is needed to define whether other new classes of antihypertensive drugs may have antiatherosclerotic effects.
6. Most hypertensive patients have only mild hypertension, and the complications of hypertension due to "pressure" have been largely eliminated by drug therapy. The prevention of atherosclerosis and atherosclerotic strokes now remains the greatest challenge.

References

1. Pickering G. *Hypertension, Causes, Consequences and Management*. London: Churchill Livingstone; 1974: pp 40–62.
2. Kannel WB, Sorlie P. Hypertension in Framingham. In: Stratton PO ed. *Epidemiology and Control of Hypertension*. New York: Intercontinental Medical Books; 1975; p 553.
3. Samuelsson O, Wilhelmson L, Andersson O, et al. Cardiovascular morbidity in relation to change in blood pressure and serum cholesterol levels in treated hypertension. *JAMA*. 1988;258:1768–1776.
4. Veterans Administration Trial on effects of antihypertensive treatment on morbidity in hypertension: II. Results in patients with diastolic blood pressure averaging 90 through 114 mm Hg. *JAMA*. 1970; 213:1143–1152.
5. Beevers DG, Fairman MJ, Hamilton T, et al. Antihypertensive treatment and the course of established cerebral vascular disease. *Lancet*. 1973;1:1407–1409.
6. Hypertension Detection and Follow-up Program Cooperative Group. Five-year findings of the Hypertension Detection and Follow-up Program: I. Reduction in mortality in persons with high blood pressure, including mild hypertension. *JAMA*. 1979; 242:2562–2571.
7. Management Committee of the Australian Therapeutic Trial in Mild Hypertension. The Australian therapeutic trial in mild hypertension. *Lancet*. 1980; 1:1261–1267.
8. Morgan T, Adam W, Carney S, et al. Treatment of mild hypertension in elderly males. *Clin Sci*. 1979; 57:255s–357s.
9. Multiple Risk Factor Intervention Trial Research Group. Multiple risk factor intervention trial: Risk factor changes and mortality results. *JAMA*. 1982; 248:1465–1477.

10. Berglund G, Sannerstedt R, Andersson O, et al. Coronary heart disease after treatment of hypertension. *Lancet*. 1978;1:1-5

11. Spence JD. Antihypertensive therapy and atherosclerosis. In: Rapaport E, ed. *Cardiology Update*. New York: Elsevier; 1986: pp 137-155.

12. Spence JD. Antihypertensive therapy and prevention of atherosclerotic stroke. *Stroke*. 1986;17:808-810.

13. Birkett NJ, Donner A. Prevalence and control of hypertension in an Ontario county. *Can Med Assoc J*. 1985;132:1019-1024.

14. Russell RWR. How does high blood pressure cause stroke? *Lancet*. 1975;2:1283-1285.

15. Giese J. Acute hypertensive vascular disease: 2. Studies on vascular reaction patterns and permeability changes by means of vital microscopy and colloidal tracer technique. *Acta Path Microbiol Scand*. 1964;62:497.

16. Skinhoj E, Strandgaard S. Pathogenesis of hypertensive encephalopathy. *Lancet*. 1973;1:461-462.

17. Strandgaard S, Olesen J, Skinhoj E, et al. Autoregulation of brain circulation in severe arterial hypertension. *Brit Med J*. 1973;1:507-510.

18. Folkow B. Structural factors: The vascular wall. Consequences of treatment. *Hypertension*. 1983; 5(suppl. III):58-62.

19. van Harten J, Burggraaf K, Danhof M, et al. Negligible sublingual absorption of nifedipine. *Lancet*. 1987; 2:1363-1365.

20. Letter to the editor. Nifedipine, hypotension and myocardial injury. *Ann Int Med*. 1988;108:305-306.

21. Spence JD, Del Maestro RF. Hypertension in acute strokes: Treat. *Arch Neurol*. 1985;42:1000-1002.

22. Hachinski VC, Norris JW. The vascular infrastructure. In: *The Acute Stroke*. Philadelphia: FA Davis; 1985: pp 27-40.

23. Gilbert JJ, Vinters HV. Cerebral amyloid angiopathy: Incidence and complications in the aging brain: I. Cerebral hemorrhage. *Stroke*. 1983;14:915-923.

24. Vinters HV, Gilbert JJ. Cerebral amyloid angiopathy: incidence and complications in the aging brain: II. the distribution of amyloid vascular changes. *Stroke*. 1983;14:924-928.

25. Fisher CM. Lacunar infarction. In: Toole JF, Sickert R, Whisnant J, eds. *Cerebral Vascular Disease* (Sixth Princeton Conference). New York, NY: Grune & Stratton; 1968: pp 232-236.

26. Hachinski VC, Potter P, Merskey H. Leuko-araiosis: an ancient term for a new problem. *Can J Neurol Sci*. 1986;13:533-534.

27. Floras JS. Antihypertensive treatment, myocardial infarction, and nocturnal myocardial ischemia. *Lancet*. 1988;2:994-996.

28. Kaplan JR, Manuck SB, Adams MR, et al. The effects of beta-adrenergic blocking agents on atherosclerosis and its complications. *Europ Heart J*. 1987;8:928-944.

29. Schwartz CJ, Mitchell JRA. Observations on localization of arterial plaques. *Circ Res*. 1962;11:63-73.

30. Glagov S, Zarins CK, Stankunavicius R, et al. Compensatory enlargement of human atherosclerotic coronary arteries. *N Engl J Med*. 1987;316:1371-1375.

31. Haust MD. Injury and repair in the pathogenesis of atherosclerotic lesions. In: Jones RJ, ed. *Atherosclerosis*. New York, NY: Springer Pub; 1970: pp 12-20.

32. Haust MD, More RH. Development of modern theories on the pathogenesis of atherosclerosis. In: Wissler RW, Geer JC, eds. *The Pathogenesis of Atherosclerosis*. Baltimore, MD: Williams and Wilkins; 1972: pp 1-19.

33. Ross R, Glomset JA. The pathogenesis of atherosclerosis. *N Engl J Med*. 1976;295:36-77.

34. Texon M. *Hemodynamic Basis of Atherosclerosis*. New York, NY: Hemisphere Publ Co; 1980.

35. Fry DL. Acute vascular endothelial changes associated with increased blood velocity gradients. *Circ Res*. 1968;22:165-167.

36. Caro CG, Fitz-Gerald JM, Schroter RC. Atheroma and arterial wall shear; observation, correlation and proposal of a shear dependent mass transfer mechanism for atherogenesis. *Proc Roy Soc Lond (Biol)*. 1971;107:109-124.

37. Nerem RM, Cornhill JF. The role of fluid mechanics in atherogenesis. *J Biomech Eng*. 1980;102:181-189.

38. Milnor WR. *Hemodynamics*. Baltimore, MD: Williams and Wilkins; 1982.

39. Stein PD, Sabbah HN. Hemorrheology of turbulence. *Biorrheology*. 1980;17:301-309.

40. Burton AC. Kinetic energy in the circulation: Streamline flow and turbulence: measurement of arterial pressure. In: *Physiology and Biophysics of the Circulation*. Chicago, IL: Year Book Medical Publishers; 1972: pp 101-113.

41. Roach MR, Scott S, Ferguson CG. The hemodynamic importance of the geometry of bifurcations in the circle of Willis (glass model studies). *Stroke*. 1972;3:255-267.

42. Yellin EL. Laminar-turbulent transition process in pulsatile flow. *Circ Res*. 1966;19L:791-804.

43. Spence JD. Spectral analysis of carotid vs femoral Doppler velocity patterns: a clue to the genesis of flow disturbances in cerebral arteries? In: Cohen, BA, ed. *Frontiers of Engineering in Health Care*; CH

1621, February 1981, 0000-0355-377. New York, NY: Institute for Electrical Engineering; 1981: pp 355–359.

44. Kannel WB, Kannel CE, Paffenbarger R. Heart rate and cardiovascular mortality in the Framingham study. *Circulation*. 1985;72 (suppl 3):111–151.

45. Kaplan JR, Manuck SB, Clarkson TB. The influence of heart rate on coronary atherosclerosis. *J Cardiovasc Pharm*. 1987;10 (suppl 2):S100–S102.

46. Friedman MH, Deters OJ, Bargeron CB, et al. Shear-dependent thickening of the human arterial intimax. *Atherosclerosis*. 1986;60:161–171.

47. Friedman MH, O'Brien B, Ehrlich LW. Calculations of pulsatile flow through a branch: implications for the hemodynamics of atherosclerosis. *Circ Res*. 1975;36:277–285.

48. Spence JD. Pathogenesis of atherosclerosis: effects of antihypertensive drugs. *J Hum Exp Hyp*. 1989; 3:63–68.

49. Lipid Research Clinics Program. The lipid research clinics coronary primary prevention trial results: II. The relationship of reduction in incidence of coronary heart disease to cholesterol lowering. *JAMA*. 1984;251:365–374.

50. Spence JD, Pesout AB, Melmon KL. Effects of antihypertensive drugs on blood velocity in rhesus monkeys. *Stroke*. 1977;8:589–594.

51. Spence JD. Effects of antihypertensive drugs on blood velocity: implications for atherogenesis. *Can Med Assoc J*. 1982;127:721–724.

52. Spence JD. Effects of hydralazine versus propranolol on blood velocity patterns in patients with atherosclerosis. *Clin Sci*. 1983;65:91–93.

53. Spence JD, Perkins DG, Kline RL, et al. Hemodynamic modification of aortic atherosclerosis: effects of propranolol vs hydralazine in hypertensive hyperlipidemic rabbits. *Atherosclerosis*. 1984;50: 325–333.

54. Scanapieco G, Pauletto P, Semplicini A, et al. Evaluation of the efficacy of various hypotensive drugs in broad-breasted white turkeys as an experimental model of arterial hypertension with high catecholamine levels. *Boll Soc Ital Biol Sper*. 1983;59:1265–1271.

55. Kaplan J, Manuck SB, Adams MR, et al. Inhibition of coronary atherosclerosis by propranolol in behaviourally predisposed monkeys fed an atherogenic diet. *Circulation*. 1987;76:1363–1372.

56. Winther K, Trap-Jensen J. Effects of three beta-blockers with different pharmacodynamic properties on platelet aggregation and platelet and plasma cyclic AMP. *Eur J Clin Pharm*. 1988;35:17–20.

57. Weinstein DB, Heider JG. Protective action of calcium channel antagonists in atherogenesis and experimental vascular injury. *Am J Hypertension*. 1989;2:205–212.

58. Fleckenstein A, Fleckenstein-Grun G, Frey M, et al. Calcium antagonism and ACE inhibition: two outstandingly effective means of interference with cardiovascular calcium overload, high blood pressure, and arteriosclerosis in spontaneously-hypertensive rats. *Am J Hypertension*. 1989;2:194–204.

9
Aspirin in Stroke Prevention

James C. Grotta

Aspirin is now standard preventive therapy in patients at risk for stroke, but many questions remain about its efficacy and use. No single trial has clearly demonstrated the efficacy of aspirin for prevention of stroke after transient ischemic attack (TIA). However, almost all studies showed some benefit in the aspirin group. Recently, meta-analysis, integrating and analyzing data from multiple studies, has attempted to clarify the picture. One such analysis[1] showed no significant benefit for aspirin alone. Another analysis was carried out in collaboration with the principal investigators of all studies of platelet antiaggregate drugs for prevention of vascular disease, and weighted the studies according to the numbers of patients in each. This represented 25 completed studies enrolling 29 000 patients with angina, myocardial infarction, TIA, or stroke. An intention-to-treat analysis demonstrated that aspirin achieved an approximate 25% reduction in the incidence of nonfatal stroke, myocardial infarction, or vascular death. Aspirin was particularly effective in preventing nonfatal vascular events, especially myocardial infarction, which occurred one third less frequently in treated patients. This was comparable to beta-blocker therapy after myocardial infarction or diuretic therapy for moderate hypertension. If only cerebrovascular trials are considered, reduction of nonfatal stroke was 22% (Fig. 9.1).[2]

Dose

The optimal dose of aspirin is still unsettled. Aspirin irreversibly inhibits platelet cyclooxygenase, thereby preventing formation of thromboxane A_2, a proaggregatory vasoconstrictor. However, in high doses, aspirin also inhibits synthesis in the vascular endothelium of prostacyclin (PGI_2), a vasodilator and inhibitor of platelet aggregation. It had been previously demonstrated in atherosclerotic patients that doses as low as 40 mg per day substantially suppressed thromboxane B_2 production, but 325 mg reduced PGI_2 significantly more than did lower doses (Fig. 9.2).[3] In patients with TIA or stroke, 40 mg significantly reduced platelet aggregation and thromboxane A_2 production in both males and females,[4] but this effect can be highly variable from patient to patient.[5] These data, therefore, indicate that 80 mg per day may be an optimal dose.

Only one clinical study has prospectively evaluated different aspirin doses for stroke prevention after TIA. The United Kingdom TIA aspirin trial demonstrated comparable results for 300 mg daily and 600 mg twice daily.[6] However, the major positive effect was on the prevention of nonvascular death, with insignificant effect on stroke incidence. Significantly fewer gastrointestinal side effects occurred with low-dose aspirin (39%) than with high-dose (52%). In a recently completed primary prevention study, 325 mg every other day reduced the incidence of nonfatal myocardial infarction compared to placebo, but this dose was not compared to other aspirin doses.[7]

A study in patients after carotid endarterectomy compared low-dose aspirin to placebo for prevention of subsequent cerebrovascular symptoms. Aspirin dose was titrated from 50 to 100 mg daily in order to achieve at least 80% inhibition of platelet aggregation.[8] Although there were 11% fewer vascular events (TIA, stroke, myocardial infarc-

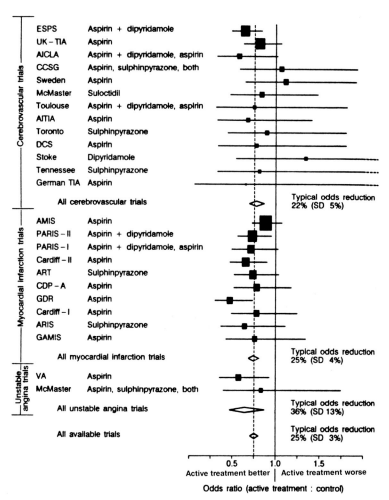

FIGURE 9.1. Odds ratios (active treatment:control) for first stroke, myocardial infarction, or vascular death during scheduled treatment period in completed antiplatelet trials. — ■ – = Trial results and 99% confidence intervals (area of ■ proportional to amount of information contributed). ◊ = Overview results and 95% confidence intervals. Dashed vertical line represents odds ratio of 0.75 suggested by overview of all trial results. Solid vertical line represents odds ratio of unity (no treatment effect). (Reprinted by permission from ref. 2.)

tion, vascular death) in the aspirin group, this difference was not significant. However, only 301 patients were entered into the study, which was designed to detect nothing less than a 50% reduction in events. This was an unrealistic expectation since no study has ever demonstrated such a substantial reduction of cerebrovascular events with any treatment. Finally, 1007 patients with nonrheumatic atrial fibrillation were randomized to receive warfarin, aspirin 75 mg daily, or placebo.[9] Significantly fewer embolic events occurred in the warfarin group, but there was no difference between low-dose aspirin or placebo.

In conclusion, while there is no reason to give more than 325 mg of aspirin daily, there is still no hard evidence to guide treatment with lower doses. An ongoing study in Holland comparing 30 mg to 300 mg, and studies in Scandinavia evaluating doses of 50 mg to 75 mg versus placebo, should provide useful data determining the efficacy of low-dose therapy.

Effect on Stroke Severity

Retrospective analysis of early stroke prevention studies suggested that patients reaching stroke end points while on aspirin therapy had less severe strokes than those on placebo.[10] In the aspirin in TIA (AITIA) study, only 1 of 12 strokes was disabling in the aspirin group, while 11 of 22 were disabling in the placebo group.[11] The European Stroke Prevention Study found 19% fatal strokes in the dipyrida-moline-aspirin group and 24% in the placebo

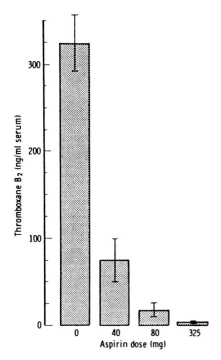

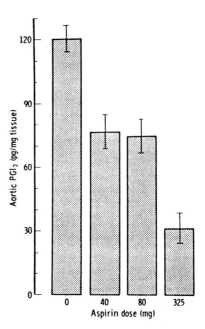

FIGURE 9.2A. Inhibition of platelet thromboxane B_2 production after aspirin ingestion. Bars represent mean levels of thromboxane B_2 ($\pm$S.E.M.) measured as nanograms per milliliter of serum after blood had clotted spontaneously at 37°C for one hour. All doses of aspirin produced significant inhibition as compared with the control pre-aspirin value. (Reprinted by permission from ref. 3.)

FIGURE 9.2B. Inhibitory effect of aspirin ingestion on arterial (aortic) production of prostacyclin (PGI_2). Bars represent mean levels of prostacyclin measured as 6-keto prostaglandin $F_{1\alpha}$ in picograms per milligram, wet weight, of tissue, after incubation as in Figure 2, but in 0.5 ml of buffer. Significant inhibition of prostacyclin formation was observed after all three doses of aspirin. (Reprinted by permission from ref. 3.)

group.[12] In a study comparing aspirin 1300 mg daily to heparin begun within a week of TIA, there was no significant difference in subsequent TIA or stroke between the two therapies during the following 2 weeks.[13] However, while the overall group had a high incidence of TIA and stroke during this interval (27% and 9%, respectively), only one of the five strokes that occurred resulted in significant neurologic deficit.

On the other hand, in the recently completed UK-TIA study, there was no difference in the distribution of nonfatal minor, nondisabling major, and disabling major strokes among the placebo, 300 mg daily, and 600 mg twice daily aspirin groups.[6] Certainly, none of these studies suggested that strokes were more severe in patients treated with platelet antiaggregates. In the primary prevention trial recently completed in a population of

American male physicians,[7] there was a comparable distribution of mild or disabling cerebral infarctions in the aspirin and placebo groups. However, 13 moderate, severe, or fatal hemorrhagic strokes occurred in the aspirin group, compared to 6 in the placebo group. While this difference was not statistically significant, this is the only study yet reported indicating a possibility of increased hemorrhage or stroke severity in patients treated with platelet antiaggregate drugs.

In conclusion, there is suggestive but inconclusive evidence that aspirin lessens the severity of cerebral infarction. Stroke severity should certainly be evaluated in any future stroke prevention trial. There is a possibility that aspirin increases the risk of hemorrhagic stroke. Consequently, it would be prudent to withhold aspirin in patients at high risk for cerebral hemorrhage, such as individuals with uncontrolled hypertension, coagulopathy, cerebral vascular malformations, or previous cerebral hemorrhage.

Prevention of Subclinical Ischemia

Studies evaluating the efficacy of aspirin and other platelet antiaggregate drugs have primarily looked at the number of clinically evident strokes as the major indicator of outcome. With the advent of magnetic resonance imaging (MRI) and computerized tomography (CT), and the recognition of periventricular abnormalities termed leukoaraiosis, renewed emphasis has been placed on dementia occurring on a vascular basis. Pathologic correlation of those MRI and CT changes usually demonstrates "innocent" etat crible probably correlating with "wear and tear,"[14] but some of these patients have more definite evidence of ischemic neuropathology and a few will demonstrate a clinical syndrome and pathologic changes consistent with Binswanger's subcortical arteriosclerotic encephalopathy. In addition, there is a correlation between leukoaraiosis and the development of dementia[15] and the presence of vascular risk factors.[16] An important question to be answered in future stroke prevention studies, therefore, is if aspirin and other platelet antiaggregate drugs can prevent the development of multiinfarct dementia and dementia associated with leukoaraiosis.

Primary Prevention

Two recent studies have evaluated aspirin for primary prevention of vascular events in individuals without any previous symptoms. In the United Kingdom, 5000 male physicians took either 500 mg of aspirin or no therapy.[17] The results of this study were negative, though there was a nonsignificant 10% decrease in mortality in the aspirin group. Twenty-two thousand male American physicians aged 40 to 84 were randomized to aspirin 325 mg every other day or placebo.[7] There was no significant reduction in the incidence of stroke, and in fact, severe hemorrhagic strokes were higher in the aspirin group (vide supra). However, there was a significant (44%) reduction in the incidence of nonfatal myocardial infarction in patients

over 50 years of age in the aspirin group. Current recommendations are that aspirin 100 to 325 mg daily be given to asymptomatic individuals over the age of 50, especially those at high risk for cerebrovascular or coronary artery disease.[18,19]

Effect on Atherogenesis

The exact pathogenetic mechanisms underlying the development of atherosclerosis are unclear but probably involve a combination of factors. While much attention has focused on serum lipids and their deposition,[20] the initiation of the atherosclerotic lesion probably results from the response of platelets and leukocytes to a disturbed luminal surface.[21] Animal and human studies have demonstrated that aspirin treatment reduces intimal hyperplasia following bypass grafting by inhibiting platelet deposition on the denuded endothelial surface,[22-25] and aspirin is now routinely recommended for maintaining graft patency after coronary artery bypass.[26]

On the other hand, Imparato and colleagues observed an association between intraplaque hemorrhage in carotid artery plaques removed at the time of endarterectomy and cerebral symptoms.[27] These investigators considered the possibility that such intraplaque hemorrhage might be aggravated by aspirin taken by the patients to prevent thromboembolic stroke. Unfortunately, this question has never been addressed in a prospective trial with pathological verification. Since carotid ultrasound cannot accurately detect or exclude intraplaque hemorrhage, this question can only be answered by careful pathological examination of plaques removed at surgery comparing plaques removed from patients treated with aspirin to those from patients not receiving the drug. Intraplaque hemorrhage may be associated with an increased incidence of cerebral symptoms,[28,29] though it is unclear if such symptoms are the direct result of plaque hemorrhage or due instead to the consequent progression to high-grade stenosis, which itself has a known association with subsequent cerebral ischemic symptoms.[30,31]

In conclusion, while aspirin slows the early development of atherosclerosis, it may lead to progression of stenosis by intraplaque hemorrhage in patients with advanced atherosclerosis. However, since most studies have demonstrated that chronic aspirin therapy reduces the incidence of cerebral symptoms,[2] the net effect of aspirin is positive, and the drug should not be withheld for fear of producing intraplaque hemorrhage.

References

1. Sze PC, Reitman D, Pincus MM, et al. Antiplatelet agents in the secondary prevention of stroke: meta-analysis of the randomized control trials. *Stroke.* 1988;19:436–442.
2. Antiplatelet Trialists' Collaboration: Secondary prevention of vascular disease by prolonged antiplatelet treatment. *Br Med J.* 1988;296:320–331.
3. Weksler BB, Pett SB, Alonso D, et al. Differential inhibition by aspirin of vascular and platelet prostaglandin synthesis in atherosclerotic patients. *N Engl J Med.* 1983;308:800–805.
4. Weksler BB, Kent JL, Rudolph D, et al. Effects of low dose aspirin on platelet function in patients with recent cerebral ischemia. *Stroke.* 1985;16:5.
5. Tohgi H, Tamura K, Kimura M, et al. Individual variation in platelet aggregability and serum thromboxane B_2 concentrations after low-dose aspirin. *Stroke.* 1988;19:700–703.
6. UK–TIA Study Group: United Kingdom transient ischaemic attack (UK–TIA) aspirin trial: interim results. *Br Med J.* 1988;296:316–319.
7. Steering Committee of the Physicians' Health Study Research Group: Final report on the aspirin component of the ongoing physicians' health study. *N Engl J Med.* 1989;321:129–135.
8. Boysen G, Sorensen S, Juhler M, et al. Danish very-low-dose aspirin after carotid endarterectomy trial. *Stroke.* 1988;19:1211–1215.
9. Petersen P, Boysen G, Godtfredsen J, et al. Placebo-controlled, randomised trial of warfarin and aspirin for prevention of thromboembolic complications in chronic atrial fibrillation. *Lancet.* 1989;1:175–179.
10. Grotta JC, Lemak NA, Gary H, et al. Does platelet antiaggregant therapy lessen the severity of stroke? *Neurol.* 1985;35:632–636.
11. Fields WS, Lemak NA, Frankowski RF, et al. Controlled trial of aspirin in cerebral ischemia. *Stroke.* 1977;8:301–316.
12. European Stroke Prevention Study Group. The European stroke prevention study (ESPS). *Lancet.* 1987; 2:1351–1353.
13. Biller J, Bruno A, Adams HP, et al. A randomized trial of aspirin or heparin in hospitalized patients with recent transient ischemic attacks. *Stroke.* 1989;20:441–447.
14. Awad IA, Johnson PC, Spetzler RF, et al. Incidental subcortical lesions identified on magnetic resonance imaging in the elderly: II. Postmortem pathological correlations. *Stroke.* 1986;17:1090–1097.
15. Steingart A, Hachinski VC, Lau C, et al. Cognitive and neurologic findings in subjects with diffuse white matter lucencies on computed tomographic scan (leuko-araiosis). *Arch Neurol.* 1987; 44:32–35.
17. Peto R, Gray R, Collins R, et al. Randomised trial of prophylactic daily aspirin in British male doctors. *Br Med J.* 1988;296:313–315.
18. Fuster V, Cohen M, and Halperin J. Aspirin in the prevention of coronary disease. *N Engl J Med.* 1989; 321:183–185.
19. Aspirin for prevention of myocardial infarctions and stroke. In: Abramswicz M, eds. *The Medical Letter.* 1989;31:77–79.
20. Grotta JC, Yatsu FM, Pettigrew LC, et al. Prediction of carotid stenosis progression by lipid and hematologic measurements. *Neurol.* 1989;39:1325–1331.
21. Ross R. The pathogenesis of atherosclerosis. An update. *N Engl J Med.* 1986;314:488–500.
22. Metke MP, Lie JT, Fuster V, et al. Reduction of intimal thickening in canine coronary bypass vein grafts with dipyridamole and aspirin. *Amer J Cardiol.* 1979;43:1144–1148.
23. Chesebro JH, Fuster V, Elveback LR, et al. Effect of dipyridamole and aspirin on late vein-graft patency after coronary bypass operations. *N Engl J Med.* 1984;310:209–214.
24. Hess H, Mietaschk A, Deichsel G. Drug-induced inhibition of platelet function delays progression of peripheral occlusive arterial disease. A prospective double-blind arteriographically controlled trial. *Lancet.* 1985;1:414–419.
25. Hansen KJ, Howe HR, Edgerton A, et al. Ticlopidine versus aspirin and dipyridamole: Influence on platelet deposition and three-month patency of polytetrafluoroethylene grafts. *J Vasc Surg.* 1986;4:174–178.
26. Verstraete M, Brown BG, Chesebro JH, et al. Evaluation of antiplatelet agents in the prevention of aorto-coronary bypass occlusion. *Eur Heart.* 1986; 7:4–13.
27. Imparato AM, Riles TS, Mintzer R, et al. The importance of hemorrhage in the relationship between gross morphologic characteristics and cerebral symptoms in 376 carotid artery plaques. *Ann Surg.* 1983;197:195–203.
28. Fisher M, Blumenfeld AM, Smith TW. The importance of carotid artery plaque disruption and hemorrhage. *Arch Neurol.* 1987;44:1086–1089.

29. Lannihan L, Kupsky WJ, Mohr JP, et al. Lack of association between carotid plaque hematoma and ischemic cerebral symptoms. *Stroke*. 1987;18:879–881.

30. Chambers BR, Norris JW. Outcome inpatients with asymptomatic neck bruits. *N Engl J Med*. 1986;315:860–865.

31. Hennerici M, Hulsbomer HB, Hefter H, et al. National history of asymptomatic extracranial arterial disease. *Brain*. 1987;110:777–791.

10
Ticlopidine: A New Drug to Prevent Stroke

William K. Hass

Two papers describing stroke prevention trials in more than 4000 patients of the drug ticlopidine hydrochloride appeared in 1989.[1,2] There was unequivocal evidence in one of a reduction of risk of the composite end point: stroke, myocardial infarction, and vascular death in patients after ischemic stroke. In the other, significant reduction of the risk of nonfatal stroke and death in patients with transient ischemic attacks (TIA), transient monocular blindness, or minor stroke was seen when ticlopidine was compared in a "horse race" to aspirin. Since ticlopidine, previously a little known drug, has proved effective in large and carefully structured clinical trials,[3] a close examination of its origin, pharmacological characteristics, and clinical safety is indicated.

Background

In 1972 Maffrand and Eloy synthesized a new series of thienopyridine derivatives,[4] including a new compound, ticlopidine, later evaluated by pharmacologists in the small firm of Castaigne (subsequently incorporated into Sanofi Recherche). Among a battery of tests to screen ticlopidine for toxicity and activity was one for platelet aggregation studied by the ex vivo method employing an old-fashioned aggregometer.[5] Unlike in vitro platelet aggregation tests, where normal platelets from an untreated individual are suspended in platelet-rich plasma to which a drug is added, the ex vivo technique employs the platelet-rich plasma from the animal or person previously given the drug for a defined period of time. The ex vivo study demonstrated that ticlopidine was particularly effective at inhibiting platelet aggregation. The addition of ticlopidine to normal platelet-rich plasma, however, did not have this effect, suggesting that a circulating ticlopidine metabolite (or a long period of exposure to the parent compound) was necessary to achieve the antiaggregate effect.

Confirmation of antiplatelet activity in humans was first described in healthy volunteers by Thebault and coworkers[6] who in 1975 established a lag time of 24 to 48 hours after an initial oral dose before antiplatelet activity appears. This effect lasted 3 days. Further, an oral daily dose of 450 mg of ticlopidine produced a 50% inhibition of adenosine diphosphate (ADP)-induced aggregation. Doses of up to 500 mg a day were well tolerated by 55 human subjects for several weeks. In 1977 Lecrubier and coworkers published the first report of a small trial of the effects of ticlopidine on ADP-, collagen-, and adrenaline-induced platelet aggregation, and on bleeding times in patients with cerebrovascular disease.[7] In 1980 members of the same group abolished TIAs in one patient with essential thrombocytosis following treatment with ticlopidine. In 1980 maintenance by ticlopidine of patent hemodialysis arterio-venous (A-V) shunts in two patients was also demonstrated.[8]

Pharmacology

Ticlopidine, 5-[2-chlorophenyl)methyl]-4,5,6,7 tetrahydrothienol[3-2-c]pyridine hydrochloride, is structurally and biochemically different from all currently employed antiplatelet agents.[9] (Figure

FIGURE 10.1. Structure of ticlopidine. (Courtesy of Dr. B. Molony.)

10.1) It is a stable, white, nonhygroscopic powder that melts and decomposes at about 200°C. It is soluble in water up to 61/mg/ml at ambient temperatures, yielding a pH of 3.58.

Apart from some effects on the cardiovascular system, ticlopidine is remarkably free from adverse pharmacologic effects.[10] In anesthetized dogs intravenous infusion at 1 mg/kg/min caused a small increase in heart rate and blood pressure lasting 30 to 60 minutes. Myocardial oxygen consumption increased after 4 minutes of injection. With a 10

mg/kg/min infusion, a brief increase in coronary blood flow and cardiac output was seen with an increase of respiratory rate. Large oral doses of ticlopidine (60 to 240 mg/kg) caused a 1 to 24 hour fall in blood pressure; this was maximal at 3 to 7 hours and was associated with a nonparallel increase in heart rate.

Large-scale screening tests for toxicity showed no effects of ticlopidine on the central nervous system except for a slight potentiation of chloral hydrate or barbiturate-induced sleep in mice. No analgesic activity was induced by ticlopidine. While intensive screening revealed significant effects on blood platelets, ticlopidine, unlike other antiplatelet agents, produced almost no other pharmacologic actions.

Studies in man and animals demonstrated up to 90% absorption of ticlopidine after an oral dose. When tagged with ^{14}C, urine samples showed <1% unchanged ticlopidine in 0 to 48 hours. Levels of unchanged ^{14}C ticlopidine at peak plasma levels

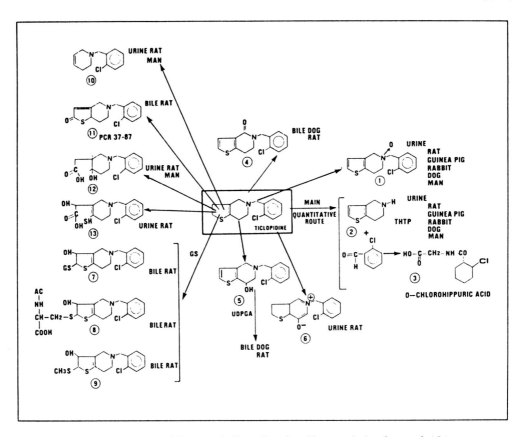

FIGURE 10.2. Ticlopidine metabolites. (Reprinted by permission from ref. 10.)

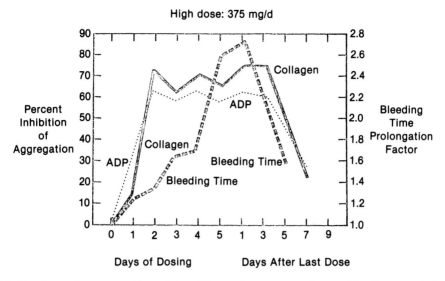

FIGURE 10.3. Ex-vivo antiaggregate effect of ticlopidine and concurrent effect on bleeding time during and after 5-day oral dosing. (Courtesy of Dr. D. Ellis.)

were 10% in the rat and 22% in man. Figure 10.2 reveals the wide variety of metabolites in man and animals observed in the urine and bile. These probably do not represent all the metabolic products; yet five major pathways of biotransformation are utilized to produce the metabolites.[10]

Most of these metabolites have been synthesized and tested for platelet antiaggregate properties. Only the 2-keto derivative of ticlopidine, PCR 3787, has exhibited antiaggregate properties. The metabolite has a more potent early effect on platelet function than ticlopidine. The onset of activity of PCR 3787 against ADP-induced aggregation after 100 mg/kg intraperitoneal administration to rats occurred in 10 minutes, in comparison to 60 minutes for ticlopidine. The 2-keto derivative, like ticlopidine, is almost inactive in vitro, suggesting that it, too, requires further biochemical transformation before exhibiting antiaggregate activity.

In summary, oxidation of the thiophen moiety of ticlopidine appears necessary for the development of antiplatelet activity. As the result of a direct effect of ticlopidine or of a metabolite, a single, large oral dose of ticlopidine is followed by ex vivo ADP-induced aggregation in the rat in only 1 hour, and in 6 hours in man. Dosing with 250 mg of ticlopidine twice a day for 21 days in man demonstrates steady-state pharmacodynamic parameters in 3 to 5 days and a maximum ex vivo ADP-induced

aggregation effect within 5 to 6 days, with recovery of the normal platelet activity after ticlopidine withdrawal within 4 to 8 days.[11] Figure 10.3 demonstrates that inhibition of aggregation reaches 60% to 70% for either a collagen or ADP challenge and that the bleeding time in man at a daily dose of 375 mg rises steadily over the first 5 days of administration. Bleeding time as well as collagen- and ADP-induced aggregation values fall rapidly in the 5 days after the last dose.

Mode and Site of Action

The antiplatelet activity of ticlopidine is based on its specific effect on exogenous ADP and, upon amplification, on released ADP from platelets after ex vivo challenge by low and high doses of collagen, thrombin at low dose, and other platelet agonists.[9] While the cellular site of the anti-ADP effect of ticlopidine remains elusive, Maffrand et al. have suggested an action near the ADP receptor inhibiting reactivity at the potential fibrinogen site, as shown diagrammatically in Figure 10.4.

The binding of ADP to its receptor, R, results in alteration and activation of the two membrane glycoproteins, GP-IIb and GP-IIIa (on the left side of the diagram). The activated complex then binds to circulating fibrinogen—shown as a black jigsawlike

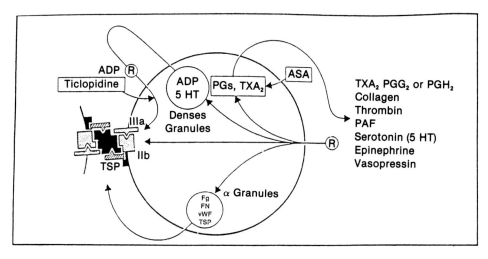

FIGURE 10.4. Diagram of platelet activation–aggregation pathways and presumed locus of ticlopidine action. (Reprinted by permission from ref. 9.)

structure—which in turn bridges to similar sites on neighboring platelets.

The agonists (on the right of the diagram) can directly activate this glycoprotein complex after each binds to its own specific receptor, or they can induce endogenous ADP secretion from platelet-dense granules. It is likely that most of these agonists work via a common pathway and hydrolyze platelet membrane phosphotidylinositol via phospholipase C to form diacylglycerol, resulting in calcium mobilization from endoplasmic reticulum. These reactions and others lead to conformational changes within the platelet associated with platelet internal contraction. A parallel reaction leads to the formation of endoperoxides (PGG$_2$, PGH$_2$) and of thromboxane TxA$_2$ from hydrolyzed arachidonic acid (AA) released from membrane phospholipids.

In this way the process of aggregation is amplified, leading to the secretion of a number of alpha granule proteins including fibrinogen (Fg), fibronectin (FN), Von-Willebrand Factor (vWF), and thrombospondin (TSP). Thrombospondin also binds to a membrane glycoprotein, GP-IV, and to fibrinogen, as drawn at the left side of the diagram. The secretion of these substances eventually serves to make the process of aggregation of platelets irreversible.

Cyclooxygenase, which catalyzes the transformation of AA to PGG$_2$ and PGH$_2$, which are then catalyzed by thromboxane synthetase to TxA$_2$, is irreversibly inhibited by aspirin within circulating platelets and reversibly inhibited by other nonsteroidal antiinflammatory drugs. Thromboxane synthetase is specifically blocked by a group of imidazole compounds, including dazoxiden. This results in reduced TxA$_2$, inhibiting platelet aggregation. An increase in cyclic adenosine monophosphate (cAMP) concentration in platelets inhibits platelet aggregation and secretion. Substances that stimulate adenylate cyclase to produce more cAMP, such as prostaglandin E$_2$ and I$_2$ (PG's), or that, like dipyridamole, inhibit phosphodiesterase, which breaks down cAMP, tend to depress to a limited degree the process of platelet aggregation.

Ticlopidine, in contrast, has no specific effect on cyclooxygenase, thromboxane synthetase, adenylate cyclase, or phosphodiesterase. It appears to function largely at the left side of the diagram as a specific inhibitor of ADP-induced aggregation. Since ticlopidine does not affect binding of ADP to its receptor,[11] Ordinas has conjectured that it seems likely that ticlopidine induces a qualitative inhibitory effect on the complexing of GP-IIb and GP-IIIa. It could also act by altering the exposure of active binding sites for either FG or vWF. This "thrombasthenic" effect is in many ways similar to the platelet abnormality present in patients with Glanzmann's thrombasthenia–type II, which is characterized by a significant diminution of platelet GP-IIb and GP-IIIa.[12,13]

Whatever the primary mechanism, ticlopidine inhibits primary and secondary aggregation induced by ADP as well as aggregation induced by collagen, epinephrine, ristocetin, TxA_2, AA, endoperoxides, thrombin, and platelet-activating factor when tested at physiological concentrations.[2] Ticlopidine's potentiation of the effects of PGI_2 and PGE_1 inhibition of platelet retention on glass beads, of inhibition of thrombin- and epinephrine-induced malonaldehyde production, and of prolongation of template bleeding time are the result of its role at the end of the platelet activation-aggregation cascade.

Clinical Studies

The antiaggregate property of this new and unusual platelet antagonist is relevant to the idea that most ischemic strokes are related to transient or persistent intraarterial thrombus.[14] Recently, Fieschi and coworkers demonstrated intraarterial occlusions in 75% of 80 patients examined by angiography within 6 hours of onset of ischemic stroke.[15] In 53 patients these arterial occlusions were intracranial. At the end of 1 week, angiography or transcranial Doppler sonography showed that 80% of the occlusions were gone, indicating that most of the occlusive lesions were thrombotic. These findings help to explain the results of studies that demonstrated reduced risk of ischemic stroke in patients on aspirin therapy[16-18] and confirmed by meta-analysis.[19]

Aspirin is not well tolerated by some patients since it is a gastric irritant like other nonsteroidal antiinflammatory drugs that act via cyclooxygenase inhibition. Ticlopidine is not a cyclooxygenase inhibitor and does not reduce the level of gastric prostaglandins that protect the gastric mucosa. Further, the secretion of the aggregation inhibitor, PGI_2, by endothelial cells is inhibited by aspirin but unaffected by ticlopidine. However, in spite of side effects, until 1980, aspirin was the only proven medication for prevention of ischemic stroke. These early trials of aspirin indicated that any drug trial for stroke prevention had to take into account the relatively small number of ischemic stroke events that occur in patients at risk as well as the relatively long time required for these events to occur.

The major problem in early clinical trials of stroke prevention was a Type II statistical error since, when sample sizes are inadequate,[20] a thera-peutic difference may be missed. Even with random allocation, patients in one group may have more favorable risk factors than the other. Larger numbers of patients provide true random allocation and a greater opportunity to reach a correct therapeutic conclusion.

Small Clinical Trials

Three clinical trials of ticlopidine designed for the prevention of cerebrovascular events were reported in 1984.[21-23] The open trial of Ono et al. compared 113 patients from 17 Japanese neurosurgical centers allocated to treatment with 300 mg/day of ticlopidine (or placebo) within 24 hours after surgery for subarachnoid hemorrhage.[21] Patients were chosen if residual subarachnoid clot was seen on computed tomography (CT). During 4 weeks on this regimen, at the 6th to 12th day, the end point of angiographic demonstration of vasospasm was achieved in 48% treated with ticlopidine and 45% treated with placebo (a nonsignificant finding). Death or persistent neurological deficit at the time of hospital discharge occurred in 14% of patients treated with ticlopidine (three deaths) and 29% of patients on placebo (nine deaths). In all, a "favorable outcome" was seen in 92% on ticlopidine and 79% on placebo. Larger numbers of patients, more precise endpoint definition, a blinded trial to eliminate bias, and a deferred ticlopidine dose of 350 to 500 mg would have achieved more general acceptance of these findings.

Tohgi described a double-blind study of 281 patients with a history of TIA allocated to treatment with ticlopidine 200 mg a day or to aspirin 500 mg a day for a period of 12 to 16 months.[22] The TIA must have occurred within 3 months of admission to the study. The composite end point of TIA/reversible neurological disease (RIND)/cerebral infarct/and myocardial infarction occurred in 29.6% of patients on aspirin therapy and 9.6% treated with ticlopidine.

Among the 50 events experienced by 145 evaluable patients on aspirin, only 6 were cerebral infarcts; only 2 cerebral infarcts occurred among 32 events in 136 evaluable patients given ticlopidine. These differences were not significant for the initial 6 months of therapy, but thereafter the ticlopidine group was significantly event free. The inclusion of TIAs in the analysis raises the question of its value as an end point in a stroke prevention study. Based on what the patient tells the investigator and not on the hard findings of a careful neurological examination, CT, or magnetic resonance imaging, the end point, TIA, may dilute the value of the study.

Thirdly, Rieger and Picho compared 118 patients after cerebral infarction. Patients were given 500 mg a day of ticlopidine and compared to a control group receiving dipyridamole at the dose level of 150 mg a day for a period of 12 months. In the ticlopidine group 13.8% suffered "relapses," compared to 21.7% in the dipyridamole group. The difference for males *and* females was not significant but there was a significant difference in favor of ticlopidine in the male patient subset.[23]

Large Clinical Trials

The Ticlopidine Aspirin Stroke Study (TASS)

Patients were recruited from February 1982 until May 1986; the follow-up period for all patients was completed by December 1987.[2] Sample size determinations called for 3000 patients for 3 years to detect a 5% difference in the rate of stroke or death between ticlopidine- and aspirin-treated patients (alpha=0.05; power=0.90). This required the combined efforts of 56 medical centers in the United States and Canada.

Following informed consent, patients were admitted to the study if they were >40 years old and if, in the previous 3 months, they had suffered:

1. One or more TIAs (a focal ischemic cerebral vascular event lasting 24 hours followed by complete recovery);
2. Transient monocular blindness (a unilateral ischemic retinal episode lasting <24 hours);
3. Reversible ischemic neurological dysfunction (RIND) (a focal ischemic cerebral vascular event lasting >24 hours but less than 3 weeks followed by complete recovery); or
4. A minor stroke (a focal ischemic cerebral vascular event resulting in minimal permanent neurological deficit with at least 80% recovery or function within 3 weeks).

Excluded were:

1. Women of childbearing potential;
2. Patients whose symptoms were due to migraine, cardiogenic embolism, and hematologic disorders;
3. Patients with a history of peptic ulcer disease, upper gastrointestinal bleeding, and/or aspirin sensitivity;
4. Those with life-threatening diseases, such as cancer.

Patient evaluations included extensive laboratory studies, including cerebral angiography in 50% of patients.

Random allocation of patients to the ticlopidine or aspirin (active control) groups was provided by the Maryland Medical Research Institute (MMRI), an unblinded nonparticipant in the study. An unblinded outside Safety Committee also provided continuous monitoring of the safety and efficacy of the medications.

This was a "triple blind" study[3] in which the investigators, the patients, and the sponsor, Syntex Research, had no knowledge of the treatment allocation. The blinding served to provide accurate, unbiased evaluations by investigators of patient eligibility and of the major end points of stroke, myocardial infarction (MI) and death from all causes.

More than 8000 patients were screened to obtain the 3069 patients for this largest of all stroke prevention trials. Eighty-nine percent of the patients took at least three fourths of their assigned medication >90% of the time. Twenty-four patients, 13 on aspirin and 11 on ticlopidine, never took their assigned drug. Only 3% of patients assigned to ticlopidine and 2% assigned to aspirin did not appear at trial's end for follow-up. The trial took nearly 6 years, during which time 52% of the ticlopidine group and 47% of the aspirin group stopped taking their study drug prematurely for various reasons.

Death occurred in 306 patients receiving ticlopidine and 349 patients on aspirin. Fatal or nonfatal strokes occurred in 172 patients taking ticlopidine and 212 taking aspirin (Table 10.1). Slightly >60% of all strokes in both ticlopidine- and aspirin-treated groups were atherothrombotic. There were fewer than expected hemorrhagic infarctions and intracerebral hemorrhages. More

TABLE 10.1. Study end points (TASS).

End point	Ticlopidine group (N = 1529)	Aspirin group (N = 1540)
Death from all causes or		
nonfatal stroke[a]	306	349
Nonfatal stroke	156	189
Fatal stroke	16	23
Death from other cause	134	137
Fatal or nonfatal stroke	172	212
Death from all causes[b]	175	196
Cerebrovascular	22	28
Cardiovascular	89	78
Acute myocardial infarction	21	14
Sudden death	44	41
Other cardiovascular	24	23
Other cause	64	90
Vascular	9	10
Nonvascular	22	32
Cancer	22	35
Unknown	11	13

Reprinted by permission from ref. 2.

[a]Only the first event was counted. Nonfatal stroke was the first event in 25 ticlopidine patients and 36 aspirin patients who subsequently died.

[b]All deaths were included, whether a first or a subsequent event.

TABLE 10.2. Adjudicated territory, type, and severity of strokes (TASS).

Characterization	Ticlopidine group (N = 1529)	Aspirin group (N = 1540)
No. of patients with strokes[a] →	172	212
Vascular distribution		
Right carotid	56	78
Left carotid	52	70
Both carotids	0	1
Vertebrobrasilar	37	38
Uncertain	27	25
Type		
Atherothrombotic	104	132
Hemorrhagic infarction	3	4
Cardioembolic	5	6
Lacunar infarction	10	17
Retinal infarction	7	11
Intracerebral hemorrhage	7	7
Uncertain	36	35
Severity		
Minor	90	116
Moderate	33	39
Major	37	48
Uncertain	12	9

Reprinted by permission from ref. 25.

[a]For patients with multiple strokes, only the first event was included. All first strokes that occurred during the course of the trial, whether the patient was taking study medication or not, are included. The number of patients in each category is indicated.

than half of all strokes in both treatment groups were minor (Table 10.2).

The large number of patients permitted life-table analysis for the combined end point of nonfatal stroke or death from any cause and the subset of fatal and nonfatal stroke by intent-to-treat analysis (Figures 10.5 and 10.6). Below the x-axis, the values in parentheses indicate the number of patients in the ticlopidine and aspirin groups in the study at the particular month of analysis. Almost from the beginning of treatment, life-table analysis reveals significantly fewer events among the ticlopidine-treated patients when compared to aspirin-treated patients.

The 3-year event rate for nonfatal stroke or death from any cause was 17% for ticlopidine and 19% for aspirin P=(0.048), representing a 12% risk reduction for ticlopidine compared to aspirin. The rates of fatal and nonfatal stroke at 3 years were 10% for ticlopidine and 13% for aspirin, representing a 21% risk reduction with ticlopidine (P=0.024). Ticlopidine was more effective than aspirin in both sexes and was more effective in

females than in males. The results of intent-to-treat analysis were echoed by the efficacy analysis, which evaluated only those events occurring while patients were taking the trial medications (and for a 10-day period thereafter).

However, side effects were more common with ticlopidine. These included diarrhea (20%), skin rash (14%), and a severe but reversible neutropenia in 0.09%. The adverse effects of aspirin included diarrhea (10%), rash (5.5%), peptic ulceration (3%), gastritis (2%), and gastrointestinal bleeding (1%). The upper gastrointestinal adverse effects of aspirin occurred in a population already carefully screened for a previous history of gastrointestinal aspirin intolerance or peptic ulcer disease. This screening removed a number of patients at risk for gastric dysfunction, perhaps unfairly weighting the side effect data against ticlopidine.

The one major side effect of ticlopidine was neutropenia. Mild to moderate neutropenias were

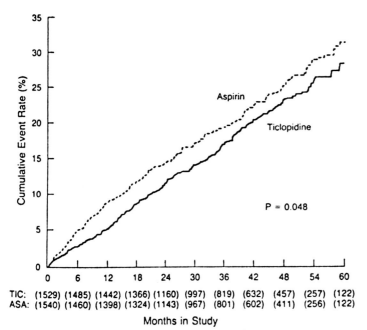

FIGURE 10.5. Cumulative event-rate curves. Compound end point, for non-fatal stroke or death from any cause. Intent-to-treat analysis. Values in parentheses are patient numbers at each interval on ticlopidine (TIC) or aspirin (ASA). (Reprinted by permission from ref. 2.)

observed in both treatment groups, 22 in those receiving ticlopidine and 12 in the aspirin group. Severe neutropenia with an absolute neutrophil count of < 450 cells/cmm occurred in eight women and five men taking ticlopidine. Their mean age was 65 (range 45 to 81). Severe neutropenia

occurred between 1 and 3 months after treatment. All severe neutropenias resolved within 3 weeks after prompt discontinuation of the medication. One patient developed systemic infection, and although this patient's neutrophil count recovered when ticlopidine was stopped and the infection

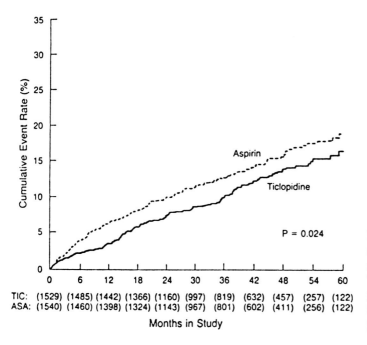

FIGURE 10.6. Cumulative event-rate curves for end point stroke-fatal or nonfatal. Intent-to-treat analysis. Values in parentheses are number of patients at each interval on ticlopidine (TIC) or aspirin (ASA). (Reprinted by permission from ref. 2.)

TABLE 10.3. Fatal and nonfatal myocardial infarction (TASS).

Event	Ticlopidine group	Aspirin group
	No. of patients (no. of men)	
No. randomized	1529 (985)	1540 (1002)
Nonfatal myocardial infarction		
Receiving study medication	44 (34)	48 (33)
Any time	83 (54)	75 (49)
Fatal myocardial infarction		
Receiving study medication	10 (6)	10 (7)
Any time	21 (12)	14 (11)

Reprinted by permission from ref. 2.

TABLE 10.4. End points–efficacy analysis (CATS)[a]

| | Placebo | | Ticlopidine | | Relative | |
	No. of events	Event rate/yr (%)	No. of events	Event rate/yr (%)	risk reduction (%)	p
Outcome						
Stroke, MI, vascular death	118	15.3	74	10.8	30.2	0.006
Stroke, MI, death	127	16.4	87	12.7	24.1	0.023
Stroke, stroke death	89	11.4	54	7.8	33.5	0.008
Vascular death	29	3.5	17	2.3	33.1	0.091
Death	38	4.5	30	4.1	9.0	0.349

Reprinted by permission from ref. 1.
[a]Excluding events that occurred >28 days after study drug was permanently discontinued.

resolved, the patient died of renal failure secondary to antibiotic toxicity.

There was an increase in total cholesterol levels in the ticlopidine group. The mean total cholesterol values were elevated at baseline (9 ± 20% in the ticlopidine group and 2 ± 16% in the aspirin group [p<0.01]). At one month, an increase in cholesterol levels was seen in patients treated with ticlopidine, but these levels stabilized by the fourth month. Subsequent analysis indicated that these elevated cholesterol levels were not predictors of cardiovascular or cerebrovascular end points.[24,25]

Nonfatal MI was four times more frequent than fatal MI. The 3-year cumulative event rates (±SE) per 100 patients for fatal or nonfatal MI were 5.55 ± 0.79 with ticlopidine and 5.53 ± 0.79 with aspirin; differences were not significant (Table 10.3).

The Canadian-American Ticlopidine Study (CATS)

This was a double-blind placebo-controlled trial of patients admitted to the study 7 to 12 days after a major stroke. Patients were given either ticlopidine 500 mg a day or placebo, as coded identical tablets. The primary analysis of efficacy was of the composite end point: recurrent stroke/MI/or vascular death. Patients were not eligible for the study if they were likely to remain bedridden or had severe comorbidity. Secondary analyses were planned for the separate outcomes of stroke, MI, and death (Table 10.4).

The study was monitored by an independent safety committee aware of the randomization code,

with an ongoing interim analysis to insure patient safety. Hematologic abnormalities, the need to remain on long-term anticoagulants, or the need for antiplatelet drugs excluded candidates from the study. Eligibility verification was provided by a blinded central adjudication committee.

Sample size determination was based upon a rate of stroke, MI, or vascular death of 25% over 2 years. Recruitment of 1000 patients would provide a 90% chance of one-sided significance at the 5% level to achieve a relative risk reduction of 30%. The analysis excluded any events that occurred >28 days after the study drug was stopped.

Of the 1072 patients enrolled by 25 clinical centers in Canada and the United States, 19 patients were ineligible, leaving 1053 patients, 528 randomized to placebo, 525 to ticlopidine. As in TASS, about two thirds of the patients were male; the mean age was 65. One third of the patients had diabetes, and almost one fifth had a previous MI. More than two thirds were hypertensive, and about 3% of patients in each group had atrial fibrillation. Slightly less than one fifth described a previous TIA. About three fourths of the qualifying atherothrombotic strokes occurred in the carotid vascular territory.

Efficacy analysis revealed an event rate per year for stroke/MI/or vascular death of 15.3% in the placebo group and 10.8% in the ticlopidine group, representing a 30.2% relative risk reduction with

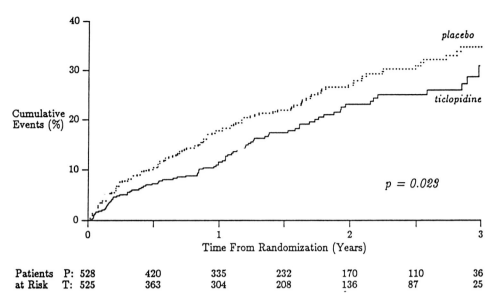

FIGURE 10.7. Cumulative event rate, efficacy analysis, for end point:stroke/MI/vascular death. (Courtesy of Professor M. Gent.)

ticlopidine (P=.006) (Figure 10.7). The relative risk reduction was 21.8% in men and 34.2% in women, both significant values. Intention-to-treat analysis gave a smaller estimate of the risk reduction for the entire group (23.3%, P=0.02). A subset efficacy analysis found the stroke risk reduction to be 33.5% (P=0.008) (Table 10.4 and Figure 10.8).

The major adverse experience with ticlopidine was severe neutropenia in about 1% of cases, while skin rash and diarrhea (severe in 2%) were the most common adverse reactions.

Critique of Large-Scale Studies

According to Warlow, efficacy analysis used in CATS as the principal form of end-point analysis provides the most optimistic estimate of treatment.[26] Bias may occur in this kind of analysis if many patients stop the trial medication as a result of a minor event, resulting in further vascular occlusive events. Further, it is difficult to know precisely when a patient stops a trial medication voluntarily.

In the CATS study, intention-to-treat analysis showed a reduced stroke/MI/vascular death risk

reduction value to 23.3%, only just statistically significant, with a wide confidence interval (1.0% to 40.5% risk reduction). Since 12% of patients stopped taking ticlopidine because of side effects, and ticlopidine is much more expensive than aspirin, Warlow suggested that aspirin may be preferable to ticlopidine if tolerated.

In the TASS study, which he reestimated to include nonfatal MI, ticlopidine was only marginally more effective than aspirin. The wide confidence levels seen when the two treatments were compared left the choice of a preferable therapy for stroke prevention after TIA or minor stroke in doubt.

Combined Therapy

No large-scale trials of aspirin *plus* ticlopidine have been reported. However, Uchiyama and coworkers recently reported the results of blood studies in patients with cerebrovascular disease.[27] Patients received either aspirin 300 mg/day (17 patients), ticlopidine 200 mg/day (24 patients), or aspirin 81 mg/day plus ticlopidine 100 mg/day (23 patients).

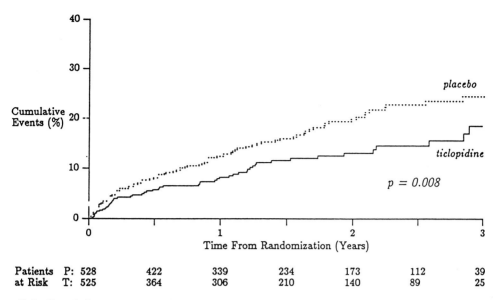

FIGURE 10.8. Cumulative event rate, efficacy analysis, for end point: stroke or stroke death. (Courtesy of Professor M. Gent.)

In the ticlopidine group, ADP- and platelet activating factors (PAF)-induced aggregation (but not AA-induced aggregation) was inhibited. Aspirin alone inhibited AA-induced aggregation, only partially inhibited ADP-induced aggregation, and did not inhibit platelet aggregation induced by PAF. In the group receiving both drugs, platelet aggregation induced by ADP, PAF, and AA was markedly inhibited.[27]

The combination of aspirin and ticlopidine also produced a more prolonged bleeding time than that with either alone. Further, plasma concentrations of beta thromboglobulin and platelet factor IV, although unchanged by aspirin and slightly reduced by ticlopidine alone, were markedly reduced when aspirin and ticlopidine were taken together.

These results suggest that combination therapy might be of value. Ordinas, however, pointed out that antiplatelet drugs that totally suppress platelet function might also induce a major risk of bleeding.[12] The ideal platelet drug should be less efficient, preventing excessive recruitment of platelets while staying within the limits of safety and patient tolerance. While the debate over the relative value of ticlopidine versus aspirin will likely continue for

some time, resolving clinical doubts with combination therapy should be accompanied by careful attention to tailoring the dose of each drug. When ticlopidine is prescribed, the potential but rare chance of absolute neutropenia requires complete blood count surveillance at 2-week intervals for the first 4 months of administration.

References

1. Gent M, Easton JD, Hachinski VC, et al. The Canadian American Ticlopidine Study (CATS) in thromboembolic stroke. *Lancet.* 1989;1:1215–1220.
2. Hass WK, Easton JD, Adams HP Jr, et al. A randomized trial comparing ticlopidine hydrochloride with aspirin for the prevention of stroke in high-risk patients. *N Engl J Med.* 1989;321:501–507.
3. Goyan JE. The "trials" of a longterm clinical trial: the ticlopidine Aspirin Stroke Study and the Canadian-American Ticlopidine Study. *Controlled Clinical Trials.* 1989;10(suppl):236–244.
4. Maffrand JP, Eloy F. Synthèse de thiénopyridines a l'étude de furopyridines d'intérêt therapeutique. *Eur J Med Chem.* 1974;9:483–486.

5. Bousser MG. Personal communication.

6. Thebault JJ, Blatrix CE, Blanchard JF, et al. Effects of ticlopidine, a new platelet aggregation inhibitor in man. *Clin Pharmacol Ther.* 1975;18:485–490.

7. Lecrubier C, Conard J, Samama M, et al. Essai randomisé d'un nouvel agent anti-aggregant: la ticlopidine. *Therapie.* 1977;32:189–194.

8. Maeda K, Usudo M, Kowaguchi S, et al. Effects of ticlopidine on thrombotic obstruction of A-V shunts and on dialysis of artificial kidneys. *Artif Organs.* 1980;4:30–33.

9. Maffrand JP, Defreyn G, Bernot A, et al. Reviewed pharmacology of ticlopidine. *Angiologie.* 1988;5 (suppl):5–13.

10. Panak E, Maffrand JP, Picard-Fraire T, et al. Ticlopidine: a promise for the prevention and treatment of thrombosis and its complications. *Haemostasis.* 1983;13(suppl 1):1–54.

11. Lips JPM, Sixma JJ, Schiphorst ME. The effect of ticlopidine administration to humans on binding of adenosine diphosphate to blood platelets. *Thromb Res.* 1980;17:19–27.

12. Ordinas A. Personal communication.

13. DeMinno G, Cerbone AM, Mattiali PL, et al. Functionally thrombasthenic state in normal patients following the administration of ticlopidine. *J Clin Invest.* 1985;75:328–338.

14. Hass WK. Aspirin for the limping brain (editorial). *Stroke.* 1977;8:299–301.

15. Fieschi C, Argentino C, Lenzi GL, et al. Clinical and instrumental evaluation of patients with ischemic stroke within the first six hours. *J Neurol Sci.* 1989; 91:311–322.

16. Canadian Cooperative Study Group. A randomized trial of aspirin and sulfinpyrazone in threatened stroke. *N Engl J Med.* 1978;299:53–59.

17. Bousser MG, Eschwege E, Haguenau M, et al. "AICLA" controlled trial of aspirin and dipyridamole in the secondary prevention of atherothrombotic cerebral ischemia. *Stroke.* 1983;14:5–14.

18. Stroke Prevention in Atrial Fibrillation Study Group Investigators. Special Report: Preliminary report of the stroke prevention in atrial fibrillation study. *N Engl J Med.* 1990;322:863–868.

19. Antiplatelet Trialists Collaboration. Open communication, April 1990.

20. Dyken ML. Transient ischemic attacks and aspirin, stroke and death; negative studies and type II error. Editorial. *Stroke.* 1983;14:2–4.

21. Ono H, Mizukami M, Kitamura K, et al. Subarachnoid hemorrhage. *Agents Actions.* 1984;15(suppl): 259–272.

22. Tohgi H. The effect of ticlopidine on TIA compared with aspirin: a double-blind twelve-month follow-up study. *Agents Actions.* 1984;15(suppl):279–282.

23. Rieger JS, Picho JLT. Effect of ticlopidine on the prevention of relapses of cerebrovascular ischemic disease. *Med Clin (Barcelona).* 1984;82:62–64.

24. Hart RG. Comparison of ticlopidine and aspirin for the prevention of stroke (letter). *N Engl J Med.* 1990;322:404–405.

25. Hass WK, Molony BA, Anderson SA, Kamm A. Comparison of ticlopidine and aspirin for the prevention of stroke (correspondence). *N Engl J Med.* 1990;322:404–405.

26. Warlow C. Ticlopidine a new antithrombotic drug: but is it better than aspirin for longterm use? (editorial). *J Neurol Neurosurg Psychiat.* 1990;53: 185–187.

27. Uchiyama S, Sone R, Nagayama T, et al. Combination therapy with low-dose aspirin and ticlopidine in cerebral ischaemia. *Stroke.* 1989;20:1643–1647.

11
Present Status of Anticoagulant Prophylaxis

J. Donald Easton

Although anticoagulation is widely used for stroke prevention, it has not been well studied and is substantially unproven in the management of cerebral vascular diseases. Even after nearly 40 years of use, major controversy questions its value in preventing infarction in patients with transient ischemic attack (TIA), in arresting progressing stroke, and in preventing cerebral reinfarction. Although most clinicians believe anticoagulants are effective in some situations, they question how well they work, and whether the bleeding risks outweigh the benefit. Anticoagulation using heparin and warfarin and the justification for its current role in the treatment of cerebral vascular disease will be reviewed in this chapter.

Mechanisms of Drug Activity

Anticoagulation therapy rests on the premise that altering coagulation diminishes the formation of intravascular thrombosis and embolism and prevents vascular obstruction and its consequences. While laboratory studies and animal models have greatly enhanced our understanding of blood clotting, they have not contributed greatly to our understanding of human thromboembolism. The mechanisms studied in vitro and in animals differ in many ways from the clinical disorders in humans. As a result, most of our information derives from clinical trials.

Thrombosis is a complex process[1,2] and differs in arteries and veins (and the left heart chambers). In arteries, circulating platelets adhere to the diseased intima. Adenosine diphosphate is released from the platelets, and aggregation of the platelets occurs. This white, or platelet, thrombus then grows, and in areas of slow flow it may occlude the lumen. Hemostasis then occurs, clotting begins, and a red thrombus forms around the white thrombus. At the site of a total arterial occlusion, one finds a mixed white and red thrombus. The initial plug formed as a result of platelet adhesion and aggregation is unstable. However, substances released at the site of the platelet mass activate the coagulation cascade, generating thrombin. Thrombin stimulates further aggregation of platelets and the formation of fibrin, which stabilizes the thrombus.

Clearly, both platelets and blood coagulation play a role in the genesis of arterial thrombi that lead to cerebral ischemia and infarction. This is the rationale for attempting to prevent and treat these processes with platelet antiaggregating agents and blood anticoagulants.

Heparin

Heparin is composed of a heterogeneous group of mucopolysaccharides that are obtained from mammalian tissue sources. Its main pharmacologic effect is to impair blood coagulation, and its effect is virtually immediate. Heparin acts indirectly by means of a naturally circulating "anticoagulant," antithrombin III, which neutralizes several activated clotting factors and thrombin. Low concentrations of heparin increase the activity of antithrombin III and form the basis for low-dose heparin therapy in certain clinical situations.

Treatment with heparin for several days causes a progressive reduction in the antithrombin III concentration in blood.[3] If treatment is then terminated abruptly, the reduced antithrombin III concentration results in a transient "hypercoagulable state" of potential clinical importance.[4] Warfarin, on the other hand, increases antithrombin III activity.

Heparin is not absorbed across the intestinal mucosa and therefore is given parenterally. Intermittent or continuous-drip intravenous infusions are the most popular mode of administration; the latter is generally preferred. A 7500 or 10 000 unit injection will produce adequate anticoagulation in the average adult with an anticoagulant half-life of about 1.5 hours. A continuous infusion of 1000 units hourly is then adjusted to maintain the activated partial thromboplastin time (aPTT) value. Since the dose of heparin required can vary considerably, it is prudent to measure the aPTT at 2 and 4 hours after treatment begins. The early hours following the event that lead to the initiation of therapy are the most important ones; so it is important to be certain early that the patient becomes, and remains, adequately anticoagulated.

New heparinoids are being developed. They are low-molecular-weight fractions that specifically enhance the neutralization of clotting factor Xa while avoiding the overall clotting effects of currently used heparins. This should maximize the antithrombotic effects while minimizing the hemorrhagic side effects. Since Protein C is a potent anticoagulant that can prevent thrombosis in primates, there is also considerable interest in producing and testing Protein C.

Warfarin

Although there are many coumarin derivatives that have anticoagulant activity, warfarin (Coumadin[R]) is the most widely used in the United States. The coumarins came into prominent use in clinical medicine in the early 1950s. The major pharmacologic effect of warfarin is inhibition of blood clotting by interference with the hepatic synthesis of the vitamin K-dependent clotting factors (II, VII, IX, and X). The effect, as measured by prolongation of the prothrombin time, begins 8 to 14 hours after oral ingestion. This is due to early depression of clotting factor VII. However, the other factors are not depressed for 5 to 7 days, and anticoagulation is not fully therapeutic until then. Some

authorities recommend an initial loading dose of 40 to 60 mg. It is probably more prudent to use 15 mg on the first day followed by 10 mg daily until the maintenance dose is determined based on prothrombin times. The prothrombin time is determined daily until it is stable at 1.3 to 1.8 times the control value (approximately 25% of normal activity). Lower level anticoagulation is effective in preventing deep vein and prosthetic heart valve thrombosis, but there are few data regarding its efficacy in stroke prevention.[5,6] Many disease states and drugs alter the effect of warfarin on blood clotting and must be taken into account.[1,7]

When heparin and warfarin are used concomitantly, heparin accentuates the warfarin-induced prolongation of the prothrombin time. Thus when heparin is discontinued, the prothrombin time will shorten and adjustment of the warfarin dosage upward is necessary.

Failure to adequately monitor heparin therapy results in failure to prevent thrombosis on the one hand, or hemorrhage on the other. Consequently, careful monitoring is mandatory if the patient is to benefit from anticoagulation.

Review of Clinical Studies

Transient Ischemic Attack (TIA)

Warfarin

Four randomized prospective studies comparing anticoagulant-treated patients with TIA to controls showed no significant difference in the incidence of stroke or death.[8-11] The data favor the view that anticoagulation reduces the number of TIA recurrences, but the evidence is weak. All of the early randomized trials involved small numbers of patients and were subject to a Type II error. Aggregate data from several other trials demonstrated a decreased incidence of stroke, but they were not randomized.[12] More recently, studies by Olsson et al.[13] and by Buren and Ygge[14] comparing coumarin anticoagulation and platelet aggregation inhibitors provided some evidence that coumarin anticoagulation prevents stroke in patients with TIA and reversible ischemic neurological deficits. Neither study's result was statistically significant, but the trend to benefit was clear. All in all, there is weak evidence that warfarin reduces the number of TIAs and decreases the risk of stroke in patients with TIA.

Heparin

Heparin is widely used for crescendo TIA, progressing stroke, and cardioembolic stroke.[15-17] While no studies prove that patients with crescendo TIA are especially prone to early stroke, the conventional wisdom is otherwise and they should be treated like patients with progressing stroke. Less commonly, heparin is used for any TIA with its onset within the previous few days. Almost no controlled-study data exist regarding the systematic use of heparin for patients with crescendo or recent-onset TIA. In most of the published studies on anticoagulation for progressing stroke, heparin was discontinued as soon as the warfarin had prolonged the prothrombin time. Many patients did not receive heparin at all.[15] For theoretical reasons, and by extrapolation from the results of studies of anticoagulation for progressing stroke, anticoagulation is used by many clinicians for "unstable TIA," that is, recent-onset and crescendo TIA.

One study is of interest in this regard. Putnam and Adams investigated heparin in recent TIA.[18] They concluded that "interim heparin, while relatively safe in supervised conditions, does not prevent recurrent TIA or cerebral infarction in high risk patients with recent TIA. The value of heparin in the interim management of recent TIA should be established by a randomized, controlled study." Still, only 2 of their 74 patients (2.7%) experienced a *spontaneous* infarction while heparinized; an excellent outcome for this group. Nevertheless, the value of this therapy needs to be proved rigorously.

Progressing Stroke

In this condition, the focal ischemia worsens from minute to minute or hour to hour, and there are stepwise, incremental increases in neurologic deficit occurring over several hours. In the vertebrobasilar circulation the stroke commonly evolves over 2 or even 3 or more days.[19] Approximately 20% of carotid territory strokes progress, compared to 40% of those in the posterior circulation.[19-21] Clearly, progressing stroke is common.

Even though heparin is the preferred treatment for progressing stroke and crescendo TIA, the data

supporting its efficacy in this situation are meager. The belief is that in these disorders there is ongoing thrombosis and that heparin will prevent the formation of large, red thrombi. The data supporting heparin's efficacy in this situation come from old and limited studies. In 1961 Whisnant reported that heparin's effect was dramatic in preventing stroke progression in patients with acute brainstem ischemia; 9% of the heparinized group died, while 59% of a similar untreated group died.[22] He emphasized that the criteria used for diagnosing progressing vertebrobasilar stroke are extremely important if one is to predict accurately the natural history of the event.

Subsequently, several other randomized and nonrandomized studies were conducted.[12] The patients were generally heparinized at the time of diagnosis and then switched over to a coumarin anticoagulant for several weeks or months thereafter. The data in aggregate suggest, but do not prove, that heparin reduces the risk of progression in progressing stroke. (Based in part on the single report by Whisnant,[22] it seems that most clinicians are inclined to heparinize patients with progressing brain-stem ischemia than those with carotid distribution ischemia.)

Duke et al. conducted a randomized, controlled trial of heparin for the prevention of stroke progression in acute partial thrombotic stroke in 225 patients.[21] Of the heparin-treated patients, 17% progressed in the first week, compared to 19.5% of the placebo-treated patients. There were no major hemorrhagic complications. They concluded: "This study does not support the use of heparin in 'acute partial stable' stroke."

In view of the large number of stroke patients and the high percentage that experience progression of their infarction,[19,20] it is astounding that a carefully controlled, definitive study of heparin for recent TIA and progressing stroke has never been conducted.

Completed Stroke

No data support the use of heparin for completed atherothrombotic stroke (see review[15]). This is true even though the probability of recurrence may be as high as 10% annually.[23,24] Nevertheless, heparin is used commonly for patients with a *minor* carotid distribution stroke that occurred within the previous 48 hours because 20% or more will have progressing, rather than completed, strokes. If a minor vertebrobasilar stroke has occurred within the previous 3 or 4 days, heparin is often used throughout the first week. The bleeding complication rate for 7 days of heparin is about 10%, with a serious bleed rate of about 2%.

Cardioembolic Stroke

The data supporting the use of anticoagulation in patients who are at risk of imminent embolization of thrombi from the left heart are not definitive but are more convincing than for atherothrombotic stroke.[16,17,25] The discussion of anticoagulation in cardioembolic stroke is best divided into prevention of recurrence and prevention of the first embolus.

Prevention of Recurrence

Based on grouped data from several studies, approximately 10% to 15% of patients with a cardioembolic stroke will experience a second embolism within 2 weeks if they are not treated.[17] Three fourths will go to the brain and one fourth to a systemic site. All types of heart disease causing nonseptic emboli have a similar rate of recurrent stroke, about 1% daily for the subsequent 2 weeks.[16] Emboli arising from the atrial or ventricular wall, as opposed to native or prosthetic valves, tend to be large and cause large infarcts. Consequently, they are especially important to prevent.

Anticoagulation has been shown (though not conclusively), to prevent embolic recurrence. In rheumatic heart disease, nonrheumatic atrial fibrillation, and acute myocardial infarction (MI), the natural recurrence rate is reduced to approximately one third to one half in the high risk period of the first few weeks. After the first few weeks following MI, anticoagulation is no longer necessary. The benefit in long-term prevention persists in rheumatic heart disease and in patients with prosthetic valves,[17] whereas long-term anticoagulation in nonrheumatic atrial fibrillation has never been studied.

While the evidence strongly suggests that early heparinization substantially minimizes the chance of early recurrent embolism, many clinicians fear brain hemorrhage in this situation. It is well known that cardioembolic infarcts are commonly hemorrhagic, and there is concern that anticoagulation will worsen the bleeding and increase the morbidity and mortality. Additionally, there is some morbidity associated with systemic hemorrhage.[16,17]

A recent review of the risks and benefits of immediate anticoagulation in patients with cardioembolic stroke indicates that the conversion of brain petechiae into purpura is probably common, but major hemorrhage is not.[17] The evidence overall suggests that immediate anticoagulation is beneficial, except in patients with computerized tomography (CT) scan evidence of blood, substantial arterial hypertension, or a large infarct. Patients with these abnormalities are at higher risk of developing clinically important hemorrhagic transformation of their infarct.

Prevention of the First Embolus

Emboli arising from the wall of the left heart produce large infarcts, and they are usually unheralded by warning TIAs. Since many potential sources of cardiac emboli are identifiable prior to stroke, emphasis should center on prevention of the first embolus. In this situation data again are very limited.

Anticoagulation prevents stroke in patients with prosthetic heart valves[17,26] and in those with severe rheumatic heart disease (that is, with mitral stenosis, an enlarged left atrium, atrial fibrillation, and congestive heart failure).[17] Most cardiologists anticoagulate prophylactically such patients. On the other hand, most do not anticoagulate young patients with mild rheumatic heart disease. The issue is where along the spectrum of severity one decides to anticoagulate patients as prophylaxis against cardioembolic stroke. Data do not exist to guide one in this regard.

Patients with nonrheumatic or nonvalvular atrial fibrillation (NVAF) have a 5 to 6 times higher likelihood of experiencing a stroke each year than their age-matched counterparts without NVAF.[17,27,28] This is a stroke risk factor of the same magnitude as new-onset TIA. Identification of subgroups of individuals with NVAF has not been accomplished except that atrial fibrillation within 1 year of onset carries an increased risk of stroke.[29-31] NVAF affects 3% to 5% of the elderly and it is the most common cause of cardioembolic stroke in America.

Prophylactic anticoagulation is beneficial for these stroke-threatened individuals. Petersen et al.[32]

first reported, based on a placebo-controlled clinical trial, a benefit for low-level anticoagulation in preventing strokes in patients with NVAF. Shortly thereafter the Stroke Prevention in Atrial Fibrillation Study Group published a preliminary report of their study.[33] The study involved 1244 patients with NVAF randomized to treatment with either warfarin (prothrombin time 1.3 to 1.8 times control), aspirin (325 mg daily) or placebo. The warfarin arm was unblinded while the aspirin and placebo were double-blind. After 17 months, the placebo arm of the trial was stopped because treatment with both aspirin and warfarin was significantly better than placebo. The trial is continuing to compare the efficacy of warfarin and aspirin. The rate of serious bleeding complications was 1.7% annually for warfarin, 1.2% for placebo and 0.9% for aspirin.

Most recently, the Boston Area Anticoagulation Trial for Atrial Fibrillation Investigators reported the results of their unblinded randomized trial to determine the effect of low-dose warfarin on the risk of stroke in patients with nonrheumatic atrial fibrillation.[34] A total of 420 patients entered the trial (212 in the warfarin group-target prothrombin time ratio, 1.2 to 1.5; and 208 in the control group-not given warfarin but could choose to take aspirin) and were followed for an average of 2.2 years. There were 2 strokes in the warfarin group and 13 in the control group (86% risk reduction). The death rate was 2.25% yearly in the warfarin group and 6% in the control group. The major hemorrhage rate was very low and equal in the two groups.

Finally, the Canadian Atrial Fibrillation Anticoagulation Study (Norris, JW, personal communication), a randomized double-blind placebo-controlled trial, recently stopped early because of the above trial results. The target range of anticoagulation was an international normalized ratio of 2.0 to 3.0. There was a risk reduction of 37% in the warfarin group for the primary outcome event cluster of non-lacunar stroke, non-CNS embolism and fatal or intracranial hemorrhage. Fatal or major bleeding occurred at annual rates of 2.5% on warfarin and 0.5% on placebo.

Clearly the presence of NVAF identifies a population at considerable risk of large, unheralded ischemic stroke and antithrombotic therapy substantially reduces the risk of stroke and death. Low-level anticoagulation with warfarin can be quite safe with careful monitoring.

About 3% of patients with acute myocardial infarction experience an ischemic stroke within 4 weeks.[17] The embolic cause of the majority of these strokes is supported by their striking relationship to the presence of left ventricular thrombi. A minority are attributable to atrial thrombi or other causes. About 90% of these strokes occur in patients with transmural infarctions. Left ventricular mural thrombi are present in about 35% of patients with a transmural anterior MI, and they are largely confined to areas of wall dyskinesis.[35-39] Consequently, it appears that the combination of an electrocardiogram (ECG) and 2-D echocardiogram can identify the 20 to 25% of patients with an acute MI who have a transmural, anteroapical infarct with wall dyskinesis.[17] This is the group at special risk for cardioembolic stroke. The 2-D echocardiogram may also demonstrate thrombus.

Several reports, old and recent, indicate that anticoagulation reduces substantially the incidence of stroke in patients with MI.[16,17] If anticoagulation is restricted to the "at risk" patients described above, it is very likely that treatment is indicated and that it should be continued for 2 or 3 months.

Cerebral embolism following MI recurs in one fourth to one third of patients, and two thirds recur within 2 weeks. For this reason, any patient with an acute MI suffering an arterial embolism should be heparinized immediately, unless the infarct is large or there are contraindications to anticoagulation.

Persistent left ventricular dyskinesis in healed MI can be a source of cardioembolic stroke. Surgical, echocardiographic, and autopsy studies demonstrate mural thrombi in about 50% of ventricular aneurysms late after infarction. However, only about 5% of such patients experience a stroke. When a ventricular aneurysm is found late after MI, with or without a mural thrombus and in the absence of embolism, chronic anticoagulation does not appear to be indicated routinely.[17,25]

There are no data regarding the efficacy of anticoagulant or platelet antiaggregation therapy in the secondary prevention of embolism for patients with a ventricular aneurysm who embolize once, but chronic anticoagulation is generally recommended empirically.

Patients with cardiomyopathies of all etiologies are also at risk for systemic embolism, especially if there is associated congestive heart failure. Mural thrombi are found at autopsy in 35 to 100% of patients who die with cardiomyopathy.[40-42] Consequently, long-term anticoagulation is recommended for patients with significant disease.

Cervicocerebral Arterial Dissections

Dissections of arteries supplying the brain occur when blood extrudes into the wall of the artery,[42-45] the intramural hematoma dilates the wall and compresses the lumen. In addition, intraluminal thrombus may occlude the lumen or produce emboli to distal arteries. Dissections may result from major or trivial head and neck trauma, or they may occur spontaneously.

While the initial event in the arterial wall is hemorrhage, the consequence of concern is thrombosis and embolism with brain infarction. This concern is based on observations at angiography, surgery, and autopsy. The treatments usually recommended are anticoagulation, surgery to open or bypass the obstruction, or nothing.[43,44]

Anecdotal reports[44-50] of heparin use in arterial dissection are encouraging, but no definitive studies have been reported. Approximately 90% of patients with extracranial carotid and vertebral artery dissections do well with no treatment. It would therefore require a very large, randomized study to show a convincing benefit for anticoagulation. Nevertheless, it is the 10% of patients who do poorly because of arterial thrombosis that lead to the recommendation to treat.

Dissection of intracranial arteries appears to be less common than extracranial cervical arteries, but the consequences are more severe. Massive stroke at the outset of the dissection is common. Additionally, rupture of the external arterial wall with subarachnoid bleeding often occurs. For these reasons the opportunity to treat is limited, and anticoagulation seems less rational. Nevertheless, the decision regarding anticoagulation is especially difficult because intracranial dissections are most often confused with arterial obstruction from an embolus, for which the treatment is typically heparin.

Cerebral Venous Thrombosis

There are many causes for cerebral vein and sinus thrombosis, and the main neurological manifestations are headache, papilledema, seizures, obtundation, and sometimes alternating focal deficits.

While the common parenchymal brain pathology is bland and hemorrhagic infarction and edema are unusual, the underlying process is thrombosis. For this reason, anticoagulation has been advocated unless the hemorrhage is substantial. This is akin to cardioembolic infarction. Again, anecdotal reports of anticoagulant use are encouraging, but no definitive studies have been reported.[51-53]

Management Recommendations

General Recommendations

The methods of initiating and maintaining treatment with heparin and warfarin are described in the section on Mechanisms of Drug Activity above. Recommendations vary on how the conversion from heparin to warfarin therapy should be accomplished. Some authors give warfarin in an initial dose of 30 to 40 mg along with heparin at the time anticoagulation is begun. In most cases this brings the prothrombin time to about twice the control value by 48 hours, at which time heparin is discontinued. Other authors recommend that warfarin be started at 10 to 15 mg daily, concomitant with the initiation of heparin therapy, and that heparin be continued for several days thereafter. The heparin is then tapered over 1 or 2 days.

A reasonable overall recommendation is to begin anticoagulation with heparin. If the decision is made to continue anticoagulation beyond 7 to 10 days, warfarin is started in a dose of 10 mg daily. The heparin should be maintained for 1 or 2 days after the prothrombin time is therapeutic; then it is tapered over 1 or 2 days.

There is also controversy over how anticoagulation should be discontinued. The existence of a "rebound hypercoagulable state" after cessation of both warfarin and heparin is controversial. Several anecdotal observations of an unduly high stroke incidence in the period following immediate cessation of anticoagulation have been reported.[54-56] Studies of rebound hypercoagulability have been undertaken for patients with prosthetic heart valves in whom warfarin was stopped briefly for elective surgery.[57,58] No untoward effects resulted. The duration of cessation averaged 2 to 6 days, a time period during which some anticoagulant effect is known to persist, and a small number of patients were involved. Others have reported several patients who experienced a stroke 5 to 7 days after discontinuing warfarin.[54] Additionally, a recent study was reported on the withdrawal of heparin in patients treated for TIA or ischemic stroke.[56] Those who were not started on aspirin or warfarin before heparin was stopped had five times as many episodes of clinical deterioration over the subsequent 24 hours as those who were. The rapidity of heparin withdrawal was not discussed. It seems reasonable, whenever possible, to discontinue anticoagulation over 1 or 2 days. This seems especially prudent for heparin since a day or two will be required for antithrombin III concentrations to return to normal.

Specific Recommendations

Atherothrombotic Stroke

There are presently limited treatments to offer the large number of people who arrive at our hospitals with progressing cerebral infarction. Many of them are heparinized, even though benefit has not been proven.

Although the data supporting coumarin anticoagulation for prevention of stroke are limited and largely derived from nonrandomized studies, the limited evidence that is available supports the use of anticoagulation in certain stroke-threatened patients.

Overall, warfarin is not widely used in North America for stroke prevention in patients with TIA because few data support its efficacy. Patients with TIA and appropriate carotid artery lesions are usually treated with carotid endarterectomy or aspirin. In some parts of the world they are treated with ticlopidine. Those with surgically inaccessible lesions and those who remain symptomatic on aspirin are often treated with anticoagulation. Since the risk of stroke is highest in the early weeks and months following the onset of TIA, and since the hemorrhagic complications of coumarin anticoagulation accumulate arithmetically over time, it seems prudent to recommend that anticoagulation be used infrequently for TIA, especially after the first 3 to 4 months. Some experts use long-term anticoagulation in patients with a tight, inoperable arterial stenosis.

Patients with crescendo TIA and progressing stroke should generally be heparinized as soon as possible. Heparin should usually be continued for 5 to 7 days. A decision can then be made about the appropriateness of angiography, surgery, aspirin,

or coumarin anticoagulation. One hopes that definitive studies will soon be undertaken to determine the value of anticoagulation in this common clinical condition.

Patients with a completed stroke should not generally be heparinized. However, an apparently completed stroke must be viewed as a potentially progressing one until it is at least 2 or 3 days out from its onset. Consequently, many patients with partial strokes are treated with heparin for several days if they are seen within the first 24 to 48 hours after onset. Obviously, 60 to 80% of these patients will be treated unnecessarily, since they are not destined to progress. Nevertheless, one cannot identify those that will progress until they actually worsen, and short-term heparin is quite safe compared to the damage done by the progression of ischemia. Again, we lack definitive information.

In synopsis, our general approach is to heparinize patients with progressing stroke, crescendo TIA, recent-onset (within the past 24 hours) TIA, and recent partial stroke. The first two groups are treated with enthusiasm. The latter two groups are treated with reluctance. We look forward to studies that will provide definitive information regarding the risks and benefits of heparin in these situations.

Cardioembolic Stroke

Heparin is used regularly in cardioembolic stroke from most causes. If the stroke is mild or the deficit is rapidly resolving and no contraindications exist, the patient is heparinized immediately to avoid recurrent embolism. In patients with moderate-sized infarcts, a CT scan is obtained after 24 hours to identify the 5% of patients with early spontaneous hemorrhagic infarction. Anticoagulation is delayed for several days in these patients and in those with large infarcts or a blood pressure higher than about 180/100 mm Hg.

Prophylactic anticoagulation at relatively low-level (prothrombin time 1.3 to 1.8 times the control value) is recommended for individuals with nonvalvular atrial fibrillation who have not had transient or permanent cerebral ischemic episodes.

Arterial Dissection

While the therapy of extracranial carotid dissection is ill-defined, it seems advisable to immediately anticoagulate most patients using heparin for about

7 days, followed by warfarin. Anticoagulation should be avoided in patients with large infarcts and in those with subarachnoid hemorrhage. Warfarin should be continued for 3 months and then discontinued. Patients with intracranial dissections may be anticoagulated also, if the ischemia is mild or progressive.

Cerebral Venous Thrombosis

This situation is virtually identical to arterial dissection. Anticoagulation makes sense, and while there are clinical suggestions that it is beneficial, it has not been properly studied. Until more definitive data are available, it seems best to anticoagulate immediately most patients using heparin for about 7 days followed by warfarin.

References

1. O'Reilly RA. Anticoagulant, antithrombotic, and thrombolytic drugs. In: Gilman AG, Goodman LS, Gilman A, eds. *The Pharmacological Basis of Therapeutics*, 6th ed. New York, NY: Macmillan Publishing Co.: 1980: pp 1347–1360.
2. Hirsh J. Anticoagulant and platelet antiaggregant agents. In: Barnett HJM, Mohr JP, Stein BM, Yatsu FM, eds. *Stroke: Pathophysiology, Diagnosis and Management*. New York, NY: Churchill, Livingstone: 1986: pp 925–966.
3. Marciniak E, Gockerman JP. Heparin-induced decrease in circulating antithrombin-III. *Lancet*. 1977; 2:581–584.
4. Schafer, AI. The hypercoagulable states. *Ann Int Med*. 1985;102:814–828.
5. Turpie AGG, Gunstensen J, Hirsh J, et al. Randomized comparison of two intensities of oral anticoagulant therapy after tissue heart valve replacement. *Lancet*. 1988;1:1242–1245.
6. Turpie AGG, Robinson JG, Doyle DJ, et al. Comparison of high-dose with low-dose subcutaneous heparin to prevent left ventricular mural thrombosis in patients with acute transmural myocardial infarction. *N Engl J Med*. 1989;320:352–357.
7. Koch-Weser J, Sellers EM. Drug interactions with coumarin anticoagulants. *N Engl J Med*. 1971;285: 487–498, 547–558.
8. Report of the Veterans Administration. Cooperative Study of Atherosclerosis, Neurology Section. An evaluation of anticoagulant therapy in the treatment of cerebrovascular disease. *Neurology*. 1961;11:132–138.
9. Baker RN, Broward JA, Fang HC, et al. Anticoagulant therapy in cerebral infarction. *Neurology*. 1962;12:823–835.
10. Pearce JMS, Gubbay SS, Walton JN. Long-term anticoagulant therapy in transient cerebral attacks. *Lancet*. 1965;1:6–9.
11. Baker RN, Schwartz W, Rose AS. Transient ischemic attacks—a report of a study of anticoagulant treatment. *Neurology*. 1966;16:841–847.
12. Easton JD, Hart RG, Sherman DG, et al. Diagnosis and management of ischemic stroke: I.-Threatened stroke and its management. *Current Probl Cardiol*. 1983;8:1–76.
13. Olsson JE, Brechter C, Backlund H, et al. Anticoagulant vs. anti-platelet therapy as prophylaxis against cerebral infarction in transient ischemic attacks. *Stroke*. 1980;11:4–9.
14. Buren A, Ygge J. Treatment program and comparison between anticoagulants and platelet aggregation inhibitors after transient ischemic attack. *Stroke*. 1981;12:578–580.
15. Byer JA, Easton JD. Therapy of ischemic cerebrovascular disease. *Ann Int Med*. 1980;93:742–756.
16. Easton JD, Sherman DG. Management of cerebral embolism of cardiac origin. *Stroke*. 1980;11:433–442.
17. Hart RG, Sherman DG, Miller VT, et al. Diagnosis and management of ischemic stroke: II- Selected controversies. *Current Probl Cardiol*. 1983;8:1–80.
18. Putnam SF, Adams HP Jr. Usefulness of heparin in initial management of patients with recent transient ischemic attacks. *Arch Neurol*. 1985;42:960–962.
19. Jones HR, Millikan CH, Sandok BA. Temporal profile (clinical course) of acute vertebrobasilar system cerebral infarction. *Stroke*. 1980;11:173–177.
20. Jones HR, Millikan CH. Temporal profile (clinical course) of acute carotid system cerebral infarction. *Stroke*. 1976;7:64–71.
21. Duke RJ, Bloch RF, Turpie AGG, et al. Intravenous heparin for the prevention of stroke progression in acute partial stable stroke: a randomized controlled trial. *Ann Int Med*. 1986;105:825–828.
22. Whisnant JP. Discussion of progressing stroke: anticoagulant therapy. In: Millikan CH, Siekert RH, Whisnant JP, eds. *Cerebral Vascular Diseases*. Third Princeton Conference. New York, NY: Grune & Stratton: 1961: pp 182–183.
23. Marquardsen J. The natural history of acute cerebrovascular disease. A retrospective study of 769 patients. *Acta Neurol Scand*. 1969;45(suppl38):1–192.
24. Gent M, Blakely JA, Easton JD, et al. The Canadian American Ticlopidine Study (CATS) in thromboembolic stroke: design, organization and baseline results. *Stroke*. 1988;19:1203–1210.
25. Sherman DG, Dyken ML, Fisher M, et al. Cerebral embolism. *Chest*. 1986;89(suppl):83S–98S.
26. Chesebro JH, Fuster V, Pumphrey CW, et al. Combined warfarin-platelet inhibitor antithrombotic

therapy in prosthetic heart valve replacement. *Circulation*. 1981;64(suppl IV)76.

27. Beer DT, Ghitman B. Embolization from the atria in arteriosclerotic heart disease, *JAMA*. 1961;177: 287–291.

28. Wolf PA, Dawber TR, Thomas HE, et al. Epidemiologic assessment of chronic atrial fibrillation and risk of stroke: the Framingham Study. *Neurology*. 1978;28:973–977.

29. Bharucha NE, Wolf PA, Kannel WB, et al. Epidemiological study of cerebral embolism: the Framingham Study. *Ann Neurol*. 1981;10:105.

30. Wolf PA, Kannel WB, McGee DL, et al. Duration of atrial fibrillation and imminence of stroke: the Framingham Study. *Stroke*. 1983;14:664–667.

31. Hart RG, Easton JD, Sherman DG. Duration of nonvalvular atrial fibrillation and stroke. *Stroke*. 1983; 14:827.

32. Petersen P, Boysen G, Godtfredsen J, et al. Placebo-controlled, randomized trial of warfarin and aspirin for prevention of thromboembolic complications in chronic atrial fibrillation. *Lancet*. 1989;1:175–179.

33. Stroke Prevention in Atrial Fibrillation Study Group Investigators. Preliminary report of the stroke prevention in atrial fibrillation study. *N Engl J Med*. 1990;322:863–868.

34. Boston Area Anticoagulation Trial for Atrial Fibrillation Investigators. The effect of low-dose warfarin on the risk of stroke in patients with nonrheumatic atrial fibrillation. *N Engl J Med*. 1990;323:1505–1511.

35. Bean WB. Infarction of the heart. III. Clinical course and morphological findings. *Ann Int Med*. 1938;12:71–94.

36. Friedman MJ, Carlson K, Marcus FI, et al. Clinical correlations in patients with acute myocardial infarction and left ventricular thrombus detected by two-dimensional echocardiography. *Am J Med*. 1982;72:894–898.

37. Asinger RW, Mikell FL, Elsperger J, et al. Incidence of left ventricular thrombosis after acute transmural myocardial infarction. *N Engl J Med*. 1981;305: 297–302.

38. Meltzer RS, et al. Intracardiac thrombi and systemic embolisation. *Ann Int Med*. 1986;104:689–698.

39. Resnekov L, et al. Antithrombotic agents in coronary artery disease. *Chest*. 1986;89:54S.

40. Demakis JG, Proskey A, Rahimatoola SH, et al. The natural course of alcoholic cardiomyopathy. *Ann Int Med*. 1974;80:293–297.

41. McDonald CD, Burch GE, Walsh JJ. Prolonged bedrest in the treatment of idiopathic cardiomyopathy. *Am J Med*. 1972;52:41–50.

42. Vost A, Wolochow DA, Howell DA. Incidence of infarcts of the brain in heart disease. *J Pathol Bacteriol*. 1964;88:463–470.

43. Hart RG, Easton JD. Dissections and trauma of cervico-cerebral arteries. In: Barnett HJM, Mohr JP, Stein BM, et al., eds. *Stroke: Pathophysiology, Diagnosis and Management*. New York, NY: Churchill, Livingstone: 1986: pp 775–788.

44. Mokri B, Sundt TM Jr, Houser OW, et al. Spontaneous dissection of the cervical internal carotid artery. *Ann Neurol*. 1986;19:126–138.

45. Biller J, Hingtgen WL, Adams HP Jr, et al. Cervicocephalic arterial dissections. A ten year experience. *Arch Neurol*. 1986;43:1234–1238.

46. Bogousslavsky J, Despland P-A, Regli F. Spontaneous carotid dissection with acute stroke. *Arch Neurol*. 1987;44:137–140.

47. Chapleau CE, Robertson JT. Spontaneous cervical carotid artery dissection: outpatient treatment with continuous heparin infusion using a totally implantable infusion device. *Neurosurg*. 1981;8:83.

48. Fisher CM, Ojemann RG, Robertson GH. Spontaneous dissection of cervicocerebral arteries. *Can J Neurol Sci*. 1978;5:9.

49. McNeill DH Jr, Dreisback J, Marsden RJ. Spontaneous dissection of the internal carotid artery: its consecutive management with heparin sodium. *Arch Neurol*. 1980;37:54.

50. Sherman DG, Hart RG, Easton JD. Abrupt change in head position and cerebral infarction. *Stroke*. 1981; 12:2.

51. Bousser M-G, Chiras J, Bories J, et al. Cerebral venous thrombosis—a review of 38 cases. *Stroke*. 1985; 16:199–213.

52. Fairburn B. Intracranial venous thrombosis complicating oral contraception: treatment by anticoagulant drugs. *Br Med J*. 1973;2:647.

53. Kalbag RM, Woolf AL. *Cerebral Venous Thrombosis*. London: University Press; 1967.

54. Hart RG, Coull BM. Hypercoagulability following coumadin withdrawal. *Am Heart J*. 1983;106:169–170.

55. Hart RG, Coull BM, Miller VT. Rebound hypercoagulability. *Stroke*. 1982;13:527.

56. Slivka AP, Levy DE. Risk associated with heparin withdrawal in ischemic cerebrovascular disease. *Stroke*. 1987;18:298. Abstract.

57. Tinker JH, Tarnahan S. Discontinuing anticoagulant therapy in surgical patients with cardiac valve prostheses. *JAMA*. 1978;239:738–739.

58. Katholi RE, Nolan SP, McGuire LB. The management of anticoagulation during noncardiac operations in patients with prosthetic heart valves. *Am Heart J*. 1978;96:163–165.

12
Prevention of Cardioembolic Stroke

David G. Sherman

It is a necessary oversimplification to emphasize that treatment decisions about a disorder are based on knowledge of its cause. This is true in stroke as in other conditions. In applying this principle to cardioembolic stroke, one must deal with several difficult clinical problems. Does the patient have a cardiac disorder that may cause a stroke via embolic mechanisms, and so be treated in an attempt to prevent the first stroke? What are the risks of treatment compared to the potential benefits? Does the patient have a cardiac disorder that could have caused the stroke? Does the patient have noncardiac potential causes for his or her stroke? Is there any way to determine which of multiple possible stroke mechanisms actually caused the stroke? If a patient suffers a cardioembolic stroke, when should treatment to prevent a recurrence begin? One of these clinical questions arises in most patients with ischemic stroke. This chapter attempts to summarize the current state of information relative to the issue of cardiac disorders and the production of embolic stroke.

Incidence/Prevalence

About 15% of all ischemic strokes are attributed to an embolus arising from the heart.[1] The importance of cardiogenic embolus may be much greater when one considers that a number of strokes are classed as of "undetermined" etiology. The Stroke Data Bank found that one third of their 1805 patients had to be classified as "infarct, unknown."[2]

About 30% of patients with an ischemic stroke have evidence of heart disease, and one third of these have atherosclerotic cerebrovascular disease sufficient to have produced the stroke.

Pathophysiology

Stasis of blood and endothelial disruption are the basic cardiac substrates for thrombus formation within the heart. In atrial fibrillation and cardiomyopathy, stasis is the predominant pathophysiology. With an acute anterior transmural myocardial infarction or a prosthetic valve, thrombosis over a damaged or nonendothelialized surface leads to thrombus, which may then embolize to the brain or elsewhere. In many patients both stasis and endothelial disruption are present, with thrombus formation further promoted by the presence of a "prothrombotic" state. Of patients dying of heart disease, one third have antemortem mural thrombi within the heart.[3] About half of patients with heart disease have an associated cerebral infarction. Forty-four percent of these have a history compatible with a stroke. There is little difference among the various types of heart disease with respect to the frequency of associated stroke.[4] Embolic material occluding a brain artery may be demonstrated pathologically, although the artery may also be unobstructed, presumably as a result of spontaneous lysis of the embolus. The brain infarction is microscopically or grossly hemorrhagic in about 65% of these cases at autopsy.[5]

Characteristics of Cardioembolic Stroke

Sudden onset of a neurologic deficit and loss of consciousness at onset are the only clinical features that distinguished a cardiac embolic stroke from other types of ischemic stroke. Specifically, no diagnostic value has been consistently noted with such traditional features as activity at onset, seizure at onset, headache, vomiting, or the presence of an isolated deficit.[6] In one series 15% of patients with an atherosclerotic cause for their first stroke had a sudden onset with maximal initial deficit, whereas 40% of patients with a presumed cardiac source of embolus had this type of onset.[7]

Transient ischemic attacks (TIA) are traditionally considered to be indicative of arterial disease rather than a cardiac embolic etiology. Bogousslavsky et al. found that 23% of 250 patients with carotid distribution TIAs had a potential cardiac source of emboli. One third of patients with TIA had known heart disease. Six percent had only a potential cardiac source of emboli, and 19% had both a cardiac and appropriate carotid lesion. Thirteen percent of the patients had neither an arterial nor a cardiac cause for their TIA.[8] While there is a tendency for TIAs of arterial origin to be of < 15 minutes duration and multiple rather than single, these features by no means exclude a cardiac cause for TIA.[8]

TIAs in the distribution of the posterior branches of the middle cerebral artery (MCA) were both longer, > 45 minutes, and more likely to be associated with a subsequent stroke due to a cardiogenic embolus than were TIAs affecting the anterior branches of the MCA.[9] Small strokes and TIAs more likely arise from a valvular or left ventricular source of emboli, whereas strokes occurring in patients with atrial fibrillation from left atrial thrombi tend to be large. About 50% of embolic strokes are associated with atrial fibrillation. In a series of 250 patients with carotid territory TIAs, only 5.6% had associated atrial fibrillation.

Cardiogenic emboli may lodge in any brain artery but are particularly common as the cause of occlusion of some vessels. More than 70% of cardiogenic emboli lodge in the MCA territory.[10] More cardiogenic causes of infarcts occur in the posterior branches of the MCA, 34% overall, than in the anterior branches, 19%. Isolated Wernicke's aphasia with or without right hemianopia and acute confusional state with left hemianopia were neurological syndromes of the temporal branches of the MCA that were particularly suggestive of an embolic source.[9]

In a study of 35 patients with occipital infarcts, 10 had a cardiac source of embolism and 11 had clinical and/or angiographic evidence to warrant the diagnosis of "unknown source of embolism." Thus 60% (21/35) of these patients with posterior cerebral artery territory ischemia had a presumed or established embolic mechanism.[11] Fisher found that 95% (43/47) of cases of distal, "top of the basilar" occlusion were due to cardiogenic emboli. One half of the patients with more distal posterior cerebral artery occlusion were believed to have their occlusion on the basis of an embolus.[12]

Subcortical lacunar infarcts in the territory of the small deep perforating arteries were evaluated in 100 patients. In 42 patients the cause of the infarct was felt to be small vessel disease. Thirty-six patients had at least one source of embolus. Twenty-seven had carotid artery stenosis or occlusion, and 17 had a cardiac source of embolus.[13] Thus no artery, no brain region, and no stroke syndrome is immune from a cardiogenic embolus.

Ambiguity in Diagnosis

Unfortunately, all too often a patient with a suspected cardioembolic stroke either has, in addition to a potential cardiac cause, cerebral atherosclerosis or has no cardiac or arterial pathology to explain the stroke. Ramirez-Lassepas found that 21% of patients with a potential cardiac source of brain embolus also had an arterial lesion that could have caused their stroke. In addition, 25% of patients with a suspected embolic stroke had neither a cardiac nor an arterial source of embolus.[6]

Computerized Tomography in Cardioembolic Stroke

Brain imaging studies such as computerized tomography (CT) or magnetic resonance imaging (MRI) scan may reveal suggestive evidence of a cardiogenic embolus such as infarction in other vascular cortical territories or occasionally visualization of embolic material within the middle cerebral or posterior cerebral artery. Hemorrhagic infarction (HI) is particularly suggestive of embolic stroke. The presumed mechanism for this phenomenon is fragmentation and distal migration of an embolus with reperfusion of ischemic and infarcted brain. This reperfusion may result in leakage of blood across ischemic damaged vascular endothelium, producing varying degrees of hemorrhagic infarction seen best pathologically but also by CT or MRI scan. Overall, about 20% of cardioembolic strokes will show hemorrhagic infarction by CT at 2 to 4 days. Hemorrhagic infarcts are more frequent with large strokes, and the anticoagulated patient is more likely to experience clinical worsening with hemorrhagic transformation.

One hundred sixty patients with a cardiogenic cerebral embolism underwent serial CT scanning. Sixty-five (40.6%) demonstrated HI within 1 month. Thirty-seven (57%) of these HIs were petechial hemorrhages, 12 (18.5%) had diffuse hemorrhages, 9 (14%) had small hemorrhages, and 7 (10%) had massive hematomas. Thus 28 (17.5%) had HIs other than petechial hemorrhage. Large infarcts, those with an infarct index of >30%, had a higher incidence of HI than those infarcts with infarct indexes of <9%. Patients over the age of 70 were at greater risk for HI (31 of 61, 50.8%) than patients <49 years old (7 of 25, 25.9%).[10]

Angiographic Features of Cardioembolic Stroke

Cerebral angiography may be of value in establishing the cause of stroke as cardioembolic. Single or multiple arterial occlusions in the absence of arterial pathology is the most characteristic feature. One is more likely to demonstrate these occlusions with early than late angiography because of the spontaneous lysis of emboli. Of 88 patients who had cerebral emboli and cerebral angiography, 33 (38%) had ipsilateral atherosclerotic carotid artery disease. Thirty-eight of the 52 (73%) angiograms done within the first 2 days of an embolic stroke demonstrated an embolic occlusion, whereas only 8 or 29 (28%) of studies done after the second day showed an embolic occlusion.[14] In another study one hundred forty-two patients with a cerebral

embolism underwent cerebral angiography at a median of 1.5 days. Complete occlusion of a cerebral artery was noted in 117 (82%) of the patients. Angiography was repeated in a median of 20 days in 59 patients, with 56 (95%) showing reopening.[10]

Cardiac Evaluation of Possible Cardioembolic Stroke

Echocardiography, electrocardiograms (ECG), and other forms of prolonged rhythm monitoring are currently the most readily available means of searching for a potential cardiac source of emboli. About 10% (range 4 to 16%) of patients with ischemic stroke will be found to have a potential cardiac source of embolus by echocardiography.[8,15-23] Most of these patients have obvious historical, physical examination, ECG, or chest X-ray evidence of cardiac disease. The yield of echocardiography in patients without the clinical heart disease is about 1.5% (range 0 to 6%).[16,17,22,24] Despite this low yield in patients without clinically obvious heart disease, young stroke patients without evidence of cerebrovascular disease should have cardiac sources vigorously pursued. Transient arrhythmias, such as atrial fibrillation and sick sinus syndrome, may be detected with prolonged ECG monitoring via telemetry or Holter monitoring with a fairly low yield, i.e., 2% (range 0 to 4%) of arrhythmias identified in these patients.[8,16,22] Standard 2D and M mode echocardiography have the additional problem of identifying common cardiac abnormalities, such as mitral valve prolapse, that may or may not be related to a patient's cerebral ischemia. Echocardiography is relatively insensitive in the detection of atrial and small intraventricular thrombi. Potentially more sensitive techniques of cardiac imaging include ultrafast CT[24-27] or MRI of the heart,[28] transesophageal echocardiography,[29-31] and isotope-labeled platelet scintigraphy.[32]

Causes of Cardioembolic Stroke: Overview

A great number of cardiac disorders may be the source of a cardiogenic embolus to the brain or systemic circulation.[33] The risk of embolization is well established in some, with clearly outlined forms of management. Unfortunately, the management of many disorders is not based on the results of well-designed clinical trials but must be left to the physician's best judgment.

Atrial Fibrillation

Atrial fibrillation (AF) is the most common dysrhythmia in the general population. Three percent of the population over the age of 65 have AF. The prevalence increases dramatically with increasing age in the elderly, with 13% of 82-year-olds having AF.[34] Population studies have consistently shown a fivefold or greater increased risk of stroke attributable to nonvalvular atrial fibrillation.[35-38] The most common coexistent cardiovascular conditions are hypertension and ischemic heart disease. The frequency of rheumatic heart disease has progressively declined until now only about 10% of patients with AF have rheumatic heart disease as the basis for their dysrhythmia. This group, however, has the greatest risk of stroke, with a 17-fold increase over comparable individuals without rheumatic valvular disease and AF.

Nonvalvular Atrial Fibrillation

Atrial fibrillation, predominantly nonvalvular AF, is the most common cardiac disorder responsible for a cardiogenic brain embolus. Nonvalvular AF is present in 6 to 24% of all ischemic strokes and accounts for 45% of all cardioembolic strokes.[33] Clinical and autopsy studies suggest that about two thirds of ischemic strokes occurring in patients with AF are cardioembolic, while the remaining third are due to large artery atherosclerosis or small arterial disease. The large population of people with AF is quite heterogeneous and undoubtedly contains subpopulations with greater and lesser stroke risk. Many physicians feel that older patients with the recent onset of sustained AF are at increased risk. Congestive heart failure seems to increase the risk of embolus. A prior stroke, embolus, or "silent" stroke on CT scan may identify a high-risk population. Several echocardiographic features, such as left atrial size, ventricular function, and the presence of atrial thrombi or mitral regurgitation, are deemed by some to identify the patient at greatest risk for stroke. It is likely that some of these features will eventually be shown to

be of prognostic value; however, at present their importance awaits appropriate clinical studies. A group of 110 elderly patients, mean age 82 years, with atrial fibrillation were analyzed for features that differentiated those with stroke (44%) and those without. Significant factors included rheumatic mitral stenosis, prior myocardial infarction, systemic hypertension, left atrial enlargement, and left ventricular hypertrophy.[34]

"Silent" and multiple strokes are common in patients with atrial fibrillation. Fifty-four of 230 (23%) patients with NVAF and an ischemic stroke had a previous stroke, and nineteen percent (38 of 194) had multiple infarcts noted on their CT scan. Nineteen percent of those evaluated for carotid artery disease (148) had atherosclerosis causing a high-grade stenosis or occlusion of a carotid or vertebral artery.[39]

In addition to the adverse effects of emboli from the left atrium to the brain, some investigators have postulated that reduction in cerebral blood flow may contribute to brain symptoms. Boysen et al. evaluated cerebral blood flow before and after cardioversion for AF. Nine patients showed a significant increase in CBF from 36 before to 40.7 the day after and 45.2 30 days after cardioversion. This increase was noted without changes in blood pressure, heart rate, or cardiac output.[39]

Lone Atrial Fibrillation

"Lone" atrial fibrillation is the term used to describe the arrhythmia present in predominantly young men without clinical, ECG, or chest radiograph evidence of heart disease. Such patients <60 years of age have a stroke risk of <0.5%/y.[37,40,41] The Framingham study reported a higher stroke risk (2.6%/y); however, the mean age of their patients was 70 years, and one third were hypertensive.[42]

Atrial Fibrillation and Thyrotoxicosis

About 15% of patients with thyrotoxicosis develop AF.[43] Patients older than 60 are more likely to develop AF in association with thyrotoxicosis than are younger patients. Less than half of these patients over 60 years of age will convert to sinus rhythm when their thyrotoxicosis is treated successfully, whereas most all of the younger patients will revert to sinus rhythm. Petersen et al. compared the stroke and TIA risk in 91 thyrotoxic patients to 519 patients without atrial fibrillation.[43] Thirteen percent of the patients with AF developed stroke (8) or TIA (4), whereas 3% of those in sinus rhythm experienced a stroke (5) or TIA (10). This apparent excess risk in patients with AF was much less impressive when the highly significant variable of increased age was taken into consideration.

Anticoagulation in Nonvalvular Atrial Fibrillation

The efficacy and safety of anticoagulation or aspirin for the prevention of stroke in patients with AF is currently being evaluated in a number of large clinical trials. One study has reported the results of a randomized trial of 1007 patients with chronic atrial fibrillation who had a mean age of 74.5 years. These patients were randomized to warfarin with an International Normalized Ratio (INR) of 2.8 to 4.2, aspirin 75 mg/d, or placebo. The study reported a significant reduction in TIAs and strokes in the warfarin-treated group. There were two major bleeds in the warfarin group and one in the aspirin group. There was a fairly high dropout rate (38%) in the warfarin group, emphasizing the difficulty of keeping a group of elderly patients on chronic warfarin therapy.[44] The Stroke Prevention in Atrial Fibrillation (SPAF) study reported an 81% reduction in stroke or systemic embolism in the 393 patients who received warfarin or aspirin (325 mg/d) compared to the 195 patients receiving placebo. There was a 49% reduction in primary events in all patients receiving aspirin (517) compared to placebo (528). The relative benefits of aspirin and warfarin are being studied in a continuation of this multicenter clinical trial.[45]

Ischemic Heart Disease

Acute Myocardial Infarction

Following an acute myocardial infarction (MI), the ventricular wall may lose its ability to contract normally; this condition, combined with the thrombogenic potential of an ischemic endocardial surface, can lead to mural thrombus formation. Anterior MIs are accompanied by a 30 to 40% prevalence of ventricular mural thrombi.[46-61]

Inferior and subendocardial MIs are much less likely to develop overlying mural thrombi and associated brain embolism. Thus it is the large, transmural anterior MI that carries the greatest risk of mural thrombus formation and embolization. Stroke complicates about 6% of anterior MIs but only about 1% of inferior MIs. The practical management question relates to which acute MI patients should be anticoagulated. Early studies of anticoagulation in all types of MI showed that the risk of embolism was reduced from 2.9% to 1.2%.[33,61] This reduction, however, was offset by an equal increase in serious bleeding complications. Thus the practice of anticoagulating all acute MIs was abandoned.

Patients most likely to benefit from anticoagulation are those with anterior MIs and dyskinetic ventricular wall with overlying mural thrombus. The management dilemma here is which of the patients with anterior MI will develop mural thrombi and when? Two-dimensional echocardiography is relatively sensitive in the detection of ventricular wall abnormalities and mural thrombi but may still miss small (<5mm) thrombi. In addition, the timing of the development of mural thrombi is such that the majority form within the first 7 days following an MI, but others continue to form in subsequent days and weeks. Therefore, if one is attempting to identify and anticoagulate only those patients with acute anterior MIs who develop mural thrombi, it may be necessary to repeat 2-D echocardiograms frequently within the first couple of weeks. While this may save some patients the added risk of anticoagulation, one may increase the costs by repeated echocardiograms by waiting until mural thrombi are visualized, and so expose those patients with mural thrombi to an increased risk of embolism until anticoagulation is initiated. Turpie et al.[62] showed in a randomized comparison of 5000 U versus 12 500 U of heparin twice daily in patients with acute anterior MI that the frequency of mural thrombus was reduced from 32% to 11% with the higher dose of heparin.

The management approach adopted by many is to anticoagulate immediately all patients with anterior MIs who do not have contraindications and only maintain long-term oral anticoagulation in those with demonstrated ventricular wall motion abnormalities.

Ventricular Aneurysm

In the months that follow an acute MI, the injured myocardial wall may form a ventricular aneurysm with or without associated mural thrombus. The risk of embolization is roughly 13% over the first year, with a wide range reported (0 to 60%).[46,52-54,59,62,63] A number of factors no doubt accounts for this wide range of embolic risk. Pedunculated, mobile, or heterogenous thrombi are more apt to embolize than flat, homogenous thrombi. Emboli occur soon after thrombus formation, and before it has become organized and adherent. Associated congestive heart failure or atrial fibrillation may identify a patient at increased risk of thrombus formation and emboli.

There are limited data about the long-term (beyond 4 to 6 months) risk of emboli and the risks and benefits of long-term anticoagulation. As in acute MI, anticoagulation of late mural thrombi reduces by about two thirds the occurrence of ventricular mural thrombi. Current practices vary widely, but generally, patients with suspected emboli are anticoagulated. Patients with ventricular aneurysms and mural thrombi are assessed, and the decision to anticoagulate is based on the patient's perceived risk from anticoagulation and the nature of the ventricle, thrombus, and associated cardiac symptoms and signs.

Nonischemic cardiomyopathy can be complicated by embolism.[64-66] As the myocardium fails, contractility decreases, congestive heart failure worsens, and intracardiac thrombi form. Thrombi visualized by echocardiography have been demonstrated in from 0 to 37% of patients with nonischemic cardiomyopathy. The risk of emboli is about 4%/y, with again a range of low to much higher risk perceived as a function of the severity of the cardiomyopathy. Most patients with severe cardiomyopathy should be treated with chronic anticoagulation.

Mitral Valve Prolapse

Emboli may originate from the valve in mitral value prolapse (MV).[67,68] Mitral value prolapse is, however, common in the general population, where it can be detected in 5% of the individuals and is especially frequent in young women. While emboli may occur in this group of individuals, they must be uncommon and are generally transient ischemic events reflecting the small size of emboli arising from this valvular anomaly. There does seem to be a subset of patients at greater risk who are older, more often men with myxomatous changes of the valve leaflets, chordae, and annulus.[69,70] They are generally given antiplatelet agents, whereas prophylactic antithrombotic therapy does not seem warranted in the group of young women without myxomatous valve changes. If MVP is discovered in a patient with TIA or stroke, other possible stroke mechanisms should still be pursued and also the possibility should be considered that the MVP is complicated by infective endocarditis or atrial fibrillation.

Prosthetic Cardiac Valves

Prosthetic cardiac valves are a potential source of emboli.[71] The greatest risk of emboli is with a mechanical valve in the mitral position. These patients need long-term anticoagulants, and if emboli occur, more intensive anticoagulation 2.0 to 2.5 times control prothrombin time and possibly the addition of dipyridamole are indicated. Patients with bioprosthetic valves are generally anticoagulated for the first few months and thereafter treated with antiplatelet agents.

Valvular Heart Disease

Embolism is a complication of mitral stenosis in about 20% of unanticoagulated patients.[72] The development of atrial fibrillation in a patient with mitral stenosis is accompanied by a dramatic 18-fold increase in a patient's risk of embolism. Recurrent embolism occurs in 30 to 75% of patients suffering an embolus. Prophylactic anticoagulation is indicated in many patients with mitral stenosis, especially those with atrial fibrillation.

Paradoxical Embolism

There has been much recent interest in searching for a mechanism for paradoxical embolism in patients with unexplained stroke. Contrast, color Doppler, and transesophageal echocardiography detect a 10 to 18% prevalence of physiologic shunting via a patent foramen ovale in normal people.[73-76] The other route for a paradoxical embolus is a pulmonary arteriovenous fistula. The most characteristic picture is the onset of stroke during a Valsalva maneuver in a patient with deep venous thrombophlebitis. A right-to-left shunt should be sought in a patient with unexplained stroke, however, if a patent foramen ovale is found, especially in the absence of venous, pulmonary, or right heart thrombi. However, a moderate skepticism should be maintained in light of the high prevalence in the general population.

Infective Endocarditis

Fifteen to 20% of patients with infective endocarditis experience an embolic stroke.[77-79] The embolic stroke may occur at any time but is most frequent early in the illness before effective antibiotic therapy is instituted. Staphylococcus aureus endocarditis seems to carry an increased risk of stroke. The risks of brain hemorrhage are such that anticoagulation is not recommended with native valve endocarditis, but with a mechanical prosthetic valve and endocarditis, however, the risk of embolization is so great that anticoagulants should be continued.

Overview of Primary Prevention

Table 12.1 summarizes the current ideas and uncertainties about the management of the most frequently encountered cardiac disorders.

Treatment of Acute Cardioembolic Stroke

Whether and when anticoagulation should be used are common questions arising when a patient has just experienced a cardioembolic stroke. The question of anticoagulation depends on the risk of recurrence; the higher the risk of recurrence, the greater the need for anticoagulation. Reports of recurrence vary widely from 0 to 22% within the first 2 weeks, with an average recurrence rate of about 12%.[33] The next question is: Is anticoagulation effective in reducing recurrence? The limited studies available suggest that anticoagulation is effective but cannot be expected to eliminate all recurrences. The recurrence rate is reduced by about two thirds from 12% to 4%.

The final question is: what is the risk of bleeding with anticoagulation? Without anticoagulation

TABLE 12.1. Cardioembolic disorders: relative risk.

High risk (>6%/y)	Management
Atrial myxoma	Surgery
Infective staph. endocarditis, mechanical PV	AC(H), antibiotics
Nonischemic cardiomyopathy + thrombus	AC(H)
Mechanical prosthetic mitral valve	AC(H)
Recent cardioembolic stroke/systemic embolus	AC(H)
Mitral stenosis with atrial fibrillation	AC(L)
Large anterior MI with thrombus	AC(L)
Intermediate or undetermined risk	
Ventricular aneurysm	?,AC(L)
Mitral stenosis without atrial fibrillation	AC(L)
Nonvalvular atrial fibrillation	ASA,AC(L)
Mitral regurgitation	–
Thyrotoxicosis with atrial fibrillation	AC(L)
Mitral valve prolapse + myxomatous changes	ASA
Nonbacterial thrombotic endocarditis	ASA,AC(L)?
Low risk (<1%/y)	
Mitral valve prolapse young women	–
Lone atrial fibrillation <60 y/o	–
Small inferior MI	–
Bioprosthetic aortic valve	ASA
Mitral annulus calcification	–

AC = anticoagulation; (H) = high dose (prothrombin time 1.5–2.0 X); (L) = low dose (prothrombin time 1.3–1.5 X); ASA = aspirin; MI = myocardial infarction.

about 1% of patients with an ischemic stroke will experience a brain hemorrhage, and with anticoagulation this risk increases to 5%. This increased risk of brain hemorrhage has prompted many physicians to withhold or delay anticoagulation in patients with a recent cardiogenic embolus. Rather than withhold anticoagulation from all patients with a cardiogenic stroke, it seems more reasonable to withhold these drugs from only those patients at the greatest risk of brain hemorrhage. Fifteen to 20% of all patients with a cardiogenic brain embolus will develop an HI.[80-87] Most of these are not associated with clinical deterioration, and the severity ranges from petechial hemorrhages (only seen pathologically) to those appearing homogeneous or hyperdense on CT scan, to the large symptomatic hematomas. There is rarely any evidence of HI on a CT scan done within the first 6 hours. On the other hand, by 48 hours 85% of embolic infarcts that are destined to undergo hemorrhagic transformation will have done so. Thus the first recommendation regarding anticoagulation is that patients with a suspected cardiogenic embolus should not be anticoagulated until a CT or MRI scan done 36 to 48 hours following stroke onset has shown no evidence of hemorrhagic infarction. The other important observation is that the patient at greatest risk for hemorrhagic transformation has the largest infarction. From this observation arises the second recommendation, namely, that patients with large embolic infarctions not be anticoagulated immediately but rather have anticoagulation delayed for 10 to 14 days. The other precautions concerning anticoagulation are to avoid bolus heparin dosing and delay or avoid anticoagulants in patients with persistently elevated blood pressure.

Summary

Stroke of cardioembolic origin is responsible for about 15% of all ischemic strokes. Cardioembolic stroke is underestimated because of the frequent coexistence of other potential stroke mechanisms. In addition, clinical features such as the nature of the stroke onset or the vascular territory involved are not highly specific for a cardioembolic mechanism. An exhaustive cardiac workup should be reserved for patients with evidence of heart disease on bedside examination or ECG and for those with unexplained cause of stroke.

The most frequent cardiac disorders causing cardioembolic stroke are atrial fibrillation with or without mitral stenosis, ischemic heart disease, and prosthetic cardiac valves. Some uncommon disorders such as infective endocarditis or atrial myxoma have a high prevalence of embolism. Other conditions such as MVP and patent foramen ovale are so common in the general population that it is often difficult to decide whether their presence is causally related to the stroke. Following a cardioembolic stroke, anticoagulation should be considered to reduce the risk of recurrent stroke. Because of the evolution of hemorrhagic transformation in 15 to 20% of embolic strokes, anticoagulation should be delayed until a CT scan done 36 to 48 hours from stroke onset has established that the patient does not have a hemorrhagic infarct. This also applies to patients with large infarcts or persistent hypertension.

References

1. Easton JD, Sherman DG. Progress in cerebrovascular disease. *Stroke.* 1980;11:433–441.
2. Foulkes MA, Wolf PA, Price TR, et al. The stroke data bank: design, methods, and baseline characteristics. *Stroke.* 1988;19:547–554.
3. Garvin CF. Mural thrombi in the heart. *Am Heart J.* 1941;21:713–720.
4. Vost A, Wolochow DA, Howell DA. Incidence of infarcts of the brain in heart disease. *J Pathol Bacteriol.* 1964;88:463–470.
5. Adams RD, Vander Eecken HM. Vascular diseases of the brain *Ann Rev Med.* 1953;4:213–252.
6. Ramirez-Lassepas M, Cipolle RJ, Bjork RJ, et al. Can embolic stroke be diagnosed on the basis of neurologic clinical criteria? *Arch Neurol.* 1987;44: 87–89.
7. Bogousslavsky J, Hachinski VC, Boughner DR, et al. Cardiac and arterial lesions in carotid transient ischemic attacks. *Arch Neurol.* 1986;43:223–228.
8. Bogousslavsky J, Van Melle FE, Regli F. The Lausanne stroke registry: analysis of 1,000 consecutive patients with first stroke. *Stroke.* 1988;19: 1083–1092.
9. Bogousslavsky J, Van Melle G, Regli F. Middle cerebral artery pial territory infarcts: a study of the Lausanne stroke registry. *Ann Neurol.* 1989;555–560.
10. Okada Y, Yamaguchi T, Minematsu K, et al. Hemorrhagic transformation in cerebral embolism. *Stroke.* 1989;20:598–603.
11. Pessin MS, Lathi ES, Cohen MB, et al. Clinical features and mechanism of occipital infarction. *Ann Neurol.* 1987;21:290–299.
12. Fisher CM. The posterior cerebral artery syndrome. *Can J Neurol Sci.* 1986;13:232–239.
13. Ghika J, Bogousslavky J, Regli F. Small deep infarct: a study of embolic sources. *Stroke.* 1989;20:158. Abstract.
14. Mohr JP, Caplan LR, Melski JW, et al. The Harvard cooperative stroke registry: a prospective registry. *Neurology.* 1978;28:754–762.
15. Biller J, Johnson MR, Adams HP, et al. Echocardiographic evaluation of young adults with nonhemorrhagic cerebral infarction. *Stroke.* 1986;17: 608–612.
16. Come PC, Riley MF, Bivas NK. Roles of echocardiography and arrhythmia monitoring in the evaluation of patients with suspected systemic embolism. *Ann Neurol.* 1983;13:527–531.
17. Fogelholm R, Melin J. Echocardiography in ischaemic cerebrovascular disease. *Brit Med J.* 1987;295:305–306.

18. Gagliardi R, Benvenuti L, Frosini F, et al. Frequency of echocardiographic abnormalities in patients with ischemia of the carotid territory—a preliminary report. *Stroke*. 1985;16:118–120.

19. Good DC, Frank S, Verhulst S, et al. Cardiac abnormalities in stroke patients with negative arteriograms. *Stroke*. 1986;17:6–11.

20. Nishide M, Irino T, Gotoh M, et al. Cardiac abnormalities in ischemic cerebrovascular disease studied by two-dimensional echocardiography. *Stroke*. 1983;14:541–545.

21. Rem JA, Hachinski VC, Boughner DR, et al. Value of cardiac monitoring and echocardiography in TIA and stroke patients. *Stroke*. 1985;16:950–956.

22. Robbins JA, Sagar KB, French M, et al. Influence of echocardiography on management of patients with systemic emboli. *Stroke*. 1988;14:546–549.

23. Todnem K, Vik-Mo H. Cerebral ischemic attacks as a complication of heart disease: the value of echocardiography. *Acta Neurol Scand*. 1986;74:323–327.

24. Foster CJ, Sekiya T, Love HG, et al. Identification of intracardiac thrombus: comparison of computed tomography and cross-sectional echocardiography. *Br J Radiol*. 1987;60:327–331.

25. Goldstein JA, Schiller NB, Lipton MJ, et al. Evaluation of left ventricular thrombi by contrast-enhanced computed tomography and two-dimensional echocardiography. *Am J Cardiol*. 1986;57:757–760.

26. Helgason CM, Chomka EV, Rich S, et al. Ultrafast cardiac CT scanning in stroke. *Stroke*. 1987;18:283. Abstract.

27. Masuda Y, Morooka N, Yoshida H, et al. Noninvasive diagnosis of thrombus in the heart and large vessels—usefulness of two dimensional echocardiography and X-ray CT. *Japanese Circ J*. 1984;48:83–89.

28. Gomes AS, Lois JF, Child JS, et al. Cardiac tumors and thrombus: evaluation with MR imaging. *AJR*. 1987;149:895–899.

29. Aschenberg W, Schluter M, Kremer P, et al. Transesophageal two-dimensional echocardiography for detection of left atrial appendage thrombus. *J Am Coll Card*. 1986;7:163–166.

30. Zenker G, Erbel R, Kramer G, et al. Transesophageal two-dimensional echocardiography in young patients with cerebral ischemic events. *Stroke*. 1988;19:345–348.

31. Seward JB, Khandheria BK, Oh JK, et al. Transesophageal echocardiography: technique, anatomic correlations, implementation, and clinical applications. *Mayo Clinic Proc*. 1988;63:649–660.

32. Kessler C, Henningsen H, Reuther R, et al. Identification of intracardiac thrombi in stroke patients with indium-111 platelet scintigraphy. *Stroke*. 1987;18:63–67.

33. Cerebral Embolism Task Force. Cardiogenic brain embolism: the second report of the cerebral embolism task force. *Arch Neurol*. 1989;46:727–743.

34. Aronow WS, Gutstein H, Fsieh FY. Risk factors for thromboembolic stroke in elderly patients with chronic atrial fibrillation. *Am J Cardiol*. 1989;63:366–367.

35. Flegel KM, Shipley MJ, Rose G. Risk of stroke in nonrheumatic atrial fibrillation. *Lancet*. 1987;1:526–529.

36. Tanaka H, Hayashi M, Date C, et al. Epidemiologic studies of stroke in Shibata, a Japanese provincial city: preliminary report on risk factors for cerebral infarction. *Stroke*. 1985;16:773–780.

37. Onundarson PT, Thorgeirsson G, Jonmundsen E, et al. Chronic atrial fibrillation—epidemiologic features and 14 year follow-up: a case-control study. *Eur Heart J*. 1987;8:521–527.

38. Wolf PA, Dawber TR, Thomas HE, et al. Epidemiologic assessment of chronic atrial fibrillation and risk of stroke: the Framingham Study. *Neurology*. 1978;28:973–977.

39. Boysen G, Petersen P, Kastrup J, et al. Cerebral blood flow during chronic atrial fibrillation and after conversion to sinus rhythm. *J Cerebral Blood Flow Metab*. 1989;9(suppl 1):S365.

40. Kopecky SL, Gerah BJ, McGoon MD, et al. The natural history of lone atrial fibrillation. *N Engl J Med*. 1987;317:669–674.

41. Close JB, Evans DW, Bailey SM. Persistent lone atrial fibrillation—its prognosis after clinical diagnosis. *J R Coll Gen Practitioners*. 1979;29:547–549.

42. Brand FN, Abbott RD, Kannel WB, et al. Characteristics and prognosis of lone atrial fibrillation. *JAMA*. 1985;254:3449–3453.

43. Petersen P, Hansen JM. Stroke in thyrotoxicosis with atrial fibrillation. *Stroke*. 1988;19:15–18.

44. Peterson P, Godtfredsen J, Boysen G, et al. Placebo-controlled, randomized trial of warfarin and aspirin for prevention of thromboembolic complications in chronic atrial fibrillation. The Copenhagen AFASAK Study. *Lancet*. 1989;1:175–179.

45. The Stroke Prevention in Atrial Fibrillation Investigators. Preliminary report of the Stroke Prevention in Atrial Fibrillation Study. *N Engl J Med*. 1990;322:863–868.

46. Johannessen KA, Nordrehaug JE, von der Lippe G, et al. Risk factors for embolization in patients with left ventricular thrombi and acute myocardial infarction. *Br Heart J*. 1988;60:104–110.

47. Johannessen KA, Nordehaug JE, von der Lippe G. Left ventricular thrombosis and cerebrovascular accident in acute myocardial infarction. *Br Heart J*. 1984;51:553–556.

48. Nordrehaug JE, Johannessen KA, von der Lippe G. Usefulness of high-dose anticoagulants in preventing left ventricular thrombus in acute myocardial infarction. *Am J Cardiol*. 1985;55:1491–1493.

49. Arvan S, Boscha K. Prophylactic anticoagulation for left ventricular thrombi after acute myocardial infarction: a prospective randomized trial. *Am Heart J*. 1987;113:688–693.

50. Domenicucci S, Bellotti P, Chiarella F, et al. Spontaneous morphologic changes in left ventricular thrombi: a prospective two-dimensional echocardiographic study. *Circulation*. 1987;75:737–743.

51. Gueret P, Dubourg O, Ferrier A, et al. Effects of full-dose heparin on the development of left ventricular thrombosis in acute transmural myocardial infarction. *J Am Coll Cardiol*. 1986;8:419–426.

52. Visser CA, Kan G, Meltzer RS, et al. Long-term follow-up of left ventricular thrombus after acute myocardial infarction. *Chest*. 1984;86:532–536.

53. Keating EC, Gross SA, Schlamowitz RA, et al. Mural thrombi in myocardial infarction. Prospective evaluation by two-dimensional echocardiography. *Am J Med*. 1983;74:989–995.

54. Asinger RW, Mikell FL, Elsperger J, et al. Incidence of left ventricular thrombosis after acute transmural myocardial infarction. *N Engl J Med*. 1981;305:297–302.

55. Friedman MJ, Carlson K, Marcus FI, et al. Clinical correlations in patients with acute myocardial infarction and left ventricular thrombus detected by two-dimensional echocardiography. *Am J Med*. 1982;72:894–898.

56. Bhatnagar SK, Hudak A, Al-Yusuf AR. Left ventricular thrombosis, wall motion abnormalities, and blood viscosity changes after first transmural anterior myocardial infarction. *Chest*. 1985;88:40–44.

57. Visser CA, Kan G, Meltzer RS, et al. Echocardiography to evaluate postinfarction left ventricular thrombi. *Clin Cardiol*. 1986;3:62.

58. Spirito P, Bellotti P, Chiarella F, et al. Prognostic significance and natural history of left ventricular thrombi in patients with acute anterior myocardial infarction: a two-dimensional echocardiographic study. *Circulation*. 1985;72:774–778.

59. Visser CA, Kan G, Meltzer RS, et al. Embolic potential of left ventricular thrombus after myocardial infarction: a two-dimensional echocardiographic study of 119 patients. *J Am Coll Card*. 1985;5:1276–1280.

60. Tramarin R, Pozzoli M, Febo O, et al. Two-dimensional echocardiographic assessment of anticoagulant therapy in left ventricular thrombosis early after acute myocardial infarction. *European Heart J*. 1986;7:482–492.

61. Chesebro JH, Ezekowitz MD, Badimon L, et al. Intracardiac thrombi and systemic thromboembolism: Detection, incidence and treatment. *Ann Rev Med*. 1985;36:579–605.

62. Turpie AGG, Robinson JG, Doyle DJ, et al. Comparison of high-dose with low-dose subcutaneous heparin to prevent left ventricular mural thrombosis in patients with acute transmural anterior myocardial infarction. *N Engl J Med*. 1989;320:352–357.

63. Weinreich DJ, Burke JF, Pauletto FJ. Left ventricular mural thrombi complicating acute myocardial infarction. Long-term follow-up with serial echocardiography. *Ann Int Med*. 1984;100:789–794.

64. Tobin R, Slutsky RA, Higgins CB. Serial echocardiograms in patients with congestive cardiomyopathies: lack of evidence for thrombus formation. *Clin Cardiol*. 1984;7:99–101.

65. Gottdiener JS, Gay JA, VanVoorhees L, et al. Frequency and embolic potential of left ventricular thrombus in dilated cardiomyopathy: assessment by two-dimensional echocardiography. *Am J Cardiol*. 1983;52:1281–1285.

66. Fuster V, Gersh BJ, Giuliani ER, et al. The natural history of idiopathic dilated cardiomyopathy. *Am J Cardiol*. 1981;47:525–531.

67. Wolf PA, Sila CA. Cerebral ischemia with mitral valve prolapse. *Am Heart J*. 1987;113:1308–1315.

68. Jackson AC. Neurologic disorders associated with mitral valve prolapse. *Can J Neurol Sci*. 1986;13:15–20.

69. Devereux RB, Hawkins I, Kramer-Fox R, et al. Complications of mitral valve prolapse. *Am J Med*. 1986;81:751–758.

70. Baddour LM, Bisno AL. Infective endocarditis complicating mitral valve prolapse: Epidemiologic, clinical and microbiologic aspects. *Reviews of Infect Dis*. 1986;8:117–136.

71. Stein PD, Kantrowitz A. Antithrombotic therapy in mechanical and biological prosthetic heart valves and saphenous vein bypass grafts. *Chest*. 1988;(suppl)95:107S–117S.

72. Levine HJ, Pauker SG, Salzman EW. Antithrombotic therapy in valvular heart disease. *Chest*. 1989;(suppl)95:98S–106S.

73. Lechat P, Mas JL, Lascault G, et al. Prevalence of patent foramen ovale in patients with stroke. *N Engl J Med*. 1988;318:1148–1152.

74. Hagen PT, Scholz DG, Edwards WD. Incidence and size of patent foramen ovale during the first 10 decades of life: an autopsy study of 965 normal hearts. *Mayo Clin Proc*. 1984;59:17–20.

75. Webster MWI, Smith HJ, Sharpe DN, et al. Patent foramen ovale in young stroke patients. *Lancet*. 1988;2:11–12.

76. Lynch JJ, Schuchard GH, Gross CM, et al. Prevalence of right-to-left atrial shunting in a healthy population: detection by Valsalva maneuver contrast echocardiography. *Am J Cardiol*. 1984;53:1478–1480.

77. Salgado AV, Furlan AJ, Keys TF, et al. Neurological complications of native and prosthetic valve endocarditis: a 12 year experience. *Neurology*. 1989;39:173–178.

78. Hart RG, Kagen-Hallet K, Joerns SE. Mechanisms of intracranial hemorrhage in infective endocarditis. *Stroke*. 1987;18:1048–1056.

79. Salgado AV, Furlan AJ, Keys TF. Mycotic aneurysm, subarachnoid hemorrhage and indications for cerebral angiography in infective endocarditis. *Stroke*. 1987;18:1057–1060.

80. Ott BR, Zamini A, Kleefield J, et al. The clinical spectrum of hemorrhagic infarction. *Stroke*. 1986;17:630–637.

81. Horning CR, Dorndorf W, Agnoli AL. Hemorrhagic cerebral infarction—a prospective study. *Stroke*. 1986;17:179–185.

82. Lodder J, Krijne-Kubat B, Broekman J. Cerebral hemorrhagic infarction at autopsy: cardiac embolic cause and the relationship to the cause of death. *Stroke*. 1986;17:626–629.

83. Hart RG, Easton JD. Hemorrhagic infarcts. *Stroke*. 1986;17:586–589.

84. Cerebral Embolism Study Group. Cardioembolic stroke, immediate anticoagulation and brain hemorrhage. *Arch Int Med*. 1987;147:636–640.

85. Sato Y, Mizoguchi K, Sato Y, et al. Anticoagulant and thrombolytic therapy for cerebral embolism of cardiac origin. *Kurume Med J*. 1986;33:89–95.

86. Gorsselink EL, Lodder J, van der Lugt PJM. Risk of early anticoagulation in patients with small deep infarcts possibly caused by cardiogenic emboli. *Clin Neurol Neurosurg*. 1987;89:157–159.

87. Krijne-Kubat B, Lodder J, van der Lugt PJM. Hemorrhagic infarction on CT in cardioembolic stroke. *Clin Neurol Neurosurg*. 1987;89:103–105.

13
Clinical Trials in Stroke: A New Approach

John A. Blakely

The Conventional Paradigm

The assessment of clinical trials data uses a paradigm (model) developed for analyses in agriculture and genetics,[1] where observations unrelated to the main endpoint were uncommon, and the predictive value of the results was implicit. The risks of the treatments and the choice of decision threshold for the particular situation were usually unimportant.

Problems in contemporary therapeutics display few of these characteristics, which is the case with trials of stroke prevention, where the use of the *conventional paradigm* has led to avoidable errors of interpretation.

The conventional paradigm incorporates several problems.

1. Clinical trials provide an excellent opportunity for systematic observations, but their real power is to validate predictions. The conclusions that can be drawn from observations and from predictions are vastly different but conventionally, the same calculations and units are used to express the results, and the distinction tends to be obfuscated. It can be difficult to know exactly what was predicted, even when the results were expected. Notwithstanding occasional warnings to exercise caution in the interpretation of data-driven analyses, calculations appropriate to the validation of predictions are often presumed to confer predictive value on observations.

2. The questions asked of the data are stereotyped and not always appropriate to the topic. "How sure?" questions tend to be formulated in terms of the null hypothesis, whether or not that is the relevant question, and it is common practice to assume that beneficial and harmful results are equivalent.

3. "Intermediate" units are used to express outcome. Relative risk, risk reduction, odds ratio, and similar units often fail to illuminate the experimental results and may be misleading. For instance, treating a thousand patients with transient ischemic attack (TIA) would not prevent the same number of strokes as treating a thousand young women, even if the risk reduction were 50% in each case. A treatment with 1% major toxicity might produce a net benefit to the patients with TIA, but a treatment with 0.1% major toxicity would probably produce a net loss in the young women.

4. Although in principle all statements incorporating "statistical shorthand" should be translatable back to the original data, in practice such translations often don't make sense.

5. Conventional analyses often display alpha preference; the risk of accepting an ineffective treatment is strenuously avoided (alpha error), while the risk of failing to recognize that a treatment may be useful is ignored, if the result is "not statistically significant." It is then a short step to confusing "not proved" with "proved not" (beta error). The practical implication is that useful treatments go unrecognized.

When the new treatment is safe and the current treatment is unsatisfactory (particularly when the disease is serious), a treatment that is more likely effective than not may be the sensible choice.

6. The conventional paradigm is categorical. (Categorical decisions are concerned with "whether?" rather than "how much?" and apply thresholds to determine the answer.) Categorical decisions are attractively simple but, as Albert Einstein said:

> Everything should be kept
> as simple as possible,
> but no simpler.

In the following example, "threshold thinking" results in the conclusions:

> A and B are the same,
>
> C and D are the same,
>
> B and C are different.

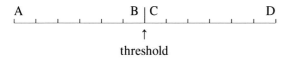

Moving the threshold by one unit (not very far, since we have assumed that a difference of five units does not matter) changes the conclusions:

> B and C and D are the same,
>
> A is different from B, C, or D.

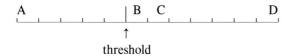

The position of the threshold has a greater effect on the conclusions than the data! Conclusions based on the application of a threshold are fraught with hazard. They are likely to make sense only to the extent that the threshold is in about the "right" place, and thresholds tend to be chosen because they have been chosen before, not because they are appropriate to the problem at hand.

7. The use of arbitrary thresholds predisposes to the confusion of "not certain" with "not true," whereby trials showing that efficacy is probable may be cited as evidence that it is absent.[2]

The Predictive Paradigm

Although use of the conventional paradigm is almost universal in current medical trials analysis, it is by no means the only possible analytic paradigm. One alternative follows; I have termed it the *predictive paradigm*, although it displays other characteristics as well. (The conventional method might be termed the *probable paradigm*.)

The predictive paradigm is a logical structure that guides the drawing of inferences from the tabulated data:

What was predicted?
Was the prediction fulfilled?
To what extent?
How sure?
How sure do you need to be?

The predictive paradigm can be used to make sense of published clinical trials by applying the following principles:

All statements must make sense in plain English.
Calculations are limited to quantitating adjectives.
The *predictive potential* and *predictive value* of an answer are defined prior to its computation.
Units used to quantitate "how much?" and "how sure?" endpoints are intuitively understandable.
The decision threshold "how sure do you need to be?" is defined by the user and is appropriate to the question and to the circumstances of application.

The steps of the predictive paradigm will be illustrated with an example:

Anticoagulant Therapy to Prevent Stroke after Acute Myocardial Infarction

While patients with acute myocardial infarction (MI) suffer stroke only occasionally, MI causes a substantial proportion of strokes, particularly those in the productive years, and an even larger proportion of strokes that might be prevented with available therapy.

About two decades ago three large, prospective, randomized trials assessed the value of anticoagulant therapy in acute MI, including efficacy in the prevention of stroke.[3-5]

At the time the first of these trials was done, various lines of evidence had suggested that anticoagulants would benefit patients with acute MI, with perhaps as much as a 50% reduction in mortality.[3,6] The expectation of such a large benefit was based on trials that were methodologically flawed or small, so direct confirmation in large, randomized, prospective trials was desirable.

Several endpoints were assessed in these trials; the hypothesis suggested that all should be affected favorably. The data were presented in various ways in the trial reports; entries, endpoints, and endpoint rates are summarized in Appendix 13.1.

The authors had expected that half the deaths might be prevented; with the exception of women in the Bronx study,[4] the absolute mortality reductions were about 2% and were not statistically significant. The reduction in thromboembolic complications, including stroke, was considered unimportant, since it was insufficient to produce a significant effect on mortality. As a result of these trials, anticoagulant therapy in acute MI was largely abandoned.

Meta-analysis of Trials of Anticoagulation in MI

In the examples that follow, the three major anticoagulant trials[3-5] have been "meta-analyzed," using a method that restricts treatment-control comparisons to patients from the same trial. The results presented are from the pooled data of the three trials (Appendix 13.2). Data regarding deaths from thromboembolism and deaths due to causes other than thromboembolism and stroke are available only for the Bronx[4] and Veterans Administration (VA)[5] trials. Answers are rounded to one place of decimals.

The five questions of the predictive paradigm need to be answered:

What was predicted?
Was the prediction fulfilled?
To what extent?
How sure?
How sure do you need to be?

What Was Predicted?

The *predictive potential* and *predictive value* of answers must be defined prior to their computation. *Predictive potential* means that a prediction

has been made. It is greatest with a single, unambiguous prior hypothesis, assessed with a single, unambiguously defined endpoint. A result may have predictive potential without having predictive value; the potential may not have been realized because of a flaw in the trial design or execution, such as bias or incomplete disclosure. Bias consists of unequal risks in the groups being compared, or selection for analysis of particular endpoints, groups, or trials. Regardless of the numerical value of the results, internal bias (selection within the trial) or external bias (selection of this particular trial) invalidate predictive calculations.

Full disclosure implies that all the questions, data, and analyses are accounted for. (All or none of patients lost to follow-up might have had endpoints.) Missing data introduce "data uncertainty" (best- and worst-case scenarios) additional to statistical uncertainty. When *predictive potential* is present, results may still be due to flaws in the trial, chance, or the treatment.

Predictive value takes into account the actual design and execution of the trial. To the extent that defects in the trial can be excluded, the result can be attributed to either chance or treatment. Since the probability that chance would produce the result can be calculated, the remaining probability is an estimate of the likelihood that treatment produced the result.

The Example

The predictions and endpoints in Table 13.1 were abstracted from the reports; mortality was the primary endpoint, but a reduction in thromboembolism was also expected. All have predictive potential.

TABLE 13.1. Anticoagulant therapy in acute MI – the analyses.

Prediction Reduction in	Fulfilled?	Control %	How much? Saves/100	ANTE[a]
Stroke	Yes	2.9	1.5	1760
Fatal emboli	Yes	1.3	0.5	1439
Fatal stroke	Yes	0.9	0.5	55
Nonfatal recurrent MI	Yes	10.8	2.1	79
Death	Yes	16.7	3.3	166
Recurrent MI + death	Yes	28.0	5.5	792

[a]ANTE = average number of trials to the estimate.

These trials have fairly high predictive value. In general, they were well designed and executed. All patients were properly randomized, accounted for at the ends of the trials, and included in the analysis.

However, treatment allocations were known to the investigators. "Soft" endpoints (decisions about the presence of stroke and recurrent MI) might be affected by expectations and have a reduced predictive value. It is a good deal less likely that mortality would be affected by lack of blinding. A treatment effect restricted to "soft" endpoints might be attributable to bias; a consistent effect on both "hard" and "soft" endpoints would suggest that the treatment prevents strokes, some being fatal.

Was the Prediction Fulfilled?

This first approach to the "how much?" answer is actually an extra "safety" step, intended to prevent the confusion of "not certain" with "not true." Did the predicted outcome occur? A "yes" or "no" answer is required (Table 13.1).

Use of evidence that suggests that efficacy is more likely present than not to support a conclusion that efficacy is absent should arouse suspicion!

To What Extent was the Prediction Fulfilled?

The results should first be described in plain English, using adjectives:

"Thromboembolism and stroke were uncommon but were greatly reduced with treatment."
"Recurrent MI and death were common, and most were not prevented by treatment."
"The absolute number of strokes prevented was small (but may represent a substantial proportion of strokes occurring in the productive years)."

Although the percentage reductions in death and recurrent MI are small, the disease is common, and the potential number of lives saved and MIs prevented in the general population is large.

In the assessment of trials of the sort involved in stroke prevention, a useful unit of "how much?" is *saves/100 treated patients*. For each 100 patients receiving the active rather than the control treatment, how many endpoints were prevented (Table 13.1)? Remember that this is a unit of "how much?"; the issue of "how sure?" is separate and has its own units. Here we are assessing the size of the estimate.

Although the numbers saved seem small with respect to the overall endpoint rates (3.3 of 16.7 deaths per 100 treated patients), this does not mean that they are not worthwhile. Suppose 3.3 of 3.3 deaths had been prevented (100 percent). We would conclude that the treatment was wonderful! But the lives saved are the same.

How Sure?

Noncategorical analysis asks "how sure?" rather than "whether." There are no "positive" trials and there are no "negative" trials; some merely constitute stronger evidence for or against efficacy than others. A zillion coincidences could produce any result. Strong evidence just consists of a low probability that either flaws in the trial or chance would produce the observed result. The object of trials analysis should be to produce accurate and understandable answers to the "how much?" and "how sure?" questions, meaning that the estimate and its certainty should be stated. This is the end of the analysis; the rest is commentary.

Average Number of Trials
to the Estimate (ANTE)

The unit of "how sure?" used for results with predictive potential is ANTE, the average number of (null) trials to the estimate. (A null trial is one with the same number of entries in the treatment and control groups and the same total number of endpoints as in the one performed, but with the endpoints apportioned equally between the treatment and control groups.)

Extreme values have more opportunity to occur in large populations. For instance, there are more Russian Olympic gold medalists than Canadian partly because there are more Russians. The probability that there is a gold medalist on your block is small; in your town or city, a little greater. In the country there are several, and in the world there are, of course, all of them. Other things being equal, the population required, on average, to contain exactly one Olympic gold medalist can be calculated. Similarly, the average number of null trials required to contain exactly one result as large as the one observed can be calculated (Table 13.1).

The ANTE values indicate that, if the treatment were ineffective, 1760 sets of three trials like these would be needed to produce, on average, one set with the observed reduction of 1.5 strokes per 100 patients treated.

How Sure Do You Need to Be?

A neglected issue in the conventional paradigm is "how sure do you need to be?". How the information supplied by the analysis should be used and the "action threshold" that governs its use depend on the situation in which it is to be applied.

Categorical evaluations usually apply the same decision threshold to a safe treatment as to a dangerous one, to a disease that is relentless as to one that is benign, to situations where there are alternatives as to where there are none. Since the trial analysts are not here now, they should not decide.

As with the issue of "how much?", it is useful to begin with ordinary English adjectives. This helps avoid the paradox that occurs when two results that are almost the same are labeled as different because they happen to lie on different sides of an arbitrary threshold (p=.05 is "statistically significant"; p=.051 is not.)

The "how sure" spectrum

| almost certainly not true | unlikely to be true | possibly true | probably true | almost certainly true |

Describing degrees of certainty first in English makes it difficult to ascribe large importance to small differences either of effect or of the probability of chance occurrence. (When you think about it, any two values can be separated by an arbitrary threshold; the issue is whether the position of the threshold is appropriate to the question being addressed—and that issue is commonly ignored.)

Risks to Consider

In deciding how sure you need to be about the trial result in order to use the treatment evaluated, it is important to consider risks arising from the disease, the data, the treatment, the benefit/risk ratio, and the statistical analysis.

Disease Risk. Sometimes it makes sense to take large risks, sometimes not. This may seem self-evident, but it is not incorporated into the conventional analytic paradigm, where the same decision thresholds are used regardless of circumstances. While evidence of efficacy is certainly an essential ingredient of any therapeutic decision, the circumstances in which the treatment is applied are equally relevant.

If the risk from the disease is great and the risk from the treatment is small, any reasonable likelihood of benefit is sufficient to justify the use of a new treatment; it is reasonable to use a low threshold.

If the established therapy is toxic and the new treatment is not, less evidence of efficacy is required than otherwise; the threshold is even lower.

If the established therapy is undoubtedly effective, more evidence of efficacy is required of a new treatment; a high threshold is appropriate.

The disease risk can be assessed by the frequency of endpoints in the control patients (Table 13.1). The risk of recurrent MI, fatal or not, was about double our current rates; by comparison, the risk of stroke was low and is likely little changed. The effect of using "intermediate" rather than absolute endpoints means that, if the same number of patients were saved in a trial with current recurrent MI and mortality rates, the treatment would appear much more effective. The value of the treatment is to those who are saved rather than those who are not.

Data Risk. "Data uncertainty" relates to the quality and quantity of the data being analyzed. The "predictive value" concept deals with data quality risks; a data quantity issue arises when there are missing data. If there are missing or doubtful data, there would still be a net benefit in a worst-case scenario.

In these trials, the principal data risk relates to the problem of the "soft" endpoints of nonfatal stroke and MI, since the studies were not blinded. This can be addressed by comparing the treatment effect on fatal and nonfatal events (Table 13.1).

The evidence suggests that preventing strokes prevents some fatal ones and that preventing recurrent MI prevents some deaths. Bias in the "soft" endpoints is not excluded, but it seems unlikely to account for the entire effect since it is implausible that fatal strokes and infarcts would be prevented if nonfatal ones were not.

Treatment Risk. All therapy carries risk. The complications of the treatment are as important as its

TABLE 13.2. Anticoagulant therapy in acute MI—benefit/risk assessment.

Fatal bleeding rates and their probability		Probability of net positive treatment effect by endpoint	
Fatal hemorrhage	Probability	Fatal stroke	All death
1.0%	0.1%	7%	93%
0.5	0.2	60	97
0.2	4	89	98
0.1	10	95	98

TABLE 13.3. Anticoagulant therapy in acute MI—other causes of death.

Prediction Reduction in	Fulfilled?	Control %	How much? Saves/100	ANTE
All stroke	Yes	2.9	1.5	1760
Fatal stroke	Yes	0.9	0.5	55
Fatal emboli	Yes	1.3	0.5	1439
Recurrent MI + death	Yes	28.0	5.5	792
Recurrent MI	Yes	10.8	2.1	79
Death	Yes	16.7	3.3	166
Nonstroke death	Yes	16.1	2.9	35
Nonthrombo-embolic or stroke death	Yes	14.2	2.6	6

efficacy. The object is a net addition to health; the degree of certainty with which the null hypothesis can be rejected with respect to the primary efficacy endpoint is often not the key issue.

The unit *saves/100 treated patients* can be compared directly with complication rates. If the estimate is that three deaths from vascular disease can be prevented by treating MI with anticoagulants and this were to produce fatal hemorrhage in 1%, the estimated net benefit would be 2%, leading directly to the issue of "how sure?" one can be about the estimates of benefit and bleeding and of the net benefit (Table 13.2).

There were no fatal hemorrhages in the three trials. The estimate of zero hemorrhages carries an uncertainty, which can be calculated. The observation of zero fatal hemorrhages in these trials means that the probability that the actual incidence is as high as 1% is only 1 in 1000.

Benefit/Risk Assessment. The benefits of treatment have been calculated, and the possibility of dying from the treatment has been estimated (it is unlikely to remain zero if enough patients are treated, regardless of the zero estimate from the 1605 patients treated in these trials). What is required now is assessment of the probability and amount of a net positive effect from treatment. The probability that the efficacy exceeds any of the plausible fatal bleeding rates can be calculated.

Table 13.2 presents the probability of a net positive effect from treatment given various rates of fatal bleeding in the treated group and the probabilities of those bleeding rates.

The top row shows that there is 1 chance in 1000 that the fatal bleeding rate is actually as high as 1% and that if that were true, it is likely that there would be more fatal hemorrhages produced than strokes prevented. This scenario is exceedingly unlikely.

A more relevant possibility is in the bottom row of the table; there is a 10% probability that the fatal bleeding rate is as high as 0.1%. If this were the case, it is 95% probable that the reduction in fatal strokes and 98% probable that the reduction in all-cause mortality would still produce a net positive treatment effect.

There is no "right" row to read; in my opinion the bottom row is more relevant to this treatment than the top one. If your treatment decision is made from a different row, that is the one for you to read.

Did the treatment prevent deaths from causes other than stroke? The last row of Table 13.3 shows that deaths from causes other than stroke are reduced by 2.9 per 100 patients treated, and that 35 sets of three trials like these would be required to produce on average one result at least this favorable.

The treatment of acute MI has changed a good deal since these trials were done, and it is possible that the nonstroke deaths being prevented were due to pulmonary emboli caused by the prolonged bedrest usual at the time. Data are available from two of the trials for deaths due to recognized pulmonary emboli (Table 13.3); since the autopsy rates were high, they are probably fairly reliable.

Excluding death from thromboembolism as well as stroke does not eliminate the benefit from treatment, so it is unlikely that thromboembolism accounted for all the reduction in deaths due to causes other than stroke.

(Users of the conventional paradigm might well apply their usual question—"Would chance produce this result more than once in 20 (or 40) times?" — discover that it would (once in six pairs of trials like these), and would be in danger of falling into the "not certain = not true" trap and construing evidence that the treatment works as evidence that it does not.)

Statistical Risk. The analysis should reflect the original prediction. If benefit from treatment was predicted and benefit was observed, then the probability should be calculated that chance alone would produce it.

The choice of endpoint should be carefully considered at the outset of the trial. Dividing MIs into fatal and nonfatal and then deciding that there are not quite enough of either to draw conclusions may be less satisfactory than counting all infarcts, fatal or not.

When several small trials have individually failed to settle an issue, it is useful to look at them together. There is a risk of "selection bias"; equally well executed "negative" trials are less published and less publicized.[7] If some were negative and some positive and you were looking only at the positive ones, you would conclude that the treatment works better than it actually does. This risk can be partly addressed by a thorough search; it is probably less for large trials. Of course, the same selection bias is present whether the trials are assessed intuitively or by formal meta-analysis.

Categorical evaluation introduces an interesting paradox. As trial after trial yield "negative" results, our conviction strengthens that the "truth" is "negative." When meta-analysis considers the same evidence together rather than separately and converts the "negative" result to "positive," it offends common sense. Since there is no magic in quantitative rather than intuitive assessment, one might suspect either that our method of deciding that the individual trials were "negative" or our understanding of the term *negative* must be flawed. The problem is that we have mistaken "not proved" for "proved not" (we have committed a beta error). Quantitative rather than categorical assessment of the trials would have led us to distinguish clearly between the estimates and their certainty; given one trial, we would observe a positive but uncertain result; as more estimates accumulate that are in themselves positive but uncertain, our confidence in the efficacy of the treatment will gradu-

ally increase. Understood in this way, it should then be no surprise that quantitative assessment by meta-analysis confirms the positive result. If assessment is to be categorical (as indeed it usually is in the published medical literature), it is necessary to distinguish between those "negative" trials that provide a confident demonstration that the treatment is ineffective and those that have merely failed to demonstrate that it works.

There are some other seemingly obvious points that are often ignored:

1. The result analyzed should address the prediction made. The probability cannot be calculated that chance would account for fulfillment of a prediction that was never made (notwithstanding frequent attempts).
2. Calculations should be appropriate to the question. The object is to quantitate the adjectives in the statement of results. It is not uncommon for a seemingly clear answer to be quantitated by calculations appropriate to a different question. This can normally be exposed by expanding the "statistical shorthand" into plain English.
3. The decision threshold should be appropriate to the question. Common practice is to use $p < 0.05$ irrespective of common sense.

The uncertainty of an estimate should be considered whether or not the treatment appeared to work.

Commentary

Anticoagulant treatment of acute MI was abandoned in most of the world shortly after publication of these trials, presumably on the basis of their evidence.

What Went Wrong?

When the trials began, it was thought that the mortality reduction might be as great as 50%[3,6]; when it proved to be less, it was considered not present or not worthwhile.

Much was made of the observation that the efficacy was far short of that predicted; the same was true of later reviews[7-9] indicating that the sample sizes were inadequate to demonstrate even a 20% reduction. Whether one expected 20 or 50% is less important than how much efficacy was actually observed. Whether the uncertainty crossed an arbitrary significance threshold is less important than whether efficacy is sufficiently probable that it is sensible to use the treatment in the circumstances, with due regard for its hazard and the availability of alternatives.

The reduction in stroke was recognized but dismissed as unimportant since it was insufficient to affect mortality.[8,9] Again, "negative" actually meant "not proved" rather than "proved not"; combining fatal and nonfatal events within trials, or fatal events across trials, would have demonstrated that the mortality reduction, although small by comparison with the disease mortality of the time, was unlikely to be a chance phenomenon, even by the measure of the statistical threshold employed. It is an interesting commentary on the "statistical" decision process that a treatment in current use was rejected on the basis of evidence that it probably worked.

The evidence was evaluated using an efficacy threshold appropriate to a dangerous treatment. If the incidence of fatal bleeding had been substantial, it would have been reasonable to insist on a high degree of certainty that the efficacy exceeded that risk. There were no deaths from bleeding in these trials. Since the treatment more likely worked than not and exceeded any reasonable estimate of the risk by a wide margin, it would seem sensible to have continued to use it.

Although the trials were undertaken with a clear expectation of benefit, the analyses employed (two-tailed) "assumed" that both benefit and harm had been predicted. This meant that the stringency of the statistical threshold, already appropriate to a dangerous treatment, was doubled.

The focus of the evaluation was on the small benefits proportionate to the total endpoint rates and on the relation to an arbitrary threshold. It should have been on the probable value of the treatment in relation to its risk. The efficacy was compared with the disease risk rather than with the treatment risk.

Another problem was that, at the time, there was no recognized method for considering evidence in the aggregate rather than within individual trials. The later trials quoted the earlier ones, but there was no attempt to combine the evidence for about a decade after their completion.[7]

The value of the treatment or, conversely, the consequences of not using it, can be roughly estimated. The Coronary Care Units associated with the Metropolitan Toronto CCU Directors' Club annually treat about 3000 patients with MI; as all have been admitted to CCUs, most could be treated. The population served by these units is roughly two million; one could therefore expect about 300 000 treatable MIs in the 200 million population of North America. Worldwide it might be reasonable to assume more than triple that number annually, or roughly one million. Extrapolation of the trial results to this population yields about 29 000 strokes annually, 9000 of them fatal, and up to 10 000 nonfatal and 5000 fatal strokes preventable by treatment each year. We have failed to prevent them for 20 years.

What Was Demonstrated?

1. The trials showed that anticoagulant treatment of acute MI, as administered, was safe. The probability that the true incidence of fatal bleeding was as great as 1 per 200 patients was about 1 in 400.
2. About half the strokes were prevented. Since fatal strokes were prevented (fairly consistently in all three trials), the reduction in nonfatal stroke is unlikely to be accounted for by bias.
3. Some deaths from causes other than stroke were prevented, and it is unlikely that these were all accounted for by thromboembolism.
4. While the reported reduction in nonfatal recurrent MI rates might be an artifact from lack of blinding, the reduction in fatal ones suggests that some recurrent MIs were actually prevented.
5. The benefits of treatment outweighed any reasonable allowance for fatal bleeding.

Present Practice

What inferences can we draw about present practice? More treatments are available, and a death or stroke can only be prevented once.

1. The problem of embolic stroke continues. Beta-blockers probably increase the incidence of intraventricular thrombus[10] and presumably increase the risk of stroke. The use of anticoagulants after fibrinolytic therapy probably decreases it.[11-13]

We now know that intraventricular thrombosis and embolic stroke are almost confined to anterior MI[14]; this means that, for the prevention of stroke, fewer patients need to be exposed to the risk of treatment, and the "benefit/risk" proportion would therefore improve.

2. Currently, three therapeutic strategies deal with the risk of embolic stroke in anterior MI:

a) Restrict anticoagulant therapy to treatment of patients with demonstrable emboli (or an additional indication). This strategy presumes that the risks of treatment should be confined to patients with the "hard" indication of embolism.

b) Confine the risk of anticoagulant prophylaxis to the smallest possible number of patients; this may be implemented by doing echocardiograms and treating patients with demonstrable thrombi, or only those with pedunculated thrombi. This strategy presupposes that there is risk without benefit from treatment of patients at low risk of embolization.

c) Treat all patients with anterior MI with anticoagulant therapy, unless there is a contraindication.

Although the old evidence might no longer apply to current patients, there is neither direct evidence that this is so, nor a plausible rationale. There *is* direct evidence that anticoagulants in anterior MI continue to reduce stroke.[15,16] The numbers involved are small, but it is no more sensible now than two decades ago to reject a treatment on the basis of evidence that it more likely works than not.

3. The assessment of clinical trials, in stroke prevention would benefit from modification of the traditional methods, as follows:

1. incorporate noncategorical analysis,

2. explicit definition of predictive potential and predictive status,

3. confinement of "null hypothesis" question formulation to circumstances where that is the relevant question,

4. abandonment of arbitrary "how sure?" thresholds in favor of assessment of the level of certainty appropriate to the question being addressed,

5. confinement of "intermediate" endpoints to intermediate calculations,

6. use of endpoints that are intuitively interpretable by the intended user, and

7. formulation of both the question and answer in meaningful English.

The rejection of anticoagulant therapy in acute MI two decades ago was an example of the confusion of "not proved" with "proved not" (beta error). The analytic paradigm by which evidence that efficacy is probable is construed to be evidence that is not is still with us.

Conclusions

1. The treatment of acute MI with oral anticoagulant therapy, particularly for the prevention of stroke, was inappropriately rejected on the basis of the original analysis of the major trials.

2. The analytic paradigm that led to the inappropriate conclusion remains in general use.

3. An alternative analytic paradigm is possible and practical; its application has been illustrated.

APPENDIX 13.1. Anticoagulant therapy in acute MI—the tabulated data.

	Treatment group		Control group			
	Endpoints	Entries	Endpoints	Entries	Treatment rate	Control rate
Stroke						
MRC	8	712	18	715	1.1%	2.5%
Bronx	13	745	9	391	1.7	2.3
VA	4	500	19	499	0.8	3.8
MI						
MRC	69	712	93	715	9.7	13.0
Bronx	88	745	51	391	11.8	13.0
VA	20	500	30	499	4.0	6.0
Death						
MRC	115	712	129	715	16.1	18.0
Bronx	111	745	83	391	14.9	21.2
VA	48	500	56	499	9.6	11.2
Fatal stroke						
MRC	3	712	7	715	0.4	1.0
Bronx	5	745	5	391	0.7	1.3
VA	0	500	3	499	0	0.6
Nonstroke death						
MRC	112	709	122	708	15.8	17.2
Bronx	106	740	78	386	14.3	20.2
VA	48	500	53	496	9.6	10.7
Thromboembolic death						
Bronx	3	745	10	391	0.4	2.6
VA	0	500	2	499	0	0.4
Nonstroke thromboembolic death						
Bronx	103	738	68	376	14.0	18.1
VA	48	500	51	499	9.6	10.3

APPENDIX 13.2. Calculations.

Saves per 100 patients = the number of endpoints prevented when 100 patients in the trial are given the active rather than the control treatment.

Saves per 100 = (control endpoint rate) − (treatment endpoint rate).

Entries per Save = the average number of patients in the trial who must be given the active rather than the control treatment in order to prevent one endpoint.

Entries per save = 100/(saves per 100).

ANTE = the average number of null trials that are required to produce one result as large as the one observed (the estimate).

ANTE = 1/p.

(A null trial is one with the same sort of patients as the one being analyzed, with the same numbers of entries in control and treatment groups and the same total numbers of endpoints but with equal endpoint rates in control and treatment groups.)

Part II
Surgical Prevention of Stroke

14
Carotid Endarterectomy: A Challenge for Scientific Medicine

H.J.M. Barnett

A Variety of Concerns About Carotid Endarterectomy

Carotid endarterectomy (CE) was introduced very shortly after cerebral angiography identified the extracranial portion of the carotid artery as a common site responsible for stroke-threatening transient ischemic attacks (TIA). On the face of it, it was, and to many remains, as logical a surgical activity as the removal of an acoustic neuroma or the clipping of a saccular intracranial aneurysm. Why, then, has the procedure fallen afoul of universal acceptance? The reasons are several:

1. In the case of a ruptured aneurysm, the mortality, let alone the morbidity, from a recurrent hemorrhage is close to 50%. The survivors have almost an equal chance of being left with a serious disability. The TIA patient has at least a 90% chance of going through each successive year after the initial event(s) without a serious outcome.

2. If a stroke does occur, there is at least a 30% chance of its being in another arterial territory from that of the artery that caused the presenting symptoms.

3. After the onset of the warning symptoms, there is as great a chance that the patient will die from heart disease, principally myocardial infarction, as there is of a disabling or fatal stroke.

4. When the procedure of CE was introduced, stroke had not shown any substantial decline in its occurrence or mortality. By contrast, 35 years later the mortality from stroke has altered substantially. In Canada stroke for men was projected to become the 6th cause of loss of potential years of life by 1989, compared with 3rd place 25 years earlier.[1] A 60% decline has been recorded over 30 years in the United States. This decline relates most importantly to the increasingly widespread recognition of the consequences of manageable predictors of stroke, especially hypertension, cigarette smoking, and excessive consumption of fats.[2-4] These predictors of stroke are being treated with reasonable aggressiveness, and their exact relationship to the decline of stroke mortality is difficult to deny or to confirm.

5. The heart, now studied by more sophisticated imaging methods, is of greater importance as a cause of stroke than was the case 20 years ago. Approximately one stroke victim in four has a cardiac condition that might have caused the stroke, and many patients have more than one potential mechanism from which they may have fallen victim to stroke. Physicians and surgeons are reluctant to submit patients to a surgical procedure with a definite risk of serious complications if other recognized potential reasons for the heralding symptoms are known to exist.

6. Aspirin prevents stroke,[5] and ticlopidine has been shown to be effective in two major, multicenter trials.[6,7] Ticlopidine may prove to be an acceptable alternative in those patients whose events persist despite aspirin or in those who cannot tolerate aspirin.

7. Endarterectomy carries a risk of stroke and death. The most able surgeons claim personal perioperative rates of risk for disabling stroke

or death between 2% and 4%. There is every reason to believe that these are accurate estimates. Nonetheless, the national average in the United States has been verified at closer to 10%.[8,9]

8. Cerebral arteriography is the prerequisite for most who perform and advise CE. Without it, the extent of obliterating atheroma in the intracranial portion of the carotid artery and in the middle cerebral artery is imperfectly known (even in the era of transcranial Doppler studies.) Also, the presence of asymptomatic cerebral aneurysms cannot be known reliably without arteriography; they are of potentially serious consequence, and this risk is aggravated by the restoration of full carotid artery flow subsequent to CE. The performance of arteriography, even in the most experienced centers, carries a small but definite risk of stroke.[10,11] Because medical management does not require arteriography, its risk must be added to the risk related to the surgical procedure.

9. Drugs introduced for serious and potentially mortal disorders are expected at times to carry some risk. In spite of this hazard, they will be accepted by the profession, the public, and the regulating agencies, but only if they are proved without equivocation by strict clinical trials to be less dangerous than the disorder for which they are administered. This type of critical thinking, which modern methodology and biostatistics have introduced into medical science, leaves many practitioners with serious concerns about the continued application of surgical procedures to which a risk is attached. This apprehension increases when these procedures have not been evaluated by properly designed trials. Radical mastectomy and extracranial-intracranial anastomosis are recent examples of the unexpected results of randomized studies that have altered substantially the acceptance of traditional or innovative surgical measures.[12,13] They raise the specter of similar concern for any conclusions about surgical claims that are based on anecdote alone.

10. Two trials have been conducted by random assignment of patients to endarterectomy versus medical care.[14,15] Neither could claim benefit for surgery, and no others have been concluded since 1970.

11. Two communications in the New England Journal of Medicine appear to have had a considerable impact on the profession's interest in carotid endarterectomy. Chambers and Norris reported on the favorable outlook for individuals followed with noninvasive studies in a large series of patients known to have stenosing carotid lesions.[16] They reported favorably on the spontaneous outcome and concluded that their data were not supportive of anything other than a very cautious application of endarterectomy. Secondly, the negative results of extracranial/intracranial (EC/IC) bypass surgery were interpreted mistakenly, but widely, as shedding doubt on the prevention of stroke by any surgical procedures.

12. Review articles and editorial comment have drawn the profession's attention to these concerns.[17-20]

The Rise and Decline of Enthusiasm for Carotid Endarterectomy

Until 1986 an annual increase was noted in the number of patients who were subjected to endarterectomy.[21] This has been true wherever extracranial carotid disease is common, especially in North America (United States and Canada), Europe, and Australia. The American enthusiasm exceeded that elsewhere by a factor of 20 in some geographical comparisons.[19] This increased enthusiasm resulted from the multiplication of surgical teams trained to carry out the procedure; from the extension to community hospitals of imaging capabilities to visualize the arteries of the brain; from the education of primary physicians to recognize the warning symptoms (TIA); and from the provision in developed countries of health-care systems capable of providing modern investigation and therapy. The number of CEs performed in the USA in 1971 was 15 000; in 1985 it peaked at 107 000. In 1986 and 1987 the number declined to 82 000 and 81 000, respectively, and the Medicare figures provide evidence that its usage continues to decline at a rate of about 3% per year.[21]

The decline of interest in this surgical procedure cannot be attributed to new data acquired by scientific methodology. None have been forthcoming that would be useful in delineating the indications for its use, or in defining situations in which its use has been convincingly negated. There are no such data. Rather, the changing practice appears to have been shaped by the concerns that we have listed.

The concerns about endarterectomy and its declining application have been accompanied by an outpouring of comments in the media and in the professional literature. Popular nationally viewed television programs have discussed the state of our knowledge and ignorance and commented about which patients, if any, should receive the operation.[22] Articles describing the lack of agreement in the profession about the appropriateness of performing CE have been featured in such widely read publications as *Time*, the *New York Times*, the *Washington Post*, and, in Canada, the *Globe* and *Mail* and the magazine *Chatelaine*.[23-27] Carotid endarterectomy has been included, rightly or wrongly, in lists of overused operations and excessively applied investigational procedures. The evidence upon which these conclusions have been based is tenuous at best. Still, it has helped to shape the public's and the profession's growing indifference and, at times, suspicion about this and other procedures.

Professional bodies have appointed committees to review the evidence and to recommend appropriate positions to be adopted. These bodies include the American Heart Association, the American College of Physicians, the Cerebral Vascular Section of the American Association of Neurological Surgeons, the American Academy of Neurology, and the American Neurological Association.[28-32] The varied recommendations of these bodies have been based on what they all acknowledge to be imperfect information. Most of these recent reviews have recommended a conservative use of the procedure, limiting it to appropriately symptomatic patients. All of those mentioned advised against the procedure being done without proven surgical skill. Most indicated that they will be prepared to make firmer recommendations at the conclusion of randomized clinical trials.

Medicare is responsible for 80% of the payments for this procedure in the United States. This reflects the average age of the patients deemed to require it. The Rand Corporation was commissioned to identify the appropriateness of its utiliza-

tion. The survey was conducted in three large geographic areas in the United States, including one where fewer than usual were done, one where more than usual were done, and one that approximated median usage.[33] The bench mark for appropriateness was constructed after consulting a committee of experts in neurology and surgery; it was applied to 1302 patients selected at random from the Medicare files. The conclusion was that 35% of the patients submitted to the operation fell within the guidelines identified by their panel of experts, 32% were outside this range of indications, and in 32% it was equivocal whether they should have been subjected to surgery.

The Health Care Financing Administration (HCFA), spurred by this survey, has issued directives about the payment policies for endarterectomy. There is an understandable disparity in the interpretation of the HCFA regulations across the member States. Some Medicare offices will accept payment for endarterectomy in the patients with severe stenosis but without symptoms. Many will pay only for patients with severe degrees of stenosis and in the presence of appropriate symptoms. The degrees of acceptable stenosis vary from 50 to 90%. Some will pay for "nonhemispheric" symptoms; some will pay for operations on arteries known to be occluded, while others specifically will not pay if the artery is occluded; some do not require confirmatory arteriography and accept non-invasive studies, while others demand conventional arteriography. These differing recommendations reflect the failure of the profession to provide scientifically sound data upon which better decisions could be based.

Responses to the Disarray

It is not an exaggeration to maintain that this procedure is in a state of disarray. Several responses are being observed in respect to this confusion. First, many primary health care providers, internists, and neurologists appear to have stopped referring their patients for CE and are treating them with conservative medical measures. It is quite possible that this is denying some patients an operation that would benefit them. Nobody can affirm or deny this because of the singular absence of hard data from acceptable evaluations.

Second, some are writing and publishing just as if there was no controversy; and some are advising the profession that there is need only for a tightening of the care with which surgical technique is applied to justify its continued usage.[34-36] No one can quarrel with the recommendation that more meticulous attention be paid to the selection of each individual patient and to the care with which the operative procedure is carried out. Unfortunately, even the best data from the series, which have made up the aggregate of the first million patients submitted to CE, have not given us a clear picture either of its appropriate use or of its benefit. It seems unlikely that we will be in a happier position after the second million have been done. We will still be lacking the denominator based on the long-term results achieved in totally comparable patients receiving modern medical care alone.

Third, we can perform randomized clinical trials. To many of us this seems the sensible answer. Three randomized trials have been launched for asymptomatic patients: one at the Mayo Clinic, one in the U.S. Veterans Administration, and one under National Institutes of Health (NIH) sponsorship,—the Asymptomatic Carotid Atherosclerosis Study (ACAS). Three multicenter, randomized trials are under way for symptomatic patients. The British Medical Research Council is funding a trial that includes 71 centers in most western European countries. Their goal is to randomly assign either best medical care or the same treatment plus surgery to 3000 symptomatic patients with appropriate carotid lesions causing their symptoms. They have passed the 2000- patient mark, continue to acquire patients, and report that the perioperative combined disabling stroke and mortality rate remains <5% (Warlow C.P. Personal communication).

The North American Symptomatic Carotid Endarterectomy Trial (NASCET) involves 45 centers in Canada and the United States. It has entered close to 1500 patients of an estimated requirement of approximately 2500. Like the European experience, the surgical skill of the carefully audited surgical participants in this trial is excellent and exceeds the demands of the protocol. The outcome events in NASCET that are of major importance are stroke, either fatal or nonfatal, and nonstroke death. A three-tier system is being used to monitor all outcome events. First, the participating neurologist and surgeon in each center agree on the event and, if a stroke, on its location

and type. For the latter they utilize computerized tomographic scanning, which is required by the protocol after a stroke occurs. Next, these data are reviewed by the neurologists and surgeons in the central office, and any differences of opinion are rationalized by communications between them and the individual centers. Finally, the outcome events are reviewed by a panel of two nonstudy neurologists, a neurosurgeon, and a vascular surgeon. The data are sent to them stripped of any information that would allow them to know of the treatment arm to which the patients were assigned.

In addition to keeping scrupulous records of the randomized patients, this trial has gathered all data pertaining to those patients who are eligible for the study but not entered into the trial in the participating centers. This information is sufficiently complete after 2 years of patient entry that the investigators can affirm that the randomized patients are identical to those who have not accepted or who have been advised against submitting to random assignment into the study. The concern expressed after the EC/IC Bypass Study that there was a possible deviation of the "most appropriate" patients away from the trial cannot be raised again in NASCET.[37-41]

The third trial of symptomatic patients is being carried out in the Veterans Administration in the United States. It has been entering patients for approximately 1 year toward its goal of 500 patients.[42]

The results of these randomized trials collectively should settle for the foreseeable future the appropriate use of carotid endarterectomy in stroke prevention. In the meantime, it would appear prudent for practitioners to continue to recommend patients for surgery if they have clearly recognizable carotid artery symptoms appropriate to an ipsilateral stenosing lesion, with at least a 50% reduction in the diameter of the lumen by linear measurement. The procedure should be carried out by a surgeon with an audited surgical record for this procedure affirming a 30-day perioperative stroke rate and mortality of no more than 5%.

Conclusion

It is essential that risk factor management and platelet-inhibiting therapy be continued indefinitely in every patient after the operative procedure. After all, the incidence of stroke decreased because of attention to risk factors.

Recently, aspirin has been confirmed also as moderately effective in the prevention of stroke. Studies are being conducted to provide even more effective antithrombotic and platelet-inhibiting drugs. The foreseeable future may provide some major breakthrough, allowing us to inhibit the development of the atheromatous plaque.

It is to be hoped, and indeed expected, that carotid endarterectomy will have an ongoing role in the secondary prevention of stroke in carefully selected patients.

References

1. Bisch L, Lee KI, Mark E. Major Causes of Death, Canada 1989. *Chronic Diseases in Canada*, Health and Welfare Canada, 1989; pp 22–24.

2. MacMahon S, Peto R, Cutler J, et al. Part 1: Prolonged differences in blood pressure: prospective observational studies corrected for the regression dilution bias. *Lancet*. 1990;335:765–774.

3. Collins R, Peto R, MacMahon HP, et al. Part 2: Short-term reductions in blood pressure: overview of randomized drug trials in their epidemiological context. *Lancet*. 1990;335:827–838.

4. Walker WJ. Change in per capita consumption in the United States 1963–1980. *N Engl J Med*. 1983;308:649–651.

5. Antiplatelet Trialists' Collaboration. Secondary prevention of vascular disease by prolonged antiplatelet treatment. *Br Med J*. 1988;296:320–331.

6. Gent M, Blakely JA, Easton JD, et al. The Canadian-American Ticlopidine Study (CATS) in thromboembolic stroke. *Lancet*. 1989;1215–1220.

7. Hass WK, Easton JD, Adams HP, et al. A randomized trial comparing Ticlopidine hydrochloride with Aspirin for the prevention of stroke in high-risk patients. *New Engl J Med*. 1989;321:501–507.

8. Dyken ML, Pokras R. The performance of endarterectomy for disease of the extracranial arteries of the head. *Stroke*. 1984;15:948–950.

9. Dyken ML. Carotid endarterectomy studies: a glimmering of science (editorial). *Stroke*. 1986;17:355–358.

10. Ernest FIV, Forbes G, Sandok BA, et al. Complications of cerebral angiography: Prospective assessment of risk. *AJNR*. 1983;4:1191–1197.

11. Dion JE, Gates PC, Fox AJ, et al. Clinical events following neuroangiography: a prospective study. *Stroke*. 1987;18:997–1004.

12. Fisher B, Bauer M, Margolese R, et al. Five-year results of a randomized clinical trial comparing total mastectomy and segmental mastectomy with or without radiation in the treatment of breast cancer. *N Engl J Med*. 1985;312:665–673.

13. The EC/IC Bypass Study Group. Failure of extracranial-intracranial arterial bypass to reduce the risk of ischemic stroke. *New Engl J Med*. 1985;393:1191–1200.

14. Fields WS, Maslenikov V, Meyer JS, et al. Joint study of extracranial arterial occlusion. *JAMA*. 1970;211:1993–2003.

15. Shaw DA, Venables GS, Cartlidge NEF, et al. Carotid endarterectomy in patients with transient cerebral ischemia. *J Neurol Sci*. 1984;64:45–53.

16. Chambers BR, Norris JW. Outcome in patients with asymptomatic neck bruits. *N Engl J Med*. 1986;315:860–865.

17. Barnett HJM, Plum F, Walton JN. Carotid endarterectomy—an expression of concern. *Stroke*. 1984;15:941–943.

18. Caplan LR. Carotid-artery disease (editorial). *N Engl J Med*. 1987;315:886–888.

19. Warlow CP. Carotid endarterectomy: does it work? *Stroke*. 1984;15:1068–1076.

20. Trobe JD. Carotid endarterectomy: who needs it? *Ophthalmology*. 1987;94:725–730.

21. Pokras R, Dyken ML. Dramatic changes in the performance of endarterectomy for diseases of the extracranial arteries of the head. *Stroke*. 1988;19:1289–1290.

22. News programs 20/20, Nightline. ABC Television, New York, New York, February 6, 1986.

23. Califano JA Jr. Billions blown on health. *New York Times*, 12 April 1989.

24. Ludtyke M. Physician, inform thyself. *New York Times Magazine*, 16 April 1989.

25. Rich S. Califano calls U.S. health bill at least $125 billion too high. *Washington Post*. 9 May 1988.

26. Surtees L. Doubts on operation make it hard to find patients for research. *Toronto Globe and Mail*, 17 June 1988.

27. Katz S. Do you really need surgery? *Chatelaine*. August 1989;65–67.

28. Beebe HG, Clagett GP, DeWeese JA, et al. Assessing risk associated with carotid endarterectomy: a statement for health professionals by an ad hoc committee on carotid surgery standards of the Stroke Council, American Heart Association. *Circulation*. 1979;2:314–315.

29. Feussner JR, Matchar DB. When and how to study the carotid arteries. *Ann Intern Med*. 1988;109:805–818.

30. Callow AD, Caplan LR, Correll JW, et al. Carotid endarterectomy—what is its current status? *Am J Med*. 1988;85:835–838.

31. Interim assessment: carotid endarterectomy: report of the American Academy of Neurology, Therapeutics and Technology Assessment Subcommittee. *Neurology.* 1990;40:682–683.
32. Committee of Health Care Issues. American Neurological Association. Does carotid endarterectomy decrease stroke and death in patients with transient ischemic attacks? *Ann Neurol.* 1987;22:72–76.
33. Winslow CM, Solomon DH, Chassin MR, et al. The appropriateness of carotid endarterectomy. *N Engl J Med.* 1988;318:721–727.
34. Lord RSA. *Surgery of Occlusive Cerebrovascular Disease.* St. Louis, MO: C.V. Mosby Company; 1986.
35. Hertzer NR. Presidential address. Carotid endarterectomy—a crisis in confidence. *J. Vasc. Surg.* 1988; 7:611–619.
36. Thompson JE. Don't throw out the baby with the bath water. A perspective on carotid endarterectomy. *J Vasc Surg.* 1986;4:543–545.
37. Goldring S, Zervas N, Langfitt T. The extracranial-intracranial bypass study: a report of the committee appointed by the American Association of Neurological Surgeons to examine the study. *N Engl J Med.* 1987;316:817–820.
38. Sundt I. Was the international randomized trial of an extracranial-intracranial arterial bypass representative of the population at risk? *N Engl J Med.* 1987; 316:814–816.
39. Relman A. The extracranial-intracranial arterial bypass study—what have we learned? *N Engl J Med.* 1987;316:809–810.
40. Barnett, HJM, Sackett D, Taylor DW, et al. Are the results of the extracranial-intracranial bypass trial generalizable? *N Engl J Med.* 1987;316:820–824.
41. Chalmers TC, Meier P, Plum F. The EC/IC bypass study (letter to the editor). *N Engl J Med.* 1987; 317:1030–1031.
42. Hobson RW II, Towne J. Carotid endarterectomy for asymptomatic carotid stenosis (editorial). *Stroke.* 1989;20:575–576.

15
Carotid Endarterectomy in Patients with Asymptomatic Carotid Stenosis

J.J. Ricotta

Surgical therapy of stroke is directed at prevention of ischemic events; in the vast majority of cases this effort involves carotid endarterectomy. As such, emphasis has been placed on identification of patients likely to suffer stroke in the future. In patients with transient cerebral ischemia or small fixed deficits, increased risk for subsequent ischemic events is recognized and the role of surgery is generally accepted. Management of patients who have had no neurologic symptoms is more controversial. The debate on this issue involves many unresolved, complex questions (See Table 15.1). Included in this list are definitions of the term *asymptomatic*, identification of clinically important lesions, natural history of carotid stenosis, and the effect of surgical intervention (i.e., carotid endarterectomy) on both short-term and long-term outcome. These questions will be examined sequentially in an attempt to define the proper role for surgery in the asymptomatic patient with carotid stenosis.

Definition of *Asymptomatic*

Precise definition of the term *asymptomatic* is extremely difficult. Review of the literature demonstrates that this term has been applied inconsistently to a number of different clinical presentations. In its broadest usage *asymptomatic* indicates absence of neurologic symptoms: focal or global, involving either the anterior or vertebral-basilar circulation. Implied in this definition is the absence of neurologic findings on physical examination. In more common clinical usage, individuals are often classified as asymptomatic with reference to a par-

ticular cerebrovascular territory. Thus a patient with symptoms of right middle cerebral artery ischemia (or a history of right carotid endarterectomy) and a left internal carotid stenosis would be considered by many to have an asymptomatic left carotid lesion. Some authors believe that vertebral-basilar territory lesions should be separated from carotid territory lesions and that patients with vertebral-basilar symptoms have asymptomatic carotid lesions.[1] The issue is more confusing when nonspecific symptoms such as dizziness, syncope, and dementia are present. Finally, recent reports that infarction, diagnosed by computed tomographic (CT) scan, may be present in up to 20% of patients with asymptomatic carotid stenosis raise the question of clinical versus anatomic definition of cerebral ischemia or infarction.[2-4] As magnetic resonance imaging (MRI) and positron emission tomography (PET) scanning become more common, such problems of definition will probably increase.

In the future, a classification similar to the one proposed by Courbier,[5] which describes both symptoms and anatomy, will probably be required to stratify patients adequately. At present it is sufficient to iterate that patients who have never had a neurologic symptom differ from those who are asymptomatic in one cerebral hemisphere and those with symptoms of "global" or vertebral-basilar insufficiency. In addition, it is likely that patients with evidence of clinically asymptomatic cerebral infarction on diagnostic studies are a different group from those without such evidence. Finally, it must be recognized that diverse groups of patients have been classified as asymptomatic at one time or another in the literature.

TABLE 15.1. Questions in asymptomatic carotid disease.

1. Is there a difference between an asymptomatic lesion and an asymptomatic patient? What are the implications of noncarotid territory symptoms, contralateral carotid lesions, and silent infarctions.
2. How is a stroke prone lesion defined? What is the importance of stenosis vs. ulceration? What is the "critical" degree of stenosis?
3. What is the natural history of asymptomatic carotid stenosis?
4. How safe is carotid endarterectomy in the asymptomatic patient?
5. Is carotid endarterectomy effective in prolonging stroke-free survival in the asymptomatic patient?
6. How to deal with subgroups of patients with asymptomatic lesions: combined coronary/carotid disease, bilateral carotid disease, lesions proximal to asymptomatic infarctions.
7. How to reduce the impact of coronary artery disease on survival of patients with asymptomatic carotid lesions.

Identification of a "Significant" Carotid Lesion

Since carotid endarterectomy is essentially a prophylactic operation, one must identify a carotid lesion that is likely to increase the patient's risk of stroke. Unless operation is limited to such lesions, it is unlikely to be of benefit in the prevention of stroke. Indeed, failure to define adequately the "stroke-prone" lesion has probably contributed to the rapid rise in carotid endarterectomy in the last decade and is a major reason for increasing scrutiny of the operation.

Carotid Bruits

Initially, "significant" asymptomatic stenoses were usually identified by auscultation of the neck. Thompson et al.[6] reported that 90% of patients with a midcervical bruit seen in their practice were subsequently found to have a stenosis of >50% diameter in the carotid bifurcation. Subsequent studies suggest that the presence of a carotid bruit is a less specific finding. Population surveys in Framingham, Massachusetts,[7] and Evans County, Georgia,[8] indicated that cervical bruits were present in 3 to 8% of the population studied and that the incidence increased with age. While presence of a bruit increased the likelihood of stroke

two to eight times over normal in both studies, many of the ischemic events were not ipsilateral to the bruit. It is now well established that presence of a neck bruit is a nonspecific indicator of generalized vascular disease that may include the carotid arteries.

Carotid Angiography

Developments in noninvasive cerebrovascular diagnosis have allowed investigators to discard the finding of a bruit in favor of a more objective measure of internal carotid disease, percent stenosis. Noninvasive studies identify carotid bifurcation lesions that result in turbulence or decrease in distal pressure or flow. Extensive correlation with angiography has allowed classification of lesions by percent stenosis.

There is currently some discrepancy between the reported methods of measuring diameter stenosis on angiograms. Barnes[9] uses the estimated diameter of the carotid bulb as the normal lumen, while others use the diameter of the "normal" internal carotid artery distal to the stenosis,[10] and still others estimate the diameter of the internal carotid artery at the point of maximal stenosis.[11] Each method has its advantages and drawbacks. However, it is clear from Figure 15.1 that when the carotid bulb diameter is used as a reference, the estimated stenosis will be higher than the number derived using the distal internal carotid artery. In general, a 50 to 60% stenosis measured using the internal carotid reference is equivalent to an 80% stenosis when the normal reference point is the carotid bulb. Noninvasive definitions reflect changes in flow velocity, not a static two-dimensional angiographic image, itself subject to variations in measurement.[11,12] Thus a significant stenosis measured noninvasively reflects reduction in lumen size sufficient to produce hemodynamic alterations. Quantification of the stenosis that results will vary with the method of measurement.

Relationship of Stenosis to Symptoms

There is general agreement that the severity of carotid stenosis is correlated with potential to produce cerebral ischemia. Riles et al.[13] showed a

FIGURE 15.1. Schematic of carotid bifurcation showing three methods of determining unobstructed lumen (UL). The percent stenosis is measured by comparing the minimal residual lumen (MRL) to the UL using the following formula: percent diameter stenosis = $(1 - MRL/UL)$ 100. It is obvious that the larger the UL, the larger the calculated percent stenosis, even though the MRL remains the same.

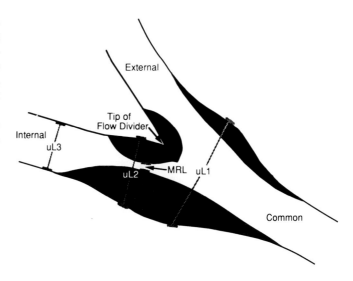

clear relationship between the degree of bifurcation stenosis and the frequency of ipsilateral ischemic symptoms. They reviewed angiographic findings in 495 patients (990 arteries) evaluated for cerebrovascular ischemic syndromes. In these patients 562 arteries were believed to be ipsilateral to a symptomatic cerebral hemisphere, while in the remaining 428 the hemisphere was asymptomatic. When arterial stenosis was measured, only one third of arteries with <40% diameter stenosis were on a "symptomatic" side, while almost three fourths of arteries with >80% stenosis were associated with ipsilateral cerebral ischemic symptoms. Similar findings by Grotta et al.[14] support the relationship of diameter stenosis to stroke risk. Pierce et al.[15] found a significantly increased incidence of carotid occlusion in patients who underwent angiography for evaluation of cerebrovascular ischemia as compared to age-matched controls evaluated for either subarachnoid hemorrhage or brain tumors. Other authors[16,17] have suggested that patients with stenosis >75 to 80% defined noninvasively are more likely to experience subsequent cerebral ischemic events than those with less severe lesions.

Presence of ulceration has also been suggested as a source of potential cerebral ischemia as a result of embolization.[18,19] Angiographically defined ulceration has been associated with cerebral and retinal embolization. Moore et al.[20] identified a group of asymptomatic patients with large ulcers who dem-onstrated an increased incidence of ischemic events on follow-up evaluation when compared with patients who lacked these angiographic characteristics. Smaller degrees of irregularity were not comparably ominous. In separate studies Imparato et al.[21] and Ricotta et al.[22] noted an increased incidence of ulceration and mural thrombi and ulceration in endarterectomy specimens of patients with symptoms of hemispheric cerebrovascular insufficiency.

The final common denominator may be plaque size. Since the dimensions of the carotid bifurcation and internal carotid artery are relatively constant, lesions that produce hemodynamic changes (i.e., 75 to 80% area stenosis) are likely to represent plaques of similar size. We have found a high correlation between plaque diameter, percent stenosis, and the presence of macroscopic ulceration and plaque hemorrhage in specimens removed at the time of carotid endarterectomy (unpublished results). Thus lesions that reduce the lumen sufficiently to cause pressure or flow changes may be dangerous by virtue of both their hemodynamic consequences and embolic potential.

It seems clear at present that any consideration of surgery in an asymptomatic patient should be limited to lesions of sufficient size to cause changes in flow or pressure and those large ulcers identified by Moore et al.[18,20] that do not otherwise produce hemodynamically significant stenosis.

Rationale for Surgery for Asymptomatic Carotid Stenosis

The argument in support of prophylactic endarterectomy for asymptomatic stenosis rests on several assumptions:

1. The risk of stroke ipsilateral to such lesions is high enough to warrant intervention;
2. Stroke occurs without warning (i.e., transient ischemic attacks [TIAs]) in a significant proportion of cases;
3. TIAs and carotid occlusion are undesirable events even when they occur without stroke;
4. The risk of carotid endarterectomy is low enough to justify prophylactic operation; and
5. Stroke-free survival is improved in patients subjected to prophylactic carotid endarterectomy.

Thus carotid endarterectomy is offered as a safe alternative to prevent stroke, transient ischemia, or carotid occlusion and improve stroke-free survival. Each of these assumptions will be examined independently.

Risk of Stroke in Patients with Asymptomatic Significant Stenosis

A number of studies supports the assertion that patients with "significant" stenosis (as defined earlier) have an increased risk of stroke (Table 15.2). This point was first emphasized by Thompson et al., who compared long-term results in 132 patients after prophylactic endarterectomy with 138 nonoperated controls.[6] Stroke occurred in 17.4% of the nonoperated group during follow-up versus 4.6% in the operated group. Objections to this study have been raised for several reasons. Patients were identified by the presence of a carotid bruit, although this was associated with a significant stenosis (>50%) in 90% of the operated group. The study was not prospective or randomized, and it was not mentioned whether late strokes were ipsilateral or contralateral to the bruit. A study in 97 patients by Dorazio et al.[23] yielded similar results. However, other population-based studies[7,8] indicated that many late strokes were not ipsilateral to the artery identified by a bruit. More recently, asymptomatic patients have been characterized on the basis of degree of stenosis.

Kartchner and McRae[24] noted a 12% stroke rate in asymptomatic patients when both oculoplethysmography and phonoangiography suggested a hemodynamically significant stenosis. Busutill et al.[25] found that patients with high grade stenoses as defined by abnormal oculopneumoplethysmography had a 16.2% increased risk of subsequent stroke and 39% risk of TIA. Again, however, the relationship of the subsequent neurologic event to the diseased artery was not specified. Most important in all these studies, the status of the extracranial vessels at the time of the event was unknown. Chambers and Norris[17] found a low rate of neurologic events in 500 patients prospectively followed with asymptomatic cervical bruits. However, when patients were identified as having severe internal carotid stenosis by noninvasive testing, the incidence of all neurologic events was 18% with a 5% incidence of stroke after 1-year follow-up. Patients who showed progression to severe stenosis were also at high risk. In this study the majority of neurologic events were ipsilateral to the stenotic carotid artery. Roederer et al.[16] reported similar findings in a prospective series of 167 patients evaluated for cervical bruits and followed for up to 36 months. Symptoms developed in 10 patients, all but one of whom demonstrated severe stenosis prior to development of symptoms. Progression to >50% stenosis occurred at an annual rate of 8%. These results were somewhat diluted by the fact that 36 patients underwent endarterectomy during the course of the study (32 prophylactic, 4 symptomatic).

Similar results have been published in a number of other studies from institutions around the world.[26-33] These results have been abstracted and summarized in Table 15.2. The general conclusion of these reports is that the occurrence of neurologic events is increased in the population with cervical bruits. The incidence of high-grade stenosis is relatively low in the population with bruits, but the risk of neurologic sequelae is virtually restricted to those patients who begin with or progress to a high-grade stenosis.

Presence of a nonfibrous degenerated or ulcerative plaque has also been associated with increased risk of neurologic events on follow-up. Moore et al. reported a stroke rate of 12.5% per year in patients with large ulcers.[20] Most of these strokes occurred either within the first year or after about 5 years of

TABLE 15.2. Neurologic events in asymptomatic patients with carotid bruit/stenosis followed without operation.[a]

Author	Year	Carotid[b] lesion	# Patients	Mean follow-up	TIA	Stroke
Thompson[6]	1978	Bruit	138	45 mo	27%	17%
Dorazio[23]	1980	Bruit	97	84 mo	11%	19%
Wolf[7]	1981	Bruit	171	96 mo	5%	12.3%
Heyman[8]	1980	Bruit	72	72 mo	–	13.9%
Kartchner[24]	1977	OPG−/CPA−	877	24 mo	–	1.9%
		OPG+/CPA+	147			11.9%
Busutill[25]	1981	OPG−	74	20 mo	8.4%	2.8%
		OPG+	71		39.2%	16.2%
Hennerici[26]	1982	Stenosis	122	18 mo	–	7%
Roederer[16]	1984	<80% stenosis	262[b]	24 mo	0.4%	0.0%
		>80% stenosis	24[b]		25.0%[c]	12.5%[d]
Moore[27]	1985	<50% stenosis		24 mo	–	35%
		>50% stenosis			–	15%
Hertzer[28]	1986	>50% stenosis	195	15 mo	–	9%
Chambers[17]	1986	<75% stenosis	387	23 mo	–	1.7%/y
		>75% stenosis	113	–	–	5.5%/y
Bogousslavsky[41]	1986	>90% stenosis	38	48 mo	10.5%/y	4.2%/y
Meissner[29]	1987	OPG−	348	40 mo	2.3%/y	1.5%/y
		OPG+	292		5.2%/y	3.4%/y
Moneta[30]	1987	>80% stenosis	73	24 mo	28%	19%
Hennerici[40]	1987	Stenosis	339	29 mo	–	12%
Taylor[31]	1988	Stenosis	203	18 mo	9.4%	5.4%[c]
Langsfeld[32]		Stenosis	130	21 mo	10.7%	1.5%

[a]In this table, lesions were identified by presence of a bruit or a variety of noninvasive tests. In some reports the degree of stenosis was not specified. In some cases only stroke and not transient ischemic attack (TIA) was noted.
[b]Analysis was by artery rather than patient.
[c]Stroke and TIA.
[d]Events were correlated with progression of stenosis.
TIA = Transient ischemic attack.
OPG = Oculoplethysmography.
CPA = Carotid phonoangiography.

follow-up, suggesting that disease progression may have played a role in those cases that became symptomatic later. In a subsequent report including 153 arteries, Dixon noted an annual stroke rate of 4.5% for large ulcers and 7.5% for complex ulcers.[34] Most of the strokes in these two studies were not preceded by warning episodes of transient cerebral ischemia. Two separate studies[35,36] failed to confirm these findings and reported a low stroke rate with large ulcers, although complex ulcers with excavation (Type "C") were not followed but subjected to prophylactic operation. Other studies have suggested that ultrasound findings often associated with ulceration or "soft plaque" were associated with increased risk of subsequent neurologic events.[32,37,38] However, the small numbers of patients, confounding effects of severe stenosis, and lack of angiographic correlation in these studies does not allow one to draw definite conclusions.

In summary, it appears that high-grade stenosis as variously defined in these papers (vide supra) is associated with a risk of neurologic events (stroke or TIA) of about 15% per year; about one third of which will be strokes. The presence of complex ulceration with excavation (Type "C" ulcers) carries a similar risk of subsequent neurologic events.[34] While some would argue that only the incidence of permanent neurologic deficit (i.e., stroke) is important, the fact that many patients are referred for endarterectomy after experiencing transient deficits (and therefore withdrawn from the study cohort) suggests that this practice would be inappropriate. Thus, the incidence of all neurologic events must be considered in determining results of nonoperative treatment.

TABLE 15.3. Frequency of stroke without warning–transient ischemic events.

Author	Year	# Patients	# Strokes (%)	Unheralded # strokes (%)	Mean follow-up
Levin[39]	1980	137[a]	0	0	1-20 y
Dorazio[23]	1980	97[a]	18 (19%)	17 (94%)	84 mo
Heyman[8]	1980	72[a]	10 (14%)	9 (90%)	72 mo
Wolf[7]	1981	171	21 (12%)	15 (71%)	96 mo
Dixon[34]	1982	153[b]	17 (11%)	17 (100%)	48 mo
Roederer[16]	1984	167	4 (2%)	3 (75%)	18 mo
Moore[27]	1985	294	26 (9%)	25 (96%)	24 mo
Chambers[17]	1986	500	12 (2%)	8 (75%)	1-5 y
Bougousslavsky[41]	1986	38	5 (13%)	2 (40%)	48 mo
Hennerici[40]	1987	339	10 (3%)	7 (70%)	29 mo
Meissner[29]	1987	292[c]	29 (10%)	25 (86%)	40 mo
Moneta[30]	1987	73	9 (12%)	9 (100%)	24 mo
Taylor[31]	1988	203	11 (5%)	5 (45%)	18 mo
Foulkes[42d]	1988	359[e]	359 (100%)	325 (91%)	–
Pierce[15f]	1989	118[g]	54 (46%)	37 (69%)	–

[a]Patients with carotid bruit.
[b]Patients with asymptomatic ulcer.
[c]Patients with +OPG only.
[d]Data from Foulkes et al.[42] are derived from a Stroke Data Bank.
[e]All patients with atheroembolic strokes.
[f]Data from Pierce et al.[15] are limited to patients found to have carotid occlusion on retrospective review.
[g]All patients had ICA occlusion.

Incidence of Stroke Without a Warning

The incidence of unheralded stroke is of vital importance in the decision whether or not to recommend prophylactic carotid endarterectomy. If all strokes were preceded by a warning recognized by the patient and appropriately treated by the physician, the argument for prophylactic surgery might well be moot. There is disagreement about the frequency with which stroke occurs without warning.[39–42] This difference of opinion has led some authors to recommend prophylactic endarterectomy and others to condemn it. Much of the disagreement revolves around distinction between the absolute incidence of stroke without warning and the relative percentage of strokes that are not preceded by transient ischemic events. In Table 15.3 it will be obvious that the overall stroke rate in asymptomatic patients is low. However, even in the studies of Hennerici et al.[40] and Bougousslavsky et al.[41] most of the strokes that did occur were not preceded by a warning transient ischemic event. Only the report of Levin et al.[39] suggests that stroke without TIA is a rare occur-

rence. This is probably a function of the degree to which both patient and physician recognize and respond to symptoms of transient ischemia. With the exception of Levin's experience, there is little support for the practice of waiting for transient ischemic events to develop in these patients before recommending endarterectomy. Decisions need to be made on the basis of the absolute stroke rate rather than the assumption that a warning event will occur. As mentioned earlier, the fact that many patients are treated surgically after transient ischemic events suggests that even reliance on absolute stroke rates will underestimate the risks of nonoperative management.

Significance of TIAs and Carotid Occlusion

The incidence of stroke alone is estimated at approximately 4 to 5% per year in patients with asymptomatic significant stenosis.[17] One must also ask about the two other events more often encountered in this group of patients—TIAs and carotid occlusion. If these are determined to be clinically

TABLE 15.4. Outcome of carotid occlusion.

Author	Year	# Patients w/occlusion	Initial stroke	Late symptoms[a]
Dyken[45]	1974	43	30 (70%)	2/25
Fields[47]	1976	1044	802 (77%)	17.3% TIA, 76/359 (21%) stroke
Barnett[46]	1978	27[b]	–	20 TIAs, 7 strokes
Furlan[48]	1980	138[c]	–	10% (2%/y)
Cote[49]	1983	47[c]	–	51% TIA, 15% stroke
Fritz[50]	1985	32	12 (38%)	4 TIAs, 1 stroke
Nicholls[51]	1986	212	111	20 strokes, 23 TIAs
Pierce[15]	1989	110	54[d]	–
Bornstein[52]	1989	19 at onset	0	0, 3 TIAs
		21 developed occlusion	0	3 strokes, 9 TIAs

[a]Excludes contralateral stroke.
[b]Retrospective selection of symptomatic patients.
[c]Only patients with minimal dysfunction were selected for F/U.
[d]Only 13% of patients had asymptomatic occlusion.

significant, then the case for prophylactic surgery is strengthened. If, however, only absolute stroke rate is important, prophylactic surgery is much more difficult to justify.

Transient ischemic events are reported with twice the frequency of stroke in most series of asymptomatic patients (see Table 15.2). Like permanent deficits, TIAs usually occur ipsilateral to the significant lesion. Once TIAs occur, most physicians would agree that the incidence of stroke is significant if they are left untreated. It is imperative that asymptomatic patients with significant carotid lesions understand the symptoms of cerebral ischemia and that close follow-up be arranged, if endarterectomy is not performed. Even with this caveat, reported experience with CT suggests ipsilateral cerebral infarction in up to 30% of patients with transient ischemic episodes and no clinical sign of permanent neurologic deficit.[2] These data suggest that TIA is not a benign phenomenon and that cerebral imaging (CT or MRI) may be important in determining the appropriateness of endarterectomy in patients without fixed deficit. Thus prevention of transient ischemia may well be an important benefit of prophylactic endarterectomy.

The importance of progression to carotid occlusion must also be evaluated. This is potentially relevant from three vantage points: (1) the association of progression to occlusion and stroke, (2) poor results of surgery once carotid occlusion occurs, (3) potential increased future stroke risk in patients who experience a carotid occlusion. There is strong evidence that lesions allowed to progress to occlusion commonly are accompanied by stroke. In a series of articles on carotid occlusion[15,43-52] 50 to 75% of patients found to have carotid occlusion when first evaluated presented with stroke, while an additional 10 to 25% presented with symptoms of transient ischemia ipsilateral to the occluded vessel (Table 15.4). Once occlusion had occurred, subsequent ipsilateral events were not infrequent. Although Dyken et al.[45] noted < 10% incidence of stroke following occlusion in 25 patients, Barnett reported 7 strokes and 21 TIAs in a similar number of cases.[46] In a later study on a larger cohort (47 patients), Cote and Barnett[49] documented an infarction rate of 5% per year ipsilateral to an occluded artery. Furlan et al[48] found approximately one half that incidence in a larger group of patients. However, most of the patients in the last series had mild residual deficits or were asymptomatic following occlusion. Nicholls et al.[51] reported a 5% per year rate of stroke after carotid occlusion, with 3% per year ipsilateral to the occluded vessel. They also noted a relationship between the patient's symptoms at the time of occlusion and subsequent neurologic symptomatology.

Bornstein and Norris[52] suggested that patients with asymptomatic carotid occlusion may have a more benign long-term prognosis than those who present with neurologic symptoms temporally related to their carotid occlusion. They followed 40 patients who either presented with carotid occlusion or developed occlusion as part of a study of 500 patients with asymptomatic bruit. While 12 of 21 patients developed symptoms (9 TIAs, 3 strokes) when an initially patent artery occluded, the clinical course of 19 patients who presented with asymptomatic occlusion was surprisingly benign; none developed symptoms ipsilateral to the carotid occlusion during the follow-up period. Thus it seems that a patient is exposed to a significant risk of stroke if allowed to progress to occlusion and that this risk is not completely eliminated once occlusion occurs. Nonetheless, if occlusion occurs *without symptoms*, the prognosis is considerably improved.

Once internal carotid occlusion occurs, surgery is rarely of benefit. This becomes important when one is considering the prognosis of patients with sympomatic occlusion, as well as that of patients with diffuse or bilateral carotid atherosclerosis. Multivessel disease has been associated with an increased frequency of subsequent neurologic events, even in initially asymptomatic patients.[26,28,40] In addition, there are several studies, although not randomized, that suggest increased stroke-free survival in patients with contralateral or "second side" endarterectomy.[53-56] While a simplistic concept, the idea that an open carotid artery may be preferable to an occluded one has some appeal and may have some merit.

Risks of Carotid Endarterectomy

Much of the current concern over endarterectomy in asymptomatic patients has quite rightly been centered on the risks of the operation itself. Reports from several large centers suggest that carotid endarterectomy can be performed with combined mortality and neurologic morbidity $<5\%$; however, several series attest to the fact that this is not always the case. Easton and Sherman[57] reported a stroke rate of 21.2% in two community hospitals in 1977, and Toole et al. reported a similarly disturbing stroke morbidity of 16%.[58] Although subsequent updates of both experiences showed improvement by 1983 to a combined complication rate of 8.9%[59] and 3.8%[60] respectively, these reports were disquieting to surgeons and physicians alike. Brott's report[1] of combined mortality-neurologic morbidity of 9.5% in a community-wide survey, including a 5.6% stroke rate for asymptomatic patients, raised cause for alarm. Although

many of these patients had nonspecific symptoms due possibly to carotid disease, it was apparent that prophylactic operation could not be recommended unreservedly with such a complication rate. Several subsequent community surveys produced more reassuring data for proponents of endarterectomy. Ruben et al. reported a combined mortality and neurologic morbidity rate of 3.7% for members of the Cleveland Vascular Society.[61] Kirshner et al.,[62] in reviewing a 2-year experience in a single community, found total mortality and neurologic morbidity of 4.8%, with 3.7% in patients with asymptomatic stenosis. All the morbidity and mortality in the asymptomatic group occurred in patients undergoing contralateral "second side" endarterectomy. Fode et al.[63] reported a retrospective multicenter review from 46 institutions encompassing 3328 cases. While overall risk of stroke or death was 6% in this report, there was considerable variation (0 to 21%) between institutions.

Despite the accepted notion that operation on asymptomatic patients is safer than on those with stroke or TIA, it has become obvious that some maximum level of complications exists, above which surgery is unlikely to benefit the patient with an asymptomatic carotid stenosis. This issue has been addressed by several investigators. Chambers and Norris[64] have suggested that benefit is unlikely to accrue to the asymptomatic patient unless a high-risk group ($>5\%$ stroke per year) can be identified and surgery is consistently performed with a complication/death rate of 3 to 5% or less. The effect of perioperative complications and mortality on potential benefit to an asymptomatic patient is graphically demonstrated in Figure 15.2. It is apparent from this figure that prophylactic endarterectomy is unlikely to benefit patients whose life expectancy is 24 months or less. However, as longevity increases, the potential benefits from surgery become greater.

Data from the literature[65,66,68] suggest that acceptable rates of mortality and stroke can be achieved in patients operated upon for asymptomatic lesions (Table 15.5). Combined morbidity and mortality rates of 5% or less have been reported from both large, single-center series[53,67,69,70] and community experiences involving large numbers of surgeons.[61,62,71] Such results are not uniformly achieved, however, and the excessive complication rates reported by some authors[1,57,73]

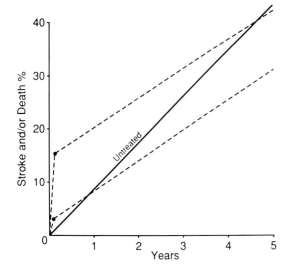

FIGURE 15.2. Relationship between operative complications and potential benefit of carotid endarterectomy. Surgery is unlikely to show benefit unless complication rates are <5% and patients live >2 years (From Chambers and Norris, *Stroke.* 1984;15:964–967. Reprinted by permission.)

would appear to negate any benefit of this operation. Success with prophylactic endarterectomy varies with the individual surgeon and appears to be related more to training and patient selection rather than to case volume or academic affiliation.[62,74] The

past performance of the individual surgeon must be considered before endarterectomy can be recommended. With this caveat, however, one can confidently state that the operation is performed with an acceptable rate of complication by a large number of surgeons in a variety of practice settings. When complication rates are acceptable, potential for long-term benefit from surgery may exist.

Prognosis After Carotid Endarterectomy

Information on expected outcome after surgery is essential before an operation can be recommended as prophylaxis. Endarterectomy for asymptomatic stenosis is performed in order to decrease the long-term risk of stroke and improve long-term survival. Therefore, data on these two questions, as well as the rate of recurrent stenoses, become important.

In appropriately selected symptomatic patients, carotid endarterectomy is reported to reduce the risk of subsequent neurologic events by 65%.[75] In a long-term study of 103 patients followed for at least 5 years, DeWeese et al.[76] reported absence of symptoms in 77% of patients (84% when only patients with "classic" cerebral ischemic symptoms were considered). Almost one quarter of patients

TABLE 15.5. Mortality and neurologic morbidity of carotid endarterectomy in asymptomatic patients.

Author	Year	# Patients	Stroke	Death	Total[a]
Moore[53]	1979	72	0%	0%	0%
Javid[65]	1971	56	4.0%	2.0%	6.0%
Kirshner[62]	1989	222	2.7%	1.2%	3.9%
Rubin[61]	1988	1055	2.8%	1.1%	3.9%
Thompson[67]	1979	132	1.5%	0%	1.5%
Lees[69]	1981	83	1.0%	4.0%	5.0%
Burke[70]	1982	57	1.0%	0%	1.0%
Fode[63]	1986	572	3.5%	3.0%	6.5%
Till[60]	1987	92	1.0%	2.0%	3.0%
Cafferata[73]	1986	92	----- 13.0% -----		13%
Modi[59]	1983	74	3.0%	3.0%	6.0%
Kremer[66]	1979	42	0%	0%	0%
Hertzer[77]	1984	655	2.0%	1.2%	3.2%
Brott[1]	1984	130	8.0%	3.0%	11.0%
Slavish[71]	1984	190	----- 26% -----		2.6%
White[68]	1984	32	0%	0%	0%
Kempczinski[74]	▶ 1986	381	2.1%	3.7%	5.3%
Easton[57]	1977	12	18.0%	0%	18.0%

[a]Some patients may have had both stroke and death.

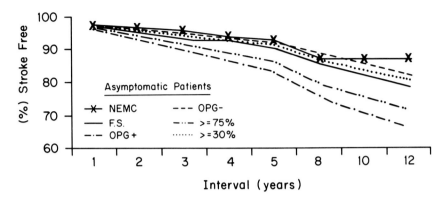

STROKE PREVENTION

(NEMC vs Optimal Medical Rx)

FIGURE 15.3. Comparison of long-term results of carotid endarterectomy for asymptomatic stenosis and reports of natural history studies. A benefit of surgery in long term prevention of stroke is seen providing operative complications are low. NEMC – New England Medical Center, FS – Framingham Study. (Reprinted from Callow and Mackey[56] with permission.)

developed new symptoms, usually associated with contralateral lesions. At the end of 5 years, 34% of patients had died, the vast majority of myocardial infarction.

In a study of >300 patients followed for 10 years, Hertzer and Aronson[77] reported a stroke-free survival of 91.8% at 5 years and 74.4% at 10 years. Most of the strokes were contralateral to the operated artery, suggesting the importance of continued follow-up of these patients. Late stroke occurred in the contralateral hemisphere of 36% of patients with uncorrected contralateral stenosis. In contrast, the stroke incidence for patients who had prophylactic contralateral endarterectomy for stenosis was only 8% over 10 years. A similar low incidence of ipsilateral stroke (~1% per year) was reported by Forsell et al.[78] and Bernstein et al.[79] in patients followed for 3 to 5 years. In all of these series the major cause of late morbidity and mortality was myocardial infarction.

Rosenthal et al.[80] reported on 42 patients followed for 10 years after endarterectomy for asymptomatic stenosis. During this time 12 patients (~29%) had contralateral endarterectomy for symptomatic or asymptomatic stenosis. Only two ipsilateral strokes occurred in this cohort—none in the first 5 years, with a cumulative stroke-free survival (ipsilateral and contralateral) of 85.3% at 10 years. Actual survival in this group at 10 years was 57%, with cardiac

disease the major cause of death. Callow[81] has recently reported on 619 patients treated in his institution since 1970 with a mean follow-up of 56.4 months. Crude annual stroke rate (including operative deficits) was 1.9%. In 179 asymptomatic patients, the crude annual stroke rate was 1.4%. These data suggest that carotid endarterectomy, when performed safely, lowers the subsequent incidence of stroke when compared to nonoperative management (Fig. 15.3).

Further support for prophylactic endarterectomy is implied in several reports that deal with the follow-up of patients who have undergone bilateral endarterectomy.[53,54,77,82] Moore et al.[53] reported on long-term survival in 39 patients subjected to prophylactic "second side" endarterectomy for large ulcers or severe stenosis and compared them to 39 patients with unilateral endarterectomy. While the survival of the operated group was decreased when compared to an age-adjusted population without carotid disease, it was superior to survival of the nonoperative patients from the Joint Study of Extracranial Occlusion. More important, they noted improved stroke-free survival in patients who had undergone prophylactic endarterectomy. Riles et al.[54] came to similar conclusions when they compared patients with unilateral and bilateral carotid endarterectomy 5 years after surgery. Cumulative stroke rates at the

TABLE 15.6. Mortality and neurologic morbidity of combined carotid and coronary procedures.*

| Author | # Patients | # Patients with CS | CABG | Complications mortality/neurologic morbidity | |
				CABG w/Asx CS	CABG w/ CEA
Jones[94]	–	–	0.6%/0.6%	–/3.3%	3.0%/1.6%
Brener[99]	4047	153 (3.8%)	4.0%/1.9%	14.5%/6.3%	10.5%/8.8%
Hertzer[95]	22 100	331 (1.5%)	1.9%/1.8%	–	5.7%/9.0%
Hertzer[97]	9714	275 (2.8%)	–	3.4%/6.9%	4.2%/2.8%
Cambria[100]	1038	72 (7.0%)	2.0%/1.0%	–	2.7%/4.2%

[a]Data on patients with symptomatic carotid disease have been excluded.
CS = carotid stenosis
CABG = coronary artery bypass graft
CEA = carotid endarterectomy

end of 5 years were 17.6% in the unilateral group versus 5.6% in the bilateral group. These results anticipated later reports[56,77,80] and emphasized the benefits of carotid surgery in prolonging stroke-free survival.

Recurrent Carotid Stenosis

The problem of recurrent stenosis after carotid endarterectomy was first addressed by Stoney and String.[83] In their series, this was a rare phenomenon, although they identified only symptomatic recurrences. As noninvasive technology and digital angiography became more available, it was appreciated that asymptomatic restenosis occurred not infrequently and that the rate of recurrence depended on how avidly it was sought.[81] Zierler et al.[84] reported a recurrence rate of 19% following endarterectomy when 89 operated arteries were followed using duplex scan technology. Less than 50% of these recurrent stenoses were symptomatic. Subsequent studies with larger patient cohorts put the recurrent stenosis rate at 8 to 15%.[81,85] Early recurrences are probably caused by thrombus deposition and intimal hyperplasia, while later recurrence is atherosclerotic.[86] The majority of early recurrent stenoses are asymptomatic, theoretically because the lesions are smooth rather than complex. Possible factors that contribute to recurrence include incomplete endarterectomy, small arteries, female gender, smoking, and failure to patch the arteriotomy in a small vessel.[81,85,87] One study[86] suggested that routine use of a patch increased the rate of restenosis.

The long-term follow-up data presented in the previous section suggest that while restenosis may occur in >10% of carotid endarterectomies, it is rarely manifest clinically since recurrent symptoms are rare. Nonetheless, when a prophylactic operation is undertaken, even an asymptomatic recurrence becomes important. This problem must be addressed and every step taken to minimize its occurrence if surgery is to be offered to asymptomatic patients with confidence.

Prophylactic Endarterectomy in Conjunction with Major Cardiovascular Surgery

Significant extracranial carotid disease is present in 5 to 10% of patients with coronary artery disease and 10 to 30% of patients with peripheral vascular disease when screened by noninvasive methods. While the overall stroke incidence following cardiac surgery is low, it appears to be increased in patients with significant extracranial carotid disease. This has stimulated efforts to reduce stroke risk by performing carotid endarterectomy prior to or simultaneous with major vascular reconstruction (coronary bypass, aortic surgery). This practice is based on the premise that hemodynamic or rheologic changes occurring in association with cardiovascular surgery predispose to stroke. While this appears to be the case in some series, clear proof is lacking that prophylactic endarterectomy will decrease neurologic morbidity in patients with unilateral asymptomatic significant stenoses (Table 15.6).

In a prospective study of 449 patients screened with Doppler before coronary or peripheral vascular surgery, Barnes et al.[88] (1981) found stenoses $\geq 75\%$ in 63 patients (14%). No patients underwent prophylactic endarterectomy. There were eight perioperative neurologic deficits in these patients (15%), but only one in the territory of the diseased vessel identified preoperatively. While these authors found an increased rate of late neurologic events and death in these patients, they did not feel that prophylactic endarterectomy would be justified prior to major cardiovascular surgery. Kartchner and McCrae[89] also found a high rate (17%) of ischemic stroke in patients with abnormal noninvasive studies but did not comment on the anatomic distribution of these deficits. Subsequent work by Turnipseed et al.[90] and Breslau et al.[91] has confirmed these findings, i.e., that patients with carotid stenosis are at increased risk for stroke, but this could not be attributed convincingly to the stenosed artery.

In view of the increased stroke rate of patients with both coronary and carotid disease, combined operation has been offered to such patients in an attempt to reduce operative morbidity and mortality.[92-100] The results have been mixed. Early reports suggested that such a combined approach could be done safely with expectation of good results.[92-94] However, while complication rates were low, they still exceeded those of patients with coronary artery disease alone. This is due, in part at least, to the fact that patients with combined disease are usually an older group and atherosclerosis is generally more diffusely distributed. In addition, the small numbers of patients (usually <5%) who might require combined procedures make it difficult to obtain sufficient numbers for statistical analysis. Several recent larger series have provided some insights.

Brener et al.[98,99] noted an incidence of severe carotid disease in 5% of >4000 patients screened prior to cardiac surgery. Stroke rate and mortality increased in this group (9.2% versus 1.9% and 13% versus 4%, respectively). When neurologic events in patients with operable disease were analyzed, no statistically significant difference emerged between those treated with simultaneous endarterectomy (8.8%) and those undergoing cardiac surgery alone (6.3%). Hertzer et al.[95,97] and Cosgrove et al.[96] from the Cleveland Clinic reported a 5.7% mortality and 9% neurologic morbidity in 331 patients with combined carotid and coronary operations. However, they noted improvement in long-term prognosis in those who survived combined surgery with long-term survival equivalent to a group of age-matched controls.[95]

More recently, the Cleveland Clinic group has divided patients with carotid and coronary disease into three groups[96,97]: patients with symptomatic or severe carotid lesions and stable coronary disease (carotid endarterectomy first), patients with asymptomatic carotid lesions and high cardiac risk (randomized simultaneous or staged procedures), and patients with symptomatic coronary and carotid disease (managed individually). In their most recent follow-up,[97] stroke rate was lowest in patients in whom endarterectomy could be performed first (4.2%) and highest in patients with symptoms in both the cerebral and coronary circulations (11%). Patients with asymptomatic carotid stenosis and symptomatic coronary disease had an overall stroke rate of 7.8%. Stroke risk was 2.8% when operations were combined versus 6.9% when coronary bypass was performed alone. When morbidity of delayed carotid endarterectomy was added, data favored a simultaneous versus "reverse staged" (i.e., bypass followed by endarterectomy) approach. However, this approach assumes that all patients with significant lesions should eventually undergo carotid endarterectomy.

Although the data are somewhat confusing, a few conclusions can be made concerning carotid endarterectomy in patients with cardiac disease. While the overall risk of stroke is low (1 to 2%) in patients following cardiac surgery, it is increased in patients with extracranial occlusive disease. At present, it is not clear that this increase can be affected significantly by performance of prophylactic carotid endarterectomy for significant stenosis.[101] This is probably due to the small numbers of patients studied and the multifactorial nature of cerebral dysfunction following cardiac surgery.[102] If carotid endarterectomy is elected in these patients, the decision should be made on the same basis that is used in patients without cardiac disease (i.e., long-term rather than perioperative protection from stroke), recognizing the increased cardiac risk these patients experience. Whenever possible, endarterectomy should be performed prior to cardiac or vascular surgery. This may be problematic in patients with unstable cardiac disease. At present there are insufficient data to support the policy of a "combined" versus "staged" surgical approach.

Patients with Asymptomatic Contralateral Stenosis

Another major area of controversy is the management of patients with an asymptomatic significant stenosis contralateral to a symptomatic or endarterectomized artery. In many series these have been classified as asymptomatic stenoses, but it should be obvious that patients with these lesions are a different group from those with no prior history of neurologic symptoms. Data from a variety of sources demonstrate that patients with bilateral carotid disease have a decreased long-term survival and increased risk of late stroke compared to patients with unilateral lesions.[26,41,54,77] Kirshner et al.[62] have suggested that the operative risk of patients subjected to a prophylactic "second side" endarterectomy is increased over that of patients with unilateral asymptomatic disease.

Several reports have addressed the fate of patients with contralateral asymptomatic significant carotid stenosis[33,39,82,103,104] (Table 15.7). These studies have reported an incidence of transient ischemia of 10 to 15% referable to the contralateral artery in patients followed after endarterectomy. The incidence of stroke varied from 0% to 7% in these series. In series reporting a low stroke rate, endarterectomy was performed in all patients who experienced TIAs. Further evidence in support of contralateral endarterectomy is provided by reports demonstrating highest long-term, stroke-free survival in patients undergoing bilateral carotid endarterectomy.[53-56,77,79]

Current Developments in Surgery for Asymptomatic Stenosis

Currently two prospective trials are evaluating the efficacy of carotid endarterectomy in patients with significant "asymptomatic stenoses." In the Veterans Administration Cooperative Study, recruitment is complete. All patients enrolled demon-

TABLE 15.7. Follow-up of asymptomatic stenosis in patients with contralateral endarterectomy.

Author	# Patients	Follow-up (years)	% TIA	% CVA
Levin[39][a]	147	0-20	12	0
Podore[103]	28	5	14	7
Johnson[104]	22	1-4	9	0
Humphries[33]	168	0-13	15	2
Durward[82][a]	67	4	13	3

[a] All patients with TIA on followup had carotid endarterectomy.

strated a ≥50% diameter stenosis by angiography. Four hundred forty-seven patients were randomized and will be followed for 5 years. Preliminary reports indicate a 1.9% mortality rate and combined mortality-neurologic morbidity of 4.3% in the operative group.[105] Toole[106] has begun a similar study involving 18 centers, including patients from independent as well as federal hospitals. Patient recruitment is ongoing in this study. Patients will be randomized on the basis of noninvasive diagnostic tests rather than angiography, and follow-up will be for 5 years with stroke, TIA, or death as end points.

In the interim, recommendations on the role of carotid endarterectomy have been published.[107] The Stroke Council of the American Heart Association suggests that for endarterectomy to be of benefit in asymptomatic patients, overall mortality should not exceed 2% and combined mortality-neurologic morbidity should not exceed 3%.[108]

Conclusions and Recommendations

The issue of indications for carotid endarterectomy in asymptomatic patients remains clouded. Some of the confusion results from inconsistent reporting in which patients with bruit, stenosis or ulceration, and unilateral and bilateral disease were included in the same groups. Until recently the lack of CT or MRI data has made it more difficult to be sure that patients being studied are indeed at comparable risk for neurologic events. Future widespread application of transcranial Doppler or cerebral blood-flow techniques may be even more important in addressing this problem. It is hoped that the two randomized studies now in progress will help to clarify this issue, although it is by no means certain that this will be the case. In the meantime, review of the available data allows one to draw some preliminary conclusions.

Extracranial carotid disease is an indiscriminate indicator of increased risk from vascular disease, especially myocardial infarction. When this extracranial disease is associated with a significant stenosis at the carotid bifurcation, the risk of subsequent ipsilateral neurologic events is increased. This increased risk is related to the severity of stenosis, progression of stenosis, and the presence of multivessel disease. Increased risk of neurologic events is also evident in patients with large ulcerations. Patients with carotid and myocardial atherosclerosis are at increased risk of stroke following cardiac surgery. At present, data are insufficient to decide whether prophylactic carotid endarterectomy reduces the risk of stroke attendant upon the cardiac procedure.

The rate of complications following carotid endarterectomy varies and is dependent on both technical expertise and patient selection. In general, patients with unilateral asymptomatic stenosis are at lowest risk of stroke or death following endarterectomy. The presence of bilateral carotid disease or significant myocardial ischemia increases operative risk. Technical expertise cannot be directly correlated with case volume but does vary between surgeons and should be an important factor in deciding whether or not endarterectomy should be performed. Neurologically intact survivors of carotid endarterectomy show reduction in long-term incidence of stroke when compared to unoperated patients with extracranial carotid stenosis.

Based on these observations, the following recommendations can be made at this time.

1. Surgical treatment of significant asymptomatic carotid stenosis (>75% area) is appropriate in asymptomatic patients with a projected life expectancy of >3 years provided combined mortality and neurologic morbidity from the procedure is <5%.
2. In patients with contralateral asymptomatic stenosis (>75% area), endarterectomy may improve long-term, stroke-free survival if surgical complications for the "second side" can be kept <5%.
3. In patients with combined carotid and coronary disease, the decision for or against prophylactic endarterectomy should be made on the basis of long-term estimate of stroke risk rather than

expectation that endarterectomy will decrease the stroke rate following cardiac surgery. Whenever possible, endarterectomy should precede cardiac or other vascular surgery.
4. Optimal treatment of patients with bilateral severe stenosis/occlusion remains to be defined. However, if operative complications can be demonstrated to be <5%, surgery is justified. Higher operative complication rates may prove to be acceptable if the natural history for patients with these lesions is worse than for patients with unilateral disease.
5. If prophylactic endarterectomy is not undertaken, thorough evaluation of patients with significant carotid stenosis, patient education, and close follow-up is necessary. Cerebral imaging may reveal the presence of silent ipsilateral infarction in up to 20% of patients. The ability of the patient and physician to recognize symptoms of cerebral ischemia, assure regular follow-up, and identify disease progression may all influence the decision whether or not to select surgery as a treatment option.
6. Patients with extracranial carotid disease should be enrolled in an aggressive program of education and behavior modification to reduce the risk of subsequent stroke and myocardial infarction. The role of prophylactic cardiac screening in these patients remains to be defined.

References

1. Brott T, Thalinger K. The practice of CEA in a large metropolitan area. *Stroke.* 1984;15(6):950–955.
2. Street DL, O'Brien MS, Ricotta JJ, et al. Observations on computerized cerebral tomography in carotid endarterectomy patients. *J Vasc Surg.* 1988; 7:798–801.
3. Berguer R, Sieggren MY, Lazo A, Hodakowski GT. The silent brain infarct in carotid surgery. *J Vasc Surg.* 1986;3:442–447.
4. Zukowski AJ, Nicolaides AN, Lewis RT, et al. The correlation between carotid plaque ulceration and cerebral infarction seen on CT scan. *J Vasc Surg.* 1984;1:782–786.
5. Courbier R. Basis for an international classification of cerebral arterial diseases. *J Vasc Surg.* 1986; 4:179–183.
6. Thompson JE, Patman RD, Talkington CM. Asymptomatic carotid bruit: long term outcome of patients having endarterectomy compared with unoperated controls. *Ann Surg.* 1978;188:308–316.

7. Wolf PA, Kannel WB, Sorlie P, McNamara P. Asymptomatic carotid bruit and risk of stroke. *JAMA*. 1981;245:1442–1445.

8. Heyman A, Wilkinson WE, Heyden S, et al. Risk of stroke in asymptomatic persons with cervical arterial bruit. *NEJM*. 1980;302:838–841.

9. Barnes RW, Bone GE, Reinertson J, et al. Noninvasive ultrasonic carotid angiography: prospective validation by contrast arteriography. *Surgery*. 1976;80:328–335.

10. O'Leary DH, Bryan FA, Goodison MW, et al. Measurement variability of carotid atherosclerosis. Real time (B mode) ultrasonography and angiography. *Stroke*. 1987;18:1011–1017.

11. DeWeese JA, May AG, Lipchick ED, et al. Anatomic and hemodynamic correlations in carotid artery stenosis. *Stroke*. 1970;1:149–157.

12. Chikos PM, Fisher LD, Hirsch HJ, et al. Observer variability in evaluating extracranial carotid artery stenosis. *Stroke*. 1983;14:885–892.

13. Riles TS, Lieberman A, Kopelmann I, Imparato AM: Symptoms, stenosis and bruit. *Arch Surg*. 1981;116:218–220.

14. Grotta JC, Bigelow RH, Hu H, et al. The significance of carotid stenosis or ulceration. *Neurology*. 1984;34:437–442.

15. Pierce GE, Keushkerian SM, Hemreck AS, et al. The risk of stroke with occlusion of the internal carotid artery. *J Vasc Surg*. 1988;8:74–80.

16. Roederer GO, Langlois VE, Jager KA, et al. The natural history of carotid arterial disease in asymptomatic patients with cervical bruits. *Stroke*. 1984;15:605–613.

17. Chambers B, Norris JW. Outcome in patients with asymptomatic neck bruits. *NEJM*. 1986;315(14):860–865.

18. Moore WS, Hall AD. Importance of emboli from the carotid bifurcation in pathogenesis of cerebral ischemic attacks. *Arch Surg*. 1970;101:708–716.

19. Ehrenfeld WK, Hoyt WF, Wylie EJ. Ulcerative lesions of the carotid artery bifurcation. *Arch Surg*. 1966;93:787–794.

20. Moore WS, Boren C, Malone JM, et al. Natural history of nonstenotic asymptomatic ulcerative lesions of the carotid artery. *Arch Surg*. 1978;113:1352–1359.

21. Imparato AM, Riles TS, Gorstein F. The carotid bifurcation plaque. Pathologic findings associated with cerebral ischemia. *Stroke*. 1979;10:238–245.

22. Ricotta JJ, Schenk EA, Ekholm SE, DeWeese JA. Angiographic and pathologic correlates in carotid artery disease. *Surgery*. 1986;99:284–292.

23. Dorazio RA, Ezzet F, Nesbitt NJ. Long-term follow up of asymptomatic carotid bruits. *Am J Surg*. 1980;140:212–213.

24. Kartchner M, McRae LP. Non-invasive evaluation and management of the "asymptomatic" carotid bruit. *Surgery*. 1977;82:840–847.

25. Busutill RW, Baker JD, Davidson RK, Machleder HI. Carotid artery stenosis: hemodynamic significance and clinical course. *JAMA*. 1981;245:1438–1441.

26. Hennerici M, Rautenberg W, Mohr S. Stroke risk from symptomless extracranial arterial disease. *Lancet*. 1982;2:1180–1183.

27. Moore DJ, Miles RD, Gooley NA, Sumner DS. Noninvasive assessment of stroke risk in asymptomatic and nonhemispheric patients with suspected carotid disease. *Ann Surg*. 1985;202:494–501.

28. Hertzer N, Flanagan R, O'Hara P, Beven E. Surgical vs. nonoperative treatment of asymptomatic carotid stenosis—290 patients documented by intravenous angiography. *Ann Surg*. 1986;204:163–171.

29. Meissner I, Wiebers DO, Whisnant JP, O'Fallon WM. The natural history of asymptomatic carotid artery occlusive lesions. *JAMA*. 1987;258:2704–2707.

30. Moneta GL, Taylor DC, Nicholls SC, et al. Operative vs. nonoperative management of asymptomatic high-grade internal carotid artery stenosis: improved results with endarterectomy. *Stroke*. 1987;18:1005–1010.

31. Taylor LM, Loboa L, Porter JM. The clinical course of carotid bifurcation stenosis as determined by duplex scanning. *J Vasc Surg*. 1988;8:255–261.

32. Langsfeld M, Lusby RJ. The spectrum of carotid artery disease in asymptomatic patients. *J Cardiovasc Surg*. 1988;29:689–691.

33. Humphries AW, Young JR, Santilli PH, et al. Unoperated asymptomatic significant internal carotid artery stenosis: a review of 182 instances. *Surgery*. 1976;80:695–698.

34. Dixon S, Pais SO, Raviola C, et al. Natural history of nonstenotic asymptomatic ulcerative lesions of the carotid artery. A further analysis. *Arch Surg*. 1982; 117:1493–1498.

35. Kroener JM, Dorn PL, Shoor PM, et al. Prognosis of asymptomatic ulcerating carotid lesions. *Arch Surg*. 1980;115:1387–1392.

36. Harward TRS, Kroener JM, Wickbom IG, Bernstein EF. Natural history of asymptomatic ulcerative plaques of the carotid bifurcation. *Am J Surg*. 1983; 146:208–212.

37. Johnson JM, Kennelly MM, DeCesare D, et al. Natural history of asymptomatic carotid plaque. *Arch Surg*. 1985;120:1010–1012.

38. O'Holleran LW, Kennelly MM, McClurken M, Johnson JM. Natural history of asymptomatic carotid plaque. *Am J Surg*. 1987;154:659–662.

39. Levin SM, Sondheimer FK, Levin JM. The contra-lateral diseased but asymptomatic carotid artery: to operate or not? *Am J Surg.* 1980;140:203–205.

40. Hennerici M, Hulsbomer HB, Hefter H, et al. Natural history of asymptomatic extracranial arterial disease. *Brain.* 1987;110:777–791.

41. Bogousslavsky J, Despland PA, Regli F. Asymptomatic tight stenosis of the internal carotid artery: long-term prognosis. *Neurology.* 1986;36:861–863.

42. Foulkes MA, Wolf PA, Price TR, et al. The stroke data bank: design methods and baseline characteristics. *Stroke.* 1988;19:541–544.

43. McDowell FH, Potes J, Grocu S. The natural history of internal carotid and vertebral-basilar artery occlusion. *Neurology.* 1961;11:153–157.

44. Marshall J. The management of occlusion and stenosis of the internal carotid artery. *Neurology.* 1966; 16:1087–1093.

45. Dyken ML, Klatte E, Kolar OJ, et al. Complete occlusion of common or internal carotid arteries. *Arch Neur.* 1974;30:343–346.

46. Barnett HJM. Delayed cerebral ischemic episodes distal to occlusion of major cerebral arteries. *Neurology.* 1978;28:764–769.

47. Fields WS, Lemak NA. Joint study of extracranial arterial occlusion. *JAMA.* 1976;235:2734–2738.

48. Furlan AJ, Whisnant JP, Baker HL. Long-term prognosis after carotid artery occlusion. *Neurology.* 1980;30:986–988.

49. Cote R, Barnett HJM, Taylor DW. Internal carotid occlusion: a prospective study. *Stroke.* 1983;14:898–902.

50. Fritz VU, Voll CL, Levien LJ. Internal carotid artery occlusion: clinical and therapeutic implications. *Stroke.* 1985;16:940–944.

51. Nicholls SC, Kohler TR, Bergelin RO, et al. Carotid artery occlusion: natural history. *J Vasc Surg.* 1986; 4:479–485.

52. Bornstein NM, Norris JW. Benign outcome of carotid occlusion. *Neurology.* 1989;39:6–8.

53. Moore WS, Boren C, Malone JM, Goldstone J. Asymptomatic carotid stenosis—immediate and long-term results after prophylactic endarterectomy. *Am J Surg.* 1979;138:228–233.

54. Riles T, Imparato AM, Mintzer R. Comparison of results of bilateral and unilateral carotid endarterectomy 5 years after surgery. *Stroke.* 1981;12:124.

55. Riles TM, Imparato AM, Kopelman I. Carotid stenosis with contralateral internal carotid occlusion: long term results in 54 patients. *Surgery.* 1980;87:363–368.

56. Callow AD, Mackey WC. Long-term follow up of surgically managed carotid bifurcation atherosclerosis. *Ann Surg.* 1989;210:308–316.

57. Easton JD, Sherman DG. Stroke and mortality rate in carotid endarterectomy: 228 consecutive operations. *Stroke.* 1977;8:565–568.

58. Toole JF, Youson CP, Janeway R, et al. Transient ischemic attacks: a prospective study of 225 patients. *Neurology.* 1978;28:746–753.

59. Modi JR, Finch WT, Sumner DS. Update of carotid endarterectomy in two community hospitals: Springfield revisited. *Stroke.* 1983;14:128.

60. Till JS, Toole JF, Howard VJ, et al. Declining morbidity and mortality of CEA. The Wake Forest University Medical Center experience. *Stroke.* 1987; 18:823–829.

61. Rubin JR, Pitluk HC, King TA, et al. Carotid endarterectomy in a metropolitan community: early results after 8535 operations. *J Vasc Surg.* 1988;7:256–260.

62. Kirshner DL, O'Brien MS, Ricotta JJ. Risk factors in community experience with carotid endarterectomy. *J Vasc Surg.* 1989;10:178–186.

63. Fode NC, Sundt TM, Robertson JT, et al. Multicenter retrospective review of results and complications of CEA 1981. *Stroke.* 1986;17:370–376.

64. Chambers B, Norris JW. The case against surgery for asymptomatic carotid stenosis. *Stroke.* 1984; 15:964–967.

65. Javid H, Ostermiller WE, Hengesh JW, et al. Carotid endarterectomy for asymptomatic patients. *Arch Surg.* 1971;102:389–391.

66. Kremer RE, Ahlquist RE. The prophylactic carotid thrombo-endarterectomy. *Am Surg.* 1979;45:703–708.

67. Thompson JJ, Talkington CM. Carotid surgery for cerebral ischemia. *Surg Clin North Am.* 1979;59:539–553.

68. White JS, Sirinek KR, Root HD, Rogers W. Morbidity and mortality of CEA: rates of occurrence in asymptomatic and symptomatic patients. *Arch Surg.* 1981;116:409–412.

69. Lees CD, Herzer NR. Postoperative stroke and late neurologic complications after carotid endarterectomy. *Arch Surg.* 1981;116:1561–1568.

70. Burke PA, Callow AD, O'Donnell TF, et al. Prophylactic carotid endarterectomy for asymptomatic bruit. *Arch Surg.* 182;117:1222–1227.

71. Slavish LG, Nicholas GG, Gee W. Review of a community experience with carotid endarterectomy. *Stroke.* 1984;15:957–959.

72. Hertzer NR, Avellone JC, Farrell CJ, et al. The risk of vascular surgery in a metropolitan community. *J Vasc Surg.* 1984;1:13–21.

73. Cafferata HT, Gainey MD. CEA in the community hospital: a continuing controversy. *J Cardiovasc Surg.* 1986;27:557–560.

74. Kempczinski RF, Brott TG, LaButta RJ. The influence of surgical specialty and caseload on the results of carotid endarterectomy. *J Vasc Surg.* 1986;3: 911–916.

75. Fields WS, Mastenikov V, Meyer JS, et al. Joint study of extracranial arterial occlusion. *JAMA.* 1970;211;23:1993–2003.

76. DeWeese JA, Rob LG, Satran R, et al. Results of carotid endarterectomy for transient ischemic attacks—5 years later. *Ann Surg.* 1973;178:258–264.

77. Hertzer NR, Aronson R. Cumulative stroke and survival 10 years after carotid endarterectomy. *J Vasc Surg.* 1985;2:661–668.

78. Forssell C, Takolander R, Bergqvist D, et al. Long-term results after carotid artery surgery. *Eur J Vasc Surg.* 1988;2:93–98.

79. Bernstein EF, Humber PB, Collins GM, et al. Life expectancy and late stroke following carotid endarterectomy. *Ann Surg.* 1983;198:80–86.

80. Rosenthal D, Rudderman R, Borrero E, et al. Carotid endarterectomy to correct asymptomatic carotid stenosis: ten years later. *J Vasc Surg.* 1987; 6:226–230.

81. Callow AD: Recurrent stenosis after carotid endarterectomy. *Arch Surg.* 1982;117:1082–1085.

82. Durward QJ, Ferguson GG, Barr HWK. The natural history of asymptomatic carotid bifurcation plaques. *Stroke.* 1982;13:459–464.

83. Stoney RJ, String ST. Recurrent carotid stenosis. *Surgery.* 1976;80:705–710.

84. Zierler RE, Bandyk DF, Thiele BL, Strandness DE. Carotid artery stenosis following endarterectomy. *Arch Surg.* 1982;117:1408–1415.

85. Ouriel K, Green RM. Clinical and technical factors influencing recurrent carotid stenosis and occluion fter endarterectomy. *J Vasc Surg.* 1987;5: 702–706.

86. Claggett GP, Robinowitz M, Youkey JR, et al. Morphogenesis and clinicopathologic characteristics of recurrent carotid disease. *J Vasc Surg.* 1986;3:10–23.

87. Claggett GP, Rich NJ, McDonald PT, et al. Etiologic factors for recurrent carotid artery stenosis. *Surgery.* 1983;93:313–318.

88. Barnes RW, Liebman PR, Marszalek PB, et al. The natural history of asymptomatic carotid disease in patients undergoing cardiovascular surgery. *Surgery.* 1981;90:1075–1083.

89. Kartchner MM, McRae LP. Carotid occlusive disease as a risk factor in major cardiovascular surgery. *Arch Surg.* 1982;117:1086–1088.

90. Turnipseed WD, Berkoff HA, Belzer FO. Postoperative stroke in cardiac and peripheral vascular disease. *Ann Surg.* 1980;192:365–368.

91. Breslau PJ, Fell G, Ivey TD, et al. Carotid arterial disease in patients undergoing coronary artery bypass operations. *J Thorac Cardiovasc Surg.* 1981;82:265–267.

92. Ennix CL, Lawrie GM, Morris GC, et al. Improved results of carotid endarterectomy in patients with symptomatic coronary disease: an analysis of 1546 consecutive carotid operations. *Stroke.* 1979;10: 122–125.

93. Crawford ES, Palamara AE, Kasparian AS. Carotid and noncoronary operations. Simultaneous, staged and delayed. *Surgery.* 1980;87:803–811.

94. Jones EL, Craver JM, Michaelik RA, et al. Combined carotid and coronary operations: when are they necessary. *J Thor Cardiovasc Surg.* 1984;87: 7–16.

95. Hertzer NR, Loop FD, Taylor PC, Beven EG. Combined myocardial revascularization and carotid endarterectomy. *J Thorac Cardiovasc Surg.* 1983;85:577–589.

96. Cosgrove DM, Hertzer NR, Loop FD. Surgical management of synchronous carotid and coronary artery disease. *J Vasc Surg.* 1986;3:690–694.

97. Hertzer NR, Loop FD, Beven EG, et al. Surgical staging for simultaneous coronary and carotid disease: a study including prospective randomization. *J Vasc Surg.* 1989;9:455–463.

98. Brener BJ, Brief DK, Alpert J, et al. A 4 year experience with preoperative noninvasive carotid evaluation of 2026 patients undergoing cardiac surgery. *J Vasc Surg.* 1984;1:326–338.

99. Brener BJ, Brief DK, Alpert J, et al. The risk of stroke in patients with asymptomatic carotid stenosis undergoing cardiac surgery: a follow-up study. *J Vasc Surg.* 1987;5:269–279.

100. Cambria RP, Ivarsson BL, Akins CW, et al. Simultaneous carotid and coronary disease: safety of the combined approach. *J Vasc Surg.* 1989;9: 56–64.

101. Barnes RW, Nix ML, Sansonetti D, et al. Late outcome of untreated asymptomatic carotid disease following cardiovascular operations. *J Vasc Surg.* 1985;2:843–849.

102. Furlan AJ, Brener AC. Central nervous system complications of open heart surgery. *Stroke.* 1984; 15:912–915.

103. Podore PC, DeWeese JA, May AG, et al. Asymptomatic contralateral carotid stenosis: a five year study following carotid endarterectomy. *Surgery.* 1980;88:748–752.

104. Johnson N, Burnham SJ, Flanigan DP, et al. Carotid endarterectomy: a follow-up study of the contralateral nonoperated carotid artery. *Ann Surg.* 1978;188:748–752.

105. Towne JB, Weiss DG, Hobson RW II. First phase report of cooperative VA asymptomatic carotid stenosis study—operative morbidity and mortality. *J Vasc Surg*. 1990;11:252–259.

106. Toole JF. Study design for randomized prospective trial of carotid endarterectomy for asymptomatic atherosclerosis. *Stroke*. 1989;20:844–849.

107. Wilson SE, Mayberg MC, Yatsu FM. Defining the indications for carotid endarterectomy. *Surgery*. 1988;104(5):932–933.

108. Beebe HG, Clagett GP, DeWeese JA, et al. Assessing risk associated with carotid endarterectomy. AHA Stroke Council special Report. 20 October 1988:472–473.

16
Does Carotid Endarterectomy Prevent Stroke?

Saran Jonas

This review of the literature on carotid endarterectomy is undertaken in an attempt to answer the following questions: Does carotid endarterectomy prevent stroke? If so, in which circumstances? I have focused on randomized controlled studies, using nonrandomized data for background and projections only.

The results of this review are not particularly satisfying, since what is needed for definitive answers — sufficient data from randomized controlled studies — is not currently available. This is distressing, considering that carotid endarterectomy has been a popular operation for >30 years.

We look forward eagerly to the results of the several well-planned controlled studies currently under way: the European study of carotid surgery after carotid transient ischemic attack (TIA),[1] the North American Symptomatic Carotid Endarterectomy Study Group Trial directed by Barnett and Peerless,[2] the Veterans Administration Cooperative Study of asymptomatic carotid stenosis directed by Hobson,[3] the Asymptomatic Carotid Atherosclerosis Study directed by Toole,[4] and the Mayo Asymptomatic Carotid Endarterectomy Study directed by Wiebers.[5]

Definitions

The lesions that are the focus of carotid endarterectomy lie at the origin of the internal carotid artery in the neck. Pathologically such a lesion can be a plaque, an ulceration, or a stenosis. Clinically, these lesions are characterized as symptomatic or asymptomatic.

The term *symptomatic carotid lesion* applies to patients with a lesion in an internal carotid artery in whose territory there has been a temporary ischemic event — TIA or reversible ischemic neurologic deficit (RIND) — or a stroke.

An asymptomatic carotid lesion is a lesion in an internal carotid artery in whose territory there has been no recognized ischemic event. The term *asymptomatic carotid stenosis* has been used by some authors in situations in which the *patient* is not asymptomatic. These include situations in which ischemic or nonischemic symptoms had occurred in another vascular territory, or when the hemisphere served by the stenotic vessel is the source of symptoms considered nonischemic.

Methods

The purpose of this review is to define the value of carotid endarterectomy (CE) in stroke prevention. This will be done in the context of the viewpoint of Warlow, who stated that the most relevant clinical question is: "What is the probability of surviving free of stroke at various points in time after surgery?"[1] Actuarial analysis of the primary data is obviously the proper way to derive this probability. Unfortunately, the studies published to date do not uniformly contain such analyses and do not tabulate the times of occurrence of end-point events so that one could carry out rigorous actuarial reanalysis. Because of this, I devised an approximation for the actuarial determination of stroke-free survival: IMPS (intact months of patient survival) analysis. The IMPS value is the area under a simplified curve of stroke-free survival.[6]

For IMPS analysis of CE results, I use stroke (S) or nonstroke death (D) as end points. I assign all operative strokes and deaths (op S+D, defined as all strokes plus all nonstroke deaths occurring within 30 days after surgery) to the day of surgery. I also assume that all strokes and deaths occurring during long-term follow-up (FU) took place on one day: the midpoint day between the day of surgery and the end of FU. For total IMPS for the entire period of observation, this assumption gives a result numerically equivalent to that derived from the assumption that the temporal distribution of the follow-up events was uniform throughout the period of observation. With this simplifying assumption, the IMPS for a cohort is:

$$m[N - op\ S+D - 0.5(follow\text{-}up\ S+D)]$$

where m is the mean length of FU in months and N is the number of patients randomized for the cohort. IMPS divided by mN gives the IMPS ratio, which is the ratio between the observed IMPS and the theoretical maximum value for IMPS: that which would have been seen had there been no operative or follow-up stroke or death.

IMPS ratio =
$$m[N - op\ S+D - 0.5(follow\text{-}up\ S+D)]/mN,$$

or:

$$[N - op\ S+D - 0.5(follow\text{-}up\ S+D])/N$$

A similar calculation can be done for the controls (early strokes and deaths, those in the first 30 days of observation, are substituted for operative stroke and death).

For CE to be useful, it is necessary that the IMPS ratio among CE patients be greater than the IMPS ratio of the controls; the area under the stroke-free survival curve for CE must be proportionally greater than that under the control curve.

IMPS analysis could be modified by the factoring out of nonstroke death during FU: stroke alone would be the end point. On the assumption that CE influences stroke rate and nonstroke death rate during surgery and in the immediate postoperative period but influences only stroke rate thereafter, one should obtain (to the effects of CE) optimal sensitivity from an analysis using stroke and death

as the end points for the operative-immediate postoperative period and using only stroke thereafter. This analysis will be called IMPS(s): IMPS stroke analysis.

For IMPS(s) analysis, stroke rate during FU after the end of the operative (or early) period is adjusted by removal from the at-risk pool those patients eliminated from further FU because of nonstroke death. This adjusted stroke rate is the net stroke rate. It is best calculated from the actual dates of the strokes and deaths occurring during long-term FU. If the dates of the events are not specified, one can approximate the net stroke rate by subtracting half of the nonstroke deaths from the at-risk pool entering long-term FU intact after the operative or early period.

Net stroke rate is thus: $S'/(N'\text{-}D'/2)$; N' is the size of the pool of patients entering long-term FU intact; S' and D' are strokes and nonstroke deaths occurring during long-term FU.

The number of net strokes is: (N') (net stroke rate). IMPS(s), that is, IMPS, with net stroke during FU substituted for S+D during FU, is then calculated as follows:

$$m[N - op\ or\ early\ S+D - 0.5(net\ strokes\ during\ follow\text{-}up)].$$

IMPS(s) ratio is:

$$[N - op\ or\ early\ S+D - 0.5(net\ strokes\ during\ follow\text{-}up)]/N$$

In all the analyses the number of patients on which the FU calculations are based is N', that is, the number originally entered into study minus op or early S+D.

The review that follows uses the following criterion as the index for successful stroke prevention: the IMPS(s) ratio for CE patients must be better than the control IMPS(s) ratio, and the CE IMPS ratio must be no worse than its control value, that is: the operated patients must have fewer strokes and must live just as long (or longer).

Outcome End Points

A final word on criteria for judging outcome should be offered. To focus on strokes or on stroke-free survival alone does not seem entirely satisfactory. Stroke-free survival with recurring TIAs is clearly not as desirable an outcome as stroke-free survival without TIAs. However, to rank TIA with a full stroke as an end point also seems unsatisfactory. Similarly, should mild strokes be counted equally with severe strokes? Also, what about the disability from a hypoglossal or recurrent laryngeal nerve injury during neck dissection? Are these not just as disabling as a mild stroke? Furthermore, should not the lost time, discomfort, and financial expense of surgery weigh in on the debit side as one compares surgical with nonsurgical treatment?

One solution is to focus not on events alone but also on the overall quality of life following treatment. Olsson et al.[7] did this partially for myocardial infarction; they looked at the number of follow-up days spent in each of seven health categories as adapted from the New York Heart Association functional state classification. Matchar and Pauker[8] have discussed in a theoretical paper how one might assign "quality factors" to months of life after CE: intact life is assigned the value 1.0; life after small stroke, 0.8; and life after large stroke, 0.2. Trudel et al.[9] did a global quality of life evaluation on 50 survivors (81 to 105 months) of CE for TIA or stroke; they did not have a control group. Regrettably, there is no way to analyze retrospectively the results of the controlled CE series currently in the literature.

Carotid Endarterectomy: Description of Six Identifiable Cohorts from Four Randomized Studies

Tables 16.1 and 16.2 summarize the results from six cohorts in four randomized studies.

Warlow pointed out in 1984,[1] and it is still true today, that the literature contains the results of only one randomized controlled study of CE for symptomatic carotid lesions: Shaw et al.[10] In this study, begun in 1965, 41 TIA or minor stroke patients were randomized for CE (20 patients) or nonsurgical (21 patients) treatment.

Op S+D (operative strokes and nonstroke deaths) was 5+2, and early S+D (during the first 30 days after randomization) for the controls was 0+0. Because of the high (35%) op S+D rate, the study was closed after 41 patients had been randomized.

TABLE 16.1. Various observed and calculated results of randomized endarterectomy studies.

Cohort	N	Mo FU	Pt-mo	Op or early S+D	S+D in FU	Net S in FU
Surgery						
Shaw[10]	20	78	1560	5+ 2	2+ 4	2.36
Clagett[11]	11	30	330	0+ 0	0+ 0	0.00
Fields[12]						
1 sten	45	42	1890	0+ 1	2+ 7	2.17
2 sten	94	42	3948	10+ 5	3+ 8	3.16
sten+oc	30	42	1260	3+ 0	1+ 5	1.10
Bauer[13]	38	33*	1254	0+ 5	5+ 7	5.59
Totals	238		10242	18+13	13+31	14.38
Fields[12]						
pooled	169	42	7098	13+ 6	6+20	6.43
Control						
Shaw[10]	21	73.2	1537	0+ 0	6+ 9	7.64
Clagett[11]	14	38	532	0+ 0	0+ 1	0.00
Fields[12]						
1 sten	49	42	2058	1+ 0	5+ 4	5.22
2 sten	73	42	3066	0+ 1	9+ 9	9.60
sten+oc	25	42	1050	0+ 0	4+ 5	4.44
Bauer[13]	40	33*	1320	0+ 0	5+13	5.97
Totals	222		9563	1+ 1	29+41	32.87
Fields[12]						
pooled	147	42	6174	1+ 1	18+18	19.19

N = number; Mo = months; FU = follow-up; Pt = patient; Op = operative; S = stroke; D = nonstroke death; 1 sten = unilateral carotid stenosis; 2 sten = bilateral carotid stenoses; oc = total carotid occlusion opposite a carotid stenosis; 33* is estimated mean FU; range was 24–42 months. See text for calculation of net stroke.

During follow-up (mean 78 months surgical, 73.2 months control), the S+D occurrence was 2+4 op and 6+9 control.

One small, controlled study of endarterectomy for asymptomatic carotid lesions has been reported. Clagett et al.[11] randomized 29 asymptomatic people (mean age 63.5 years) who had mid-cervical bruit and abnormal ophthalmoplethysmography (OPG). The arms of the study were intervention: arteriography preparatory to prophylactic CE (15 persons), and nonintervention unless symptoms developed during follow-up (14 persons); all 29 were given 1300 mg of aspirin (ASA) daily. The study was therefore immediate CE versus no or delayed CE.

Of the 15 randomized for intervention, one person refused arteriography, and died of myocardial

TABLE 16.2. Summary of analyses of outcomes of randomized endarterectomy studies.

Cohort	Op or early S+D: % per pt	% per y of FU:		IMPS ratio	IMPS ratio × pt-mo	IMPS(s) ratio	IMPS(s) ratio × pt-mo
		S+D	Net S				
Surgery							
Shaw[10]	35.0	7.1*	2.8*	0.500	780	0.591	922
Clagett[11]	0.0	0.0*	0.0	1.000*	330	1.000	330
Fields[12]							
1 sten	2.2	5.8	1.5	0.878	1659	0.954*	1803
2 sten	16.0**	4.0*	1.2*	0.782	3087	0.824	3253
sten+oc	10.0**	6.3*	1.3*	0.800	1008	0.882	1111
Bauer[13]	13.2**	13.2*	6.9	0.711	892	0.795	997
Totals	13.0	5.2*	1.7*	0.757	7756	0.822	8416
Fields[12]							
pooled	11.2	5.0*	1.2*	0.811	5754	0.869	6165
Control							
Shaw[10]	0.0	11.7	6.0	0.643	988	0.818	1257
Clagett[11]	0.0	2.3	0.0	0.972	517	1.000	532
Fields[12]							
1 sten	2.0	5.4	3.2	0.888	1828	0.926	1906
2 sten	1.4	7.1	4.1	0.863	2646	0.921	2824
sten+oc	0.0	10.3	5.6	0.820	861	0.911	957
Bauer[13]	0.0	16.4	6.5	0.775	1023	0.925	1221
Totals	0.9	8.8	4.1	0.822	7863	0.909	8697
Fields[12]							
pooled	1.4	7.1	3.8	0.864	5334	0.921	5687

Op = operative; y = year; FU = follow-up; S = stroke; D = nonstroke death; IMPS = intact months of patient survival (See text); IMPS(s) = intact months of patient survival calculated for net stroke in follow-up (see text); × pt-mo = multiplied by patient-months; 1 sten = unilateral carotid stenosis; 2 sten = bilateral carotid stenoses; oc = total carotid occlusion opposite a carotid stenosis; * indicates that the surgical results are better than the control results. Example of calculations: under "Totals" for "Surgery": (18+13)/238 = 13.0%; (13+31)(12)/10242 = 5.2%; (14.38)(12)/10242 = 1.7%, 7756/10242 = 0.757; 8416/10242 = 0.822. The various values are found in the "Totals" for "Surgery" in Tables 16.1 and 16.2. The analogous values under "Totals" for "Control" are calculated in an analogous manner.
**: The 94 "2 sten" patients had 110 CE and 10 VE = 120 operations. S+D rate per operation was (10+5)/120 = 12.5%. The 30 "sten+oc" patients had 39 operations. The S+D rate per operation was (3+0)/39 =7.7%. The 38 patients of Bauer et al.[13] were from a group of 89 who apparently had 108 CE and 10 VE; the authors give the number of S+D for the 38, but not the number or type of operations.

infarction two years later. The other 14 had arteriography. One of these 14 had a myocardial infarction during arteriography; he did not have CE. He died a year later of a myocardial infarction. Of the remaining 13, one had a completely occluded carotid artery, and one had no lesion (false positive OPG; apparently, this person died during FU). The remaining 11 had advanced carotid stenoses and had prophylactic CE; op S+D occurrence was nil, and there were no strokes or deaths among these 11 during a mean of 30 months of FU.

Among the 14 randomized for nonintervention, there were no early S+D. Mean FU was 38 months. During FU one person died of heart disease. Three others had TIAs and had carotid surgery. Two others had nonfocal symptoms; one of these two also had CE. There were no strokes among the 14

"nonintervention" patients. (The angiographic complication in the "intervention" group is noted; it is clear that failure to include angiographic complications in evaluation of outcome in surgical series is a potential source of error in cost/benefit analysis. On the other hand, failure to obtain angiography may lead to errors in the assembling of a control series: see the false positive OPG case described above.)

The two papers just described present separately the results of carotid surgery in symptomatic and in asymptomatic people. There are two randomized controlled endarterectomy studies in which the results in the symptomatic and the asymptomatic groups cannot be separated.

Fields et al.[12] randomized 316 TIA or minor stroke patients with carotid stenoses for carotid surgery or for nonsurgical management between 1962 and

1968. Every patient in the surgical cohort of 169 had carotid surgery. Some had bilateral carotid surgery, and in 10 patients vertebral endarterectomy (VE) was also performed (total of 194 carotid and 10 vertebral operations among 169 patients). Since at least 73 of the operated patients had ischemia in the vertebrobasilar territory only (authors' table 4); it is clear that many of the operated lesions were asymptomatic; their results are not identified separately in the presentation of the outcomes.

The report describes the results by angiographic criteria: unilateral carotid stenosis, bilateral carotid stenosis, and carotid stenosis opposite carotid occlusion.

In the unilateral stenosis cohort, 45 patients had carotid surgery. In the bilateral carotid stenosis cohort, 94 patients had 110 CE; 10 patients also had VE. In patients with carotid stenosis opposite carotid occlusion, 30 patients had procedures on 19 stenotic vessels and on 20 occluded vessels (back flow was obtained in 4).

The results in these three cohorts of Fields et al.[12] are summarized in Tables 16.1 and 16.2.

Bauer et al.[13] accepted into a randomized study of endarterectomy versus nonsurgical management (begun in 1962) 183 patients who had TIA, RIND, or stroke. Endarterectomy was carried out in 89 (54 had one CE, 11 had bilateral CE, 6 had CE + vertebral endarterectomy, and 18 had vertebral endarterectomy only; apparently, the total was 82 CE + 26 VE). The outcomes for the patients entered for TIA or RIND are apparently included in the results of Fields et al. (as part of a multi-institution study), reviewed above.[12] Bauer et al. gave FU outcomes for 78 of the completed stroke patients whom they followed for at least two years (range 24 to 42 months).[13] Thirty-eight of these completed stroke patients had endarterectomy. (It is not clear that all had CE; it is possible that some had VE alone); 40 were controls. Results are given in Tables 16.1 and 16.2.

Results of Analysis of the Randomized Studies and Projections from Nonrandomized Data

Table 16.1 summarizes the observations. Table 16.2 summarizes event rates, IMPS ratios, and IMPS(s)

ratios. Entries marked * indicate that the CE result was superior to the control result.

In both the Shaw and Bauer studies[10,13] and in two groups of the Fields study,[12] both IMPS and IMPS(s) ratios among the operated patients were worse than among the controls (lower values meaning less stroke-free survival). These studies therefore showed no benefit from surgery.

The unilateral stenosis group in the Fields study[12] also failed to show overall benefit. Although IMPS(s) ratio was increased in the CE patients, the IMPS ratio was reduced. The study of Clagett et al.[11] failed because there was no reduction in stroke: IMPS ratio was higher in the surgical group but IMPS(s) ratio was the same in the two groups.

Thus, there was no overall benefit from endarterectomy in any randomized study or in the pooled results: 238 operated and 222 control patients.

Before dismissing endarterectomy, however, one should look at the array of asterisks in Table 16.2. For the annual rates of stroke and death and of net stroke in long-term FU, 9 of 12 surgical results from the six cohorts of the four studies were more favorable than the control results. On pooled analysis, these reductions among the intact survivors of surgery were statistically significant: annual stroke and death rates: 5.2% surgical, 8.8% control (p < 0.05); net stroke rates: 1.7% surgical, 4.1% control (p < 0.02). The problem was the very poor early outcome for surgery: 13.0% op stroke and death rate per patient versus 0.9% early rate in the controls (p < 0.00005).

This raises an important question: If op rates had been lower and stroke and death rates and net stroke rates among the intact survivors unchanged from those originally observed during long-term FU, would surgical IMPS and IMPS(s) ratios equal to or better than the control values have occurred? One could raise this question because all the randomized studies were begun before 1979; Table 16.3 suggests that op stroke and death risks among patients with prior TIA or stroke may, overall, be lower now (although the results of CE for asymptomatic stenosis are contradictory).

In the case of Shaw et al.[10] the break-even op stroke and death rate is 10.0% (IMPS ratio = 0.692 versus control 0.643, IMPS(s) ratio = 0.818 versus control 0.818); any S+D rate below the break-even level would have successfully prevented strokes (considerations of sample size and statistical significance aside).

TABLE 16.3. Strokes and deaths after carotid endarterectomy performed in U.S. hospitals.

Studies	Number of operations	op S+D S + D	%
Studies begun before 1979			
Asymptomatic carotid stenosis			
21 studies: Till,[14] table 4	902	14 + 11	
Clagett[11]	13	2 + 0	
Asymptomatic Stenosis totals			3.0
TIA: 30 studies: Till,[14] table 5	3348	150 + 73	6.7
Established cerebral infarction			
19 studies: Till,[14] table 6	1259	88 + 91	14.2
Pre-1979 pooled	5522	254 + 175	7.8
Surgery performed 1979–86			
Asymptomatic carotid stenosis			
4 studies: Till,[14] table 4	839	31 + 24	
AbuRahma[15]	151	6	
Moneta[16]	56	1	
Asymptomatic stenosis totals			5.9
TIA: 4 studies: Till,[14] table 5	2091	80 + 26	5.1
Established cerebral infarction			
4 studies: Till,[14] table 6	639	38 + 8	7.2
1979–86 pooled	3776	214	5.7

Op = operative; S = stroke; D = death; TIA = transient ischemic attack. The data taken from Till et al.[14] are from tables 4, 5, and 6 of those authors; excluded from the present table are those entries of Till et al. that lack either stroke or death data. The data from Clagett et al.[11] are from only the nonrandomized cases.

For the pooled cohorts of Fields et al.,[12] the break-even op S+D rate is 5.0% per patient (169 patients; there were 204 operations, including 10 VE; the 5.0% rate per patient would be 4.1% per operation); this would project an IMPS ratio of 0.864 (control 0.864) and an IMPS(s) ratio of 0.938 (control 0.926).

For the cohort of Bauer et al.,[13] an op S+D rate of 0.0% would project an IMPS ratio of 0.818, better than the control value of 0.775, but the resulting IMPS(s) ratio of 0.915 would still be inferior to the 0.925 control level.

Since the op S+D rate in the asymptomatic stenosis study of Clagett et al.[11] was 0.0%, the failure to demonstrate benefit was not a consequence of operative complications. Projection as done for Shaw et al., Fields et al., and Bauer et al. is not relevant.[10,12,13]

Thus, for Shaw et al.[10] and for Fields et al.,[12] an op S+D level that projects favorable surgical IMPS and IMPS(s) values can be found. This is not true for Bauer et al.[13]; even an op S+D rate of 0.0 results in an unfavorable IMPS(s) projection. Projection is irrelevant for Clagett et al.[11]

Is there any basis for thinking that the op S+D rates identified in the projections can be obtained? With respect to Shaw et al.,[10] Table 16.3 shows that the op S+D rate for 2091 carotid endarterectomies performed 1979–1986 for TIA in uncontrolled cohorts was 5.1%. Thus, it appears that the needed op S+D rate of 10.0% or lower can reasonably be expected.

The pooled cohorts of Fields et al.[12] would need an S+D rate per operation no higher than 4.1% to show benefit. These patients had surgery for a mixture of symptomatic and asymptomatic lesions. According to Table 16.3, in the period 1979–1986 TIA surgery (2091 operations) had an op S+D rate of 5.1%, and asymptomatic stenosis surgery (639 operations) a rate of 5.9%. If these figures reflect current surgical results, then the average contemporary surgeon could not provide benefit to a group of patients like those of Fields et al.[12]

Follow-up Medical Management After Endarterectomy

Can the results of CE be improved by aspirin (ASA) treatment during long-term FU? Two randomized studies are available.

Fields, Lemak et al.[17] randomized (1972–1975) for ASA 1300 mg daily or for placebo 125 patients who had recently had CE for TIA or minor stroke. No op S+D data are given. The authors give (their tables 6 and 7) cumulative probabilities for stroke and death for 6-month intervals during 2 years of FU (ASA 65 patients, placebo 60 patients). From the averages for these intervals, one can calculate IMPS and IMPS(s) ratios. IMPS ratio = 0.898 for ASA and 0.858 for placebo (p = 0.70, according to the authors). IMPS(s) ratio = 0.988 ASA and 0.857 placebo (p = 0.03).

Boysen et al.[18] gave ASA 50–100 mg or placebo daily to 301 patients who 1 week to 3 months earlier (1982–1986) had had CE for stroke or TIA (292 patients), or for asymptomatic lesions

(9 patients). Treatment averaged 21 months. Strokes plus vascular deaths for 150 ASA patients came to 9 + 12 = 14%; for 151 placebo patients the values were 11 + 6 = 11%. Net stroke rate was 0.06 ASA and 0.07 placebo. Chi-square values were nonsignificant.

Thus the use of ASA 1300 mg daily was associated with a statistically significant reduction in strokes in FU after CE (the intact survival was also enhanced, but not to a statistically significant degree); ASA 50 to 100 mg daily had no value.

These results address only the issue of placebo versus ASA after CE and give no information on the issue of CE plus ASA versus nonsurgical management plus ASA.

Discussion

Although the Shaw study[10] showed no overall evidence of benefit from carotid endarterectomy, reasonable projections suggest that groups of patients with TIAs or minor strokes who have appropriate carotid lesions could benefit from carotid surgery if the immediate operative stroke and death rate is low enough.

There is no evidence from the study of Bauer et al. that patients who already have had a completed stroke can benefit from endarterectomy.[13] With respect to the value of *carotid* endarterectomy in this setting, it should be recognized that some of the patients of Bauer et al. may have had vertebral and not carotid surgery. Whether this is true, and if so, the direction and magnitude of the consequent bias cannot be ascertained from the published data.

The Clagett study showed no evidence of stroke reduction in asymptomatic patients who had CE at the time of identification of a carotid stenosis (when compared with controls who did not have CE or who had it after having specific or nonspecific symptoms during FU), and provides no basis for projecting circumstances in which such benefit could be expected.[11]

Fields et al. reported on the results of 194 CE in 169 patients with TIA or minor stroke.[12] Perhaps half of the CE were on asymptomatic vessels. In one group, 10 patients had vertebral endarterectomy as well as CE. As in the case of Bauer et al.,[13] one cannot evaluate the effect of asymptomatic vessel surgery on outcome, since no specific data

are given; also, one has no choice but to ignore the possible vertebral endarterectomy effects.

The study of Fields et al.[12] showed no overall benefit from surgery—the operated cohort did worse overall than the 147 controls—and no basis for projecting such. Analysis of the results of the Shaw study[10] suggests that benefit can be obtained from surgery on symptomatic carotid lesions, while analysis of the results of Clagett et al.[11] suggests that CE does not benefit asymptomatic people. In these terms, one could conclude that in the Fields study[12] the potential beneficial effects from CE on symptomatic vessels was diluted by the lack of benefit from CE on asymptomatic vessels; so that no overall benefit was seen or could be projected (none of the *patients* of Fields et al.[12] were asymptomatic, although many of the operated carotid arteries were).

With respect to the issue of surgery for asymptomatic carotid lesions, one might wish to emphasize again that the situation would be simpler if the first symptom to develop in the territory of such a vessel is always a TIA and never a stroke. That seemed true in the small control group of Clagett et al.[11] On this point, reports from various nonrandomized studies are reviewed below.

Levin et al.[19] followed for 5 years 142 patients with an ulcerated plaque or a stenosis of 50% or greater (or both) in an asymptomatic carotid artery contralateral to a vessel on which surgery had been performed because of symptoms. Sixteen eventually had carotid surgery on the originally asymptomatic vessel. None of the 142 had strokes. However, Durward et al.[20] followed for 4 years 73 patients with an ulcerated plaque or a stenosis of 50% or greater in an asymptomatic carotid artery contralateral to a vessel treated with CE because of symptoms. During follow-up 12 patients had ischemic episodes in the originally asymptomatic carotid territory; in 2 the first episode was a stroke and in 10 a TIA (uneventful CE was performed in 9 of the 10). Also, Podore et al.[21] followed for 5 years 28 patients with asymptomatic 50 to 99% internal carotid artery stenosis in the vessel contralateral to a CE for symptomatic stenosis; there were apparently two strokes without TIA, and four TIAs for which CE was done, in the originally asymptomatic carotid territories. Furthermore, Moneta et al.[16] noted a 19% 2-year cumulative stroke rate among 73 initially nonsymptomproducing 80 to 99% stenotic internal carotid arteries; no stroke was preceded by a TIA.

Thus, deferring carotid surgery until an asymptomatic lesion becomes symptomatic, as in the control group in the small randomized study of Clagett et al.,[11] is not ipso facto optimal; the nonrandomized observations make it clear that asymptomatic stenosis can lead to stroke without warning TIA. The issue of initial intervention is clearly one of cost/benefit ratio; the reduction in stroke risk versus the hazards of intervention. The recent op S+D data (see Table 16.3: $31+24+6+1 = 62$ S+D in $839+151+56 = 1046$ CE for asymptomatic stenosis 1979–1986; op S+D rate = 5.9%) are sobering.

To summarize, the scanty randomized data currently available do not favor surgical intervention for asymptomatic carotid lesions; one looks forward to the several large, randomized studies currently under way for definitive answers.

On medical management during long-term follow-up, two controlled studies give useful data: high-dose aspirin treatment (1300 mg daily) reduces strokes after CE[17]; low-dose (50 to 100 mg daily) aspirin treatment does not.[18]

Summary

1. No benefit was seen from carotid endarterectomy in six cohorts from four randomized studies.
2. Projections suggest that surgery on a carotid lesion appropriate to a TIA or minor stroke could be helpful if carried out at a suitably low operative stroke plus death rate. Extensive data from uncontrolled studies suggest that such rates are obtainable.
3. There is no evidence that surgery after completed stroke has value.
4. From the results in the asymptomatic cohort, and in the cohort composed of patients operated for symptomatic and asymptomatic lesions, there is no evidence of potential benefit from surgery on asymptomatic carotid lesions.
5. Long-term treatment with aspirin 1300 mg daily reduces strokes after carotid surgery; 50 to 100 mg daily does not.
6. We look forward to the results of the several large, randomized studies now under way to replace with definitive answers the above projections and inferences concerning carotid endarterectomy.

References

1. Warlow CP. Carotid endarterectomy: does it work? *Stroke.* 1984;15:1068–1076.
2. North American Symptomatic Carotid Endarterectomy Study Group. Carotid endarterectomy: three critical evaluations. *Stroke.* 1987;18:987–989.
3. Veterans Administration Cooperative Study. Role of carotid endarterectomy in asymptomatic carotid stenosis. *Stroke.* 1986;17:534–539.
4. Asymptomatic Carotid Atherosclerosis Study Group. Study design for randomized prospective trial of carotid endarterectomy for asymptomatic atherosclerosis. *Stroke.* 1989;20:844–849.
5. Mayo Asymptomatic Carotid Endarterectomy Study Group. Effectiveness of carotid endarterectomy for asymptomatic carotid stenosis: design of a clinical trial. *Mayo Clin Proc.* 1989;64:897–904.
6. Jonas S. IMPS (intact months of patient survival): an analysis of the results of carotid endarterectomy. *Stroke.* 1986;17:1329–1334. [Corrective correspondence regarding paper: *Stroke.* 1987;18:1173–1175; *Stroke.* 1988;19:1054,1180–1181].
7. Olsson G, Lubsen J, Van Es G-A, et al. Quality of life after myocardial infarction: effect of long term metoprolol on mortality and morbidity. *Brit Med J.* 1986;292:1491–1493.
8. Matchar DB, Pauker SG. Endarterectomy in carotid artery disease: a decision analysis. *JAMA.* 1987; 258:793–798.
9. Trudel L, Fabia J, Bouchard J-P. Quality of life of 50 carotid endarterectomy survivors: a long-term follow-up study. *Arch Phys Med Rehabil.* 1984;65: 310–312.
10. Shaw DA, Venables GS, Cartlidge NEF, et al. Carotid endarterectomy in patients with transient cerebral ischaemia. *J Neurol Sci.* 1984;64:45–53.
11. Clagett PG, Yourkey JR, Brigham RA, et al. Asymptomatic cervical bruit and abnormal ocular pneumoplethysmography: a prospective study comparing two approaches to management. *Surgery.* 1984;96:823–830.
12. Fields WS, Maslenikov V, Meyer JS, et al. Joint study of extracranial arterial occlusion: V. Progress report of prognosis following surgery or nonsurgical treatment for transient cerebral ischemic attacks and cervical carotid artery lesions. *JAMA.* 1970;211: 1993–2003.

13. Bauer RB, Meyer JS, Gotham JE, et al. A controlled study of surgical treatment of cerebrovascular disease; forty-two months' experience with 183 cases. In: Millikan CH, Siekert RG, Whisnant JP, eds. *Cerebral Vascular Diseases.* New York, NY: Grune & Stratton; 1966:pp 254–272.

14. Till JS, Toole JF, Howard VJ, et al. Declining morbidity and mortality of carotid endarterectomy: the Wake Forest University Medical Center study. *Stroke.* 1987;18:823–829.

15. Abu Rahma AF, Robinson P. Indications and complications of carotid endarterectomy as performed by four different surgical specialty groups. *J Cardiovasc Surg.* 1988;29:277–282.

16. Moneta GL, Taylor DC, Nicholls SC, et al. Operative versus nonoperative management of asymptomatic high-grade internal carotid artery stenosis: improved results with endarterectomy. *Stroke.* 1987;18:1005–1010.

17. Fields WS, Lemak NA, Frankowski RF, et al. Controlled trial of aspirin in cerebral ischemia. II: Surgical group. *Stroke.* 1978;9:309–319.

18. Boysen G, Sorensen PS, Juhler M, et al. Danish very-low-dose-aspirin after carotid endarterectomy trial. *Stroke.* 1988;19:1211–1215.

19. Levin SM, Sondheimer FK, Levin JM. The contralateral diseased but asymptomatic carotid artery: to operate or not? An update. *Am J Surg.* 1980;140:203–205.

20. Durward QJ, Ferguson GG, Barr HWK. The natural history of asymptomatic carotid bifurcation plaques. *Stroke.* 1982;13:459–464.

21. Podore PC, DeWeese JA, May AG, et al. Asymptomatic contralateral carotid artery stenosis: a five-year follow-up study following carotid endarterectomy. *Surgery.* 1980;88:748–752.

17
Balloon Transluminal Angioplasty of the Carotid Artery in the Head and Neck

Fong Y. Tsai and Randall Higashida

Percutaneous transluminal angioplasty (PTA) for vascular occlusive disease was first described by Dotter and Judkins more than 25 years ago. However, the technique was not popularized until the introduction of the Gruntzig and Hopff method of double-lumen balloon catheterization approximately 10 years after the introduction of the original concept of PTA in 1964.[1-3]

Over the past decade, PTA has been widely used in the nonsurgical treatment of coronary, iliofemoral and most other stenotic arteries in the body. However, the use of PTA in the treatment of brachiocephalic arteries progressed very slowly and cautiously because of the potential risk of cerebral catastrophe from dislodging emboli distally. Hence, the carotid territory was thought to be the most dangerous among the brachiocephalic arteries, and balloon angioplasty of the carotid artery did not start until later.[4-59]

In 1980 Kerber et al. reported successful transluminal angioplasty in stenosis of the proximal common carotid artery via distal endarterectomy.[4] Later, Mathias et al. reported successful angioplasty from the percutaneous approach.[34] Since then, reports of successful PTA for carotid stenosis have intensified.[4-59] This chapter will describe the practical aspects of PTA as an alternative procedure for the treatment of extracranial carotid artery stenosis and for vasospasm of the intracranial proximal carotid branches. (See Figs. 17.1–17.5.)

Balloon Angioplasty of the Extracranial Carotid Artery

Mechanism of Balloon Angioplasty

The angioplastic balloon dilatation produces splitting and disruption of the intima, with stretching of the media rather than compression of atheromatous plaque. Right after the dilatation, platelets start to deposit in areas denuded of endothelium, and a layer of fibrin covers the site of vascular injury. The healing process occurs with retraction of the intimal flaps, with neointimal formation and scar tissue similar to those seen after endarterectomy.[1,3,29,60-62]

Technique

Patients undergoing PTA of the carotid artery are maintained on oral and parenteral anticoagulants for at least 1 week prior to the procedure. Those with carotid bifurcation stenosis are given atropine 0.3 mg intravenously prior to the PTA to avoid sudden falls in blood pressure from compression of the carotid body. Oral Decadron 10 mg is administered twice daily for 2 days prior to the procedure. With use of the Seldinger technique, a 5 to 7.5 French sheath is placed intraarterially via the femoral artery. Then 3000 units of heparin is given for systemic anticoagulation. All patients are monitored by electroencephalogram (EEG).

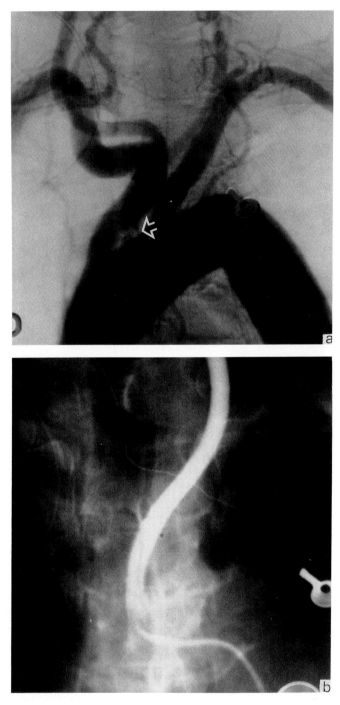

FIGURE 17.1. (a) Arch angiogram showed severe stenosis of left proximal common carotid artery (arrow).
(b) Postangioplastic carotid and arch angiography demonstrated good restoration of left proximal common
carotid artery.

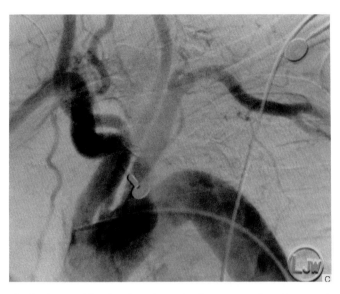

FIGURE 17.1. (c) Postangioplastic carotid and arch angiography demonstrated good restoration of left proximal common carotid artery.

A 5-French catheter is then advanced to the stenotic site under fluoroscopic guide. A 260 inch exchange guide wire is then advanced beyond the stenotic area to be treated. The 5-F catheter is removed immediately, and the angioplastic balloon catheter is passed over the guide wire. The EEG is checked continuously to detect signs of early cerebral ischemia due to passing the balloon catheter. If the EEG shows slowing of cerebral activity, fresh heparinized arterial blood is injected continuously during and after the catheter is passed through the stenosis. Balloon dilatation is performed one or two times across the atheromatous plaque or stenosis under fluoroscopic observation. The balloon is inflated very slowly and gently. Once the balloon is fully inflated, it is deflated immediately. During inflation, the guide wire is removed to allow continuous injection of heparinized fresh arterial blood to avoid an ischemic attack due to inflation of the balloon, which interrupts the cerebral circulation. The patient is rechecked neurologically in addition to the continuous EEG monitoring. Postangioplastic digital subtraction angiography (DSA) is performed to assess patency of the vessel and to evaluate the intracranial circulation.

Patients are then closely monitored by EEG and neurological examination for 24 hours and discharged on aspirin 325 mg/day for 3 weeks, as well as oral steroids for 1 week. Patients are closely followed clinically at 3- and 12-month intervals.[26,27,33,57]

Indications

1. Any severe carotid artery stenosis suitable for surgical treatment or in patients with severe cardiopulmonary disease that contraindicates carotid surgery.
2. Stenosis in a smooth, angiographic segment without evidence of ulceration by angiography or Doppler examination.
3. Failure of anticoagulant treatment in symptomatic patients.

Results

Percutaneous transluminal angioplasty of the carotid artery for stenotic lesions due to atherosclerosis, fibromuscular hyperplasia, Takayasu's disease, and myointimal fibrosis after endarterectomy

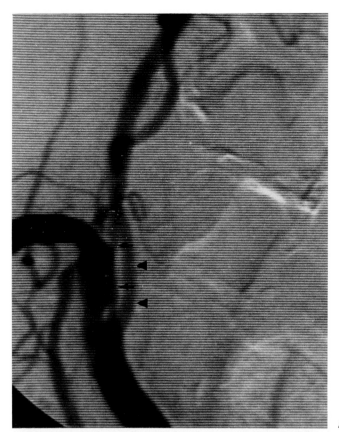

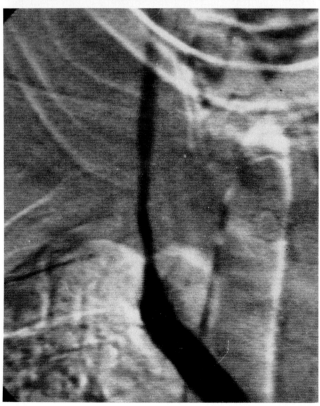

FIGURE 17.2. (A) Right innominate and common carotid angiography demonstrated a long segment stenosis of right proximal common carotid artery (arrows) and stenosis of right subclavian artery just distal to vertebral artery (arrowheads). (B) Right innominate and common carotid angiography demonstrated a long segment stenosis of right proximal common carotid artery (arrows) and stenosis of right subclavian artery just distal to vertebral artery (arrowheads).

FIGURE 17.2 (C) Postangioplastic angiography showed good restoration of right common carotid artery.

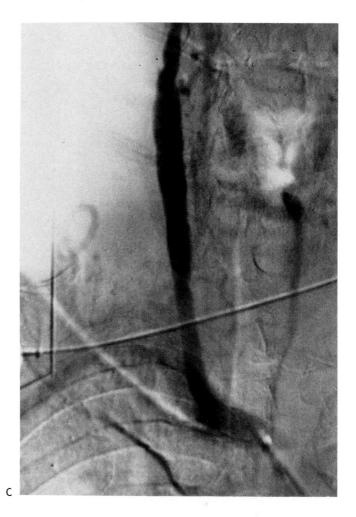

C

has been successfully performed in the following segments (reported from our centers)[26,27,33,57]:

Common carotid	58
Carotid bifurcation	11
Internal carotid	29
External carotid	11

A total of 109 procedures has been performed without any permanent morbidity or mortality. Two patients had sudden falls in blood pressure and transient cerebral ischemia during inflation of the balloon at the carotid bifurcation prior to routine administration of Atropin. Seven patients showed slow waves on EEG during inflation of the balloon.

These problems have not recurred since we introduced injection of heparinized arterial blood during the procedure.

Discussion

Surgical procedures, either endarterectomy or bypass, have been the customary treatment for carotid artery disease.[59,60-71] Transluminal angioplasty of the carotid artery, often believed to start after the introduction of balloon catheter, actually started much earlier. It was first described by Morris et al. in 1968 using a bile duct dilator for the treatment of a surgically inaccessible fibromuscular hyperplasia of the internal carotid artery during operation.[60-63]

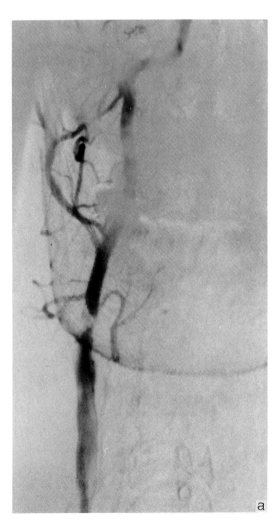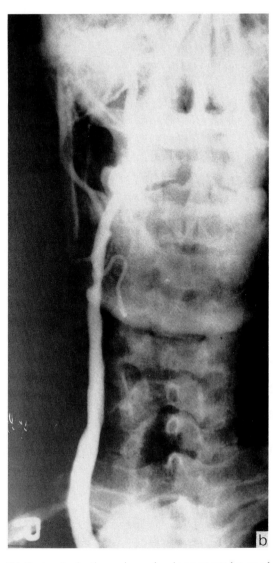

FIGURE 17.3. (a) Common carotid angiography demonstrated severe stenosis of left carotid bifurcation and
proximal internal carotid artery.

(b) Postangioplastic angiography demonstrated a good
restoration of proximal internal carotid lumen.

The current use of PTA for treatment of the carotid
artery was started at the turn of this decade by
Kerber and Mathias.[4,17,34] According to the literature and to our experience over the past decade,
nearly 300 cases of carotid stenosis have been successfully treated by PTA.

Most PTA procedures were performed similar
to our technique.[4-59,72] A modified technique

reported recently utilizes an extraprotective balloon distal to the angioplastic balloon. This newly
developed technique is designed specially for carotid bifurcation and ulcerative plaques.[54] However,
most PTAs of the carotid artery are performed
without this additional balloon. The primary problem we encountered was transient cerebral ischemia during inflation of the balloon or on passing

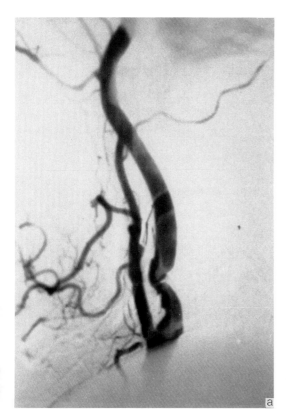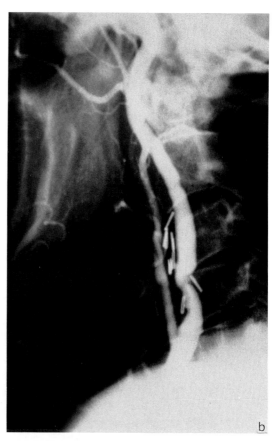

FIGURE 17.4. (a) Common carotid angiography showed postsurgical stenosis at proximal internal carotid artery.

(b) Postangioplastic angiography showed better caliber of proximal internal carotid artery.

through the stenosis. We prefer to inject fresh heparinized arterial blood through the inner lumen during inflation without the guide wire to avoid temporary cessation of blood flow. This situation is more critical in patients with multiple stenoses or occlusions.[56]

From past experience, PTA is a feasible alternative procedure for treatment of carotid stenosis. So far, this technique appears to be highly effective and has a very low associated morbidity or reported mortality. The most controversial issue of the use of PTA in the carotid artery is long-term patency; it does need further study to determine its longevity. Prevention of restenosis is essential to maintain the successful results of PTA.[73-75] To this end, we have used steroids, hoping to prevent excessive fibrosis and collagen disposition.[74,75] A recent report also indicates that inhibitors of angiotensin-converting enzyme may suppress the vascular response to injury by interfering with the conversion of angiotensin I to active angiotensin II to prevent myointimal proliferation in animals.[73]

Further studies are needed to establish the use and effectiveness clinically of this technique. We believe that gentle inflation of the balloon can avoid overstretching and damage to the media. We also believe anticoagulant treatment prior to PTA is important to prevent restenosis.

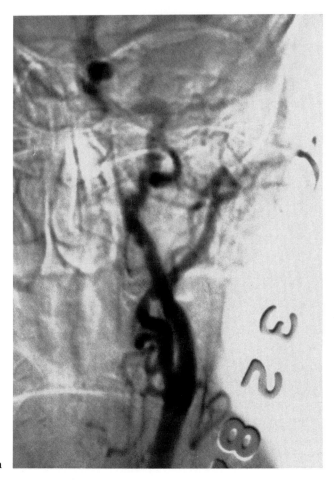

a

FIGURE 17.5. (a) Frontal view of common carotid angiography showed extensive fibromuscular dysplasia at mid-segment of left internal carotid artery.

Treatment of Intracranial Arterial Vasospasm by Transluminal Angioplasty

Intracranial arterial vasospasm from subarachnoid hemorrhage (SAH) remains the leading cause of serious morbidity and mortality from rupture of a cerebral aneurysm. Despite extensive research over the past decades with countless pharmacological agents alleged to prevent or reverse the neurological complications of vasospasm (including adrenergic blocking agents, sympathomimetic and parasympathomimetic amines, prostaglandins and calcium channel blockers), no agent has been found to be effective consistently.[76-102]

Mechanical intraluminal dilatation was developed subsequent to the unsatisfactory results of previous pharmacological treatment over the last two to three decades. In 1984 Zubkov et al. first reported 105 dilatations in 33 patients in which they effectively treated spastic intracranial arteries by balloon.[103] They concluded that focal or diffuse areas of vasospasm could be effectively dilated, so improving cerebral perfusion. More recently, Hieshima et al. and Higashida et al. reported successful dilatation of 35 arterial segments in

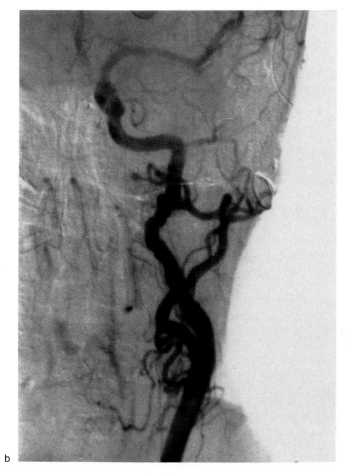

b

FIGURE 17.5. (b) Postangioplastic angiography demonstrated elimination of beading appearance of dysplastic segment.

in 13 patients and 40 vascular territories in 14 patients.[104-107] Patient selection is extremely important to avoid complications of reperfusion.

The indications for transluminal angioplasty in SAH are as follows:

1. Failure to respond to conventional medical and pharmacological therapy with clinical evidence of continued neurological deterioration and angiographic vasospasm.
2. No radiographic evidence of cerebral infarction in the spastic arterial distribution demonstrated by computerized tomography or magnetic resonance imaging.

Technique

Transluminal angioplasty of the intracranial cerebral artery was performed with a custom-made device consisting of a nondetachable silicone microballoon attached to a 2.0-F catheter. The balloon is delivered by a coaxial 2 F/4 F polyethylene set passed through a 7.3-F untapered, thin-walled catheter. Balloons utilized measured 0.85 mm for most anterior, middle, or posterior cerebral arteries and 1.5 mm for basilar or distal carotid artery in the noninflated state. The balloon is dilated very gently and slowly. Digital subtraction angiography is used to monitor the progression of the procedure.[104-107] (See Fig. 17.6.)

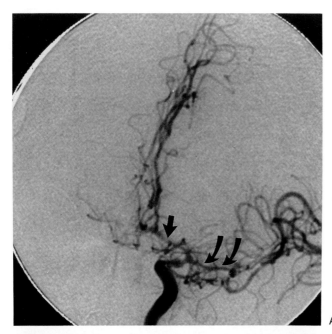

FIGURE 17.6. (A) Acute vasospasm with narrowing of the left middle cerebral artery (curved arrows) and left anterior cerebral artery (straight arrow) due to subarachnoid hemorrhage. (B) Following transluminal angioplasty with the ITC silicone balloon, there is return of normal luminal diameter of the left middle cerebral artery (curved arrows). The left anterior cerebral artery, which was not dilated, remains in spasm (straight arrow). (© American Society of Neuro-radiology. Reprinted by permission.)

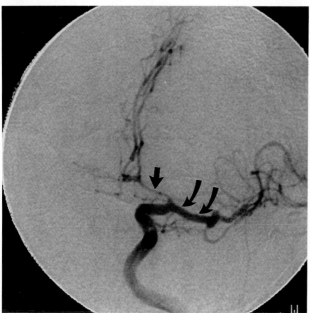

Discussion

The transluminal angioplastic technique for vasospastic intracranial artery due to subarachnoid hemorrhage is quite feasible. Although more research is needed, this technique has been reported as the most effective treatment for vaso-spastic intracranial proximal cerebral arteries in patients in whom pharmacological treatment had failed. The timing of angioplasty is very important; it must be performed before cerebral infarction has occurred to avoid hemorrhage from reperfusion into infarcted brain. If angioplasty is performed too late, successful angiographic evidence of patency does not guarantee clinical recovery.[104-107] We prefer to perform angioplasty in the acute stage when the patient is experiencing rapid clinical deterioration but without cerebral infarction and in whom clinical treatment has failed.

Transluminal angioplasty is usually performed after the aneurysm is clipped. If it is performed in those with nonclipped aneurysms, however, extra caution must be taken to avoid the risk of rupture of the aneurysm due to transmission of pressure or increasing perfusion. If the aneurysm is proximal to the angioplastic segment, there is a higher risk of rupture than in those aneurysms distal to the angioplasty.[104-108]

Two large centers have found that dilatation of vasospastic arteries is possible and reverses the immediate cerebral ischemia of the major cerebral arteries at the base of the brain.[103,104-107]

Conclusion

Percutaneous transluminal balloon angioplasty improves the cerebral circulation and reverses extracranial and intracranial carotid stenosis. Although there is a potential risk of cerebral embolization, vascular rupture, arterial spasm, and cerebral hemorrhage, no significant complications have yet been experienced. Patient selection plays a very important role in achieving this result. A close working relationship among neurologist, neurovascular surgeon, and interventional neuroradiologist is essential. The future of PTA of carotid artery disease rests upon further studies of the long-term results, with effective prevention of restenosis and with comparison to the results of surgery.

Acknowledgments. We would like to take this opportunity to thank Linda Ehlers for her time and effort in typing this chapter.

References

1. Dotter CT, Judkins MP. Transluminal treatment of arteriosclerotic obstruction: description of a new technique and preliminary report of its application. *Circulation.* 1964;30:654-670.
2. Portsman W. Ein neuer korsett Balloon Katheter zur transluminalen Rekanalisation nach doter unter besonderer berucksichtigung von Obliterationen an den Beckenarterien. *Radiol Diagn.* 1973;14: 239-241.
3. Gruntzig A, Hopff H. Perkutane Rekanalisation chronischer Arterieller verschluse mit einem neuen Dilatations-Katheter. *Dtsch Med Wochenschr.* 1974;99:2502-2505.
4. Kerber CS, Cromwell LD, Lehden OL. Catheter dilatation of proximal carotid stenosis during distal bifurcation endarterectomy. *Am J Neurolog Radiol.* 1980;1:348-349.
5. Zeitler E, Holki B. Angiographische diagnostik. In: Raithel D, ed. *Zerebrale Insuffizienz durch Extrakranielle Gefabverschusse.* Erlangen: Permid; 1977:359-363.
6. Backman DM, Kim RM. Transluminal dilatation for subclavian steal syndrome. *Am J Radiol.* 1980;135: 995-996.
7. Basche S, Ritter H, Gaerisch F, et al. Percutaneous transluminal angioplasty of the subclavian artery. *Zentralbl Chir.* 1983;108(3):142-149.
8. Courtheoux P, Theron J, Maiza D, et al. Endoluminal angioplasty for atheromatous stenosis of supra-aortic trunks. The brachiocephalic arterial trunk, subclavian arteries. *J Radiol.* 1984;65(12):845-851.
9. Damoth HD Jr, Diamond AB, Rappoport AS, et al. Angioplasty of subclavian artery stenosis proximal to the vertebral origin. *Am J Neurolog Radiol.* 1983;4(6):1239-1242.
10. Galich JP, Bajaj AK, Vine DL, et al. Subclavian artery stenosis treated by transluminal angioplasty: six cases. *Cardiovasc Intervent Radiol.* 1983;6(2): 78-81.
11. Gordon RL, Haskell L, Hirsch M, et al. Transluminal dilatation of the subclavian artery. *Cardiovasc Intervent Radiol.* 1985;8(1):14-19.
12. Grote R, Greyschmidt J, Walterbusch G. Percutaneous transluminal angioplasty in proximal subclavian stenoses. *ROFO.* 1983;138(6):660-664.
13. Hodgins GW, Dutton JW. Subclavian and carotid angioplasties for Takayasu's arteries. *J Can Assoc Radiol.* 1982;33(3):205-207.
14. Kichikawa K, Nakagawa H, Yoshiya K, et al. Percutaneous transluminal angioplasty in a case of left subclavian and brachiocephalic artery stenosis due to aortitis syndrome. *Rinsho Hoshasen.* 1985; 30(1):121-124.
15. Levien LJ, Fritz VU. Intra-operative transluminal angioplasty in the management of symptomatic aortic arch vessel stenosis. *S Afr J Surg.* 1985; 23(2):49-52.
16. Lowman BG, Queral LA, Holbrook WA, et al. The correction of cerebrovascular insufficiency by transluminal dilatation: a preliminary report. *Am Surg.* 1983;49(11):621-624.
17. Mathias K, Staiger J, Thron A, et al. Perkutane Katheterangioplastik der Arteria subclavia. *Dtsch Med Wochenschr.* 1980;105:16-31.

18. Moore TS, Russell WF, Parent AD, et al. Percutaneous transluminal angioplasty in subclavian steal syndrome: recurrent stenosis and retreatment in two patients. *Neurosurgery*. 1982;11(4):512–517.

19. Motarjeme A, Keifer JW, Zuska AJ. Percutaneous transluminal angioplasty of the brachiocephalic arteries. *AJR*. 1982;138(3):457–462.

20. Motarjeme A, Keifer JW, Zuska AJ, et al. Percutaneous transluminal angioplasty for treatment of subclavian steal. *Radiology*. 1985;155(3):611–613.

21. Obert F, Mendel H, Muzika N, et al. Percutaneous transluminal vasodilatation. Long-term results and report on experience with a new system of catheters: transaxillary technic. *Wien Klin Wochenschr*. 1983; 95(15):528–536.

22. Pernes JM, Brenot P, Seuro M, et al. Percutaneous endoluminal angioplasty of the supra-aortic arterial trunks. Immediate and remote results. *Presse Med*. 1984;12(17):1075–1078.

23. Rabkin IKH, Matevosov AL, Shekhter IUI. X-ray endovascular dilatation of the subclavian artery. *Grudn Khir*. 1984;2:76–78.

24. Schlosser V. Subclavian steal syndrome: correction by transthoracic or extra-anatomic repair. *Vasc Surg*. 1984;18:289–293.

25. Theron J, Courtheoux P, Henriet JP, et al. Angioplasty of supra-aortic arteries. *J Neuroradiol*. 1984; 11(3):187–200.

26. Theron J, Melancon D, Ethier R. Subclavian steal syndromes and their treatment by angioplasty. Hemodynamic classification of subclavian artery stenoses. *Neuroradiology*. 1985;27(3):265–270.

27. Tsai FY, Hieshima G, Mehringer CM, et al. Arterial digital subtraction angiography with particulate intravascular embolization and angioplasty. *Surg Neurol*. 1984;22:204–212.

28. Tsai FY, Yoon JW, Hieshima G, et al. Percutaneous transluminal angioplasty of subclavian steals. Presented at RSN November 28, 1985; Radiological Society of North America.

29. Zeitler E, Berger G, Schemitt-Ruth R. Percutaneous transluminal angioplasty of the supra-aortic arteries. In: Dotter CT, Gruntzig A, Schoop W, et al., eds. Berlin: Springer-Verlag; 1983:245–261.

30. Lowman B, Queral L, Holbrook W, et al. The treatment of innominate artery stenosis by intraoperative transluminal angioplasty. *Surgery*. 1981;5: 565–568.

31. Garrido E, Garofola J. Intraluminal dilatation of the innominate artery before extracranial-intracranial bypass: case report. *Neurosurgery*. 1983; 12(5):581–583.

32. Kobinia G, Bergmann H Jr. Angioplasty in stenosis of the innominate artery. *Cardiovasc Intervent Radiol*. 1983;6:82–85.

33. Tsai FY, Matovich V, Hieshima G, et al. Percutaneous transluminal angioplasty of the carotid artery. *Am J Neurolog Radiol*. 1986;7:349–358.

34. Mathias K, Mitlermeyer C, Ensinger H, et al. Percutane Katherdilatation von Karotisstenosen. *Fortschr Roetgenstr*. 1980;133:348–361.

35. Mullan S, Duda EE, Petro NAS. Some examples of balloon technology in neurosurgery. *J Neurosurg*. 1980;52:321–329.

36. Belan A, Vesela M, Vanek I, et al. Percutaneous transluminal angioplasty of fibromuscular dysplasia of the internal carotid artery. *Cardiovasc Intervent Radiol*. 1982;5:79–81.

37. Tievsky AL, Dray EM, Mardiat JG. Transluminal angioplasty in postsurgical stenosis of the extracranial carotid artery. *Am J Neurolog Radiol*. 1980;1:348–349.

38. Hasso AN, Bird CR, Zinek DE, et al. Fibromuscular dysplasia of the internal carotid artery. Percutaneous transluminal angioplasty. *Am J Neurolog Radiol*. 1981;2:175–180.

39. Hodgins GW, Dutton JW. Subclavian and carotid angioplasties for Takayasu's arteritis. *J Can Assoc Radiol*. 1982;33:305–307.

40. Wiggli U, Gratzl O. Transluminal angioplasty of stenotic carotid arteries: case report and protocol. *Am J Neurolog Radiol*. 1983;4:793–795.

41. Vitek JJ. Percutaneous transluminal angioplasty of the external carotid artery. *Am J Neurolog Radiol*. 1983;4:796–799.

42. Pritz MB, Smolin MF. Treatment of tandem lesions of the extracranial carotid artery. *Neurosurgery*. 1984;15:233–236.

43. Freitag G, Freitag J, Koch RD, et al. Percutaneous angioplasty of carotid artery stenoses. *Neuroradiology*. 1986;28:126–127.

44. Kachel R, Ritter H, Grossmann K, et al. Ergebnisse der perkutanen transluminalen Dilatation (PTD) von Hirngefabstenosen. *Fortschr Roentgenstr*. 1986;144:338–342.

45. Namaguchi Y, Puyau FA, Provenza LJ, et al. Percutaneous transluminal angioplasty of the carotid artery. *Neuroradiology*. 1984;26:527–530.

46. Tsai FY, Matovich VB, Hieshima GB, et al. Practical aspects of percutaneous transluminal angioplasty of the carotid artery. *Acta Radiol*. 1986;369: 127–139.

47. Courtheoux P, Tournade A, Theron J, et al. Transcutaneous angioplasty of vertebral artery atheromatous ostial stricture. *Neuroradiology*. 1985; 27:259–264.

48. Bockenheimer SAM, Mathias K. Percutaneous transluminal angioplasty in arteriosclerotic internal carotid artery stenosis. *AJNR*. 1983;4:791–792.

49. Motarjeme A, Keifer JW, Zuska AJ. Percutaneous transluminal angioplasty of the vertebral arteries. *Radiology.* 1981;139:715–717.

50. Schultz H, Yeung HP, Chin MC, et al. Dilatation of vertebral artery stenosis. *N Engl J Med.* 1981;304: 733.

51. Higashida RT, Hieshima GB, Tsai FY, et al. Percutaneous transluminal angioplasty of the subclavian and vertebral arteries. *Am J Neurolog Radiol.* 1986;369:124–126.

52. Higashida RT, Hieshima GB, Tsai FY, et al. Transluminal angioplasty of the vertebral and basilar artery. *Am J Neurolog Radiol.* 1987;8:745–750.

53. Sundt TM Jr, Smith HC, Campbell JK, et al. Transluminal angioplasty for basilar artery stenosis. *Mayo Clin Proc.* 1980;55:673–680.

54. Theron J, Courtheoux P. New system for the angioplasty of the internal carotid artery. Presented at the Annual Meeting of ASNR; March 19–24, 1989; Orlando, FL.

55. Giorgio B, Giuseppe B, Luca M, et al. PTA of atherosclerotic carotid arteries—16 patients, 1 dissection, 4 hypotension. Presented at the Annual Meeting of ASNR; March 19–24, 1989; Orlando, FL.

56. Tsai FY. How to prevent transient ischemia during PTA of brachiocephalic artery. Presented at the Annual Meeting of the Western Neuroradiologic Society; October 12–15, 1989; Monterey, CA.

57. Tsai FY, Hieshima GB, Higashida RT. Percutaneous transluminal angioplasty for the treatment of stroke. In: Fisher M, ed. *Medical Therapy of Acute Stroke.* New York, NY: Marcel Dekker, Inc., 1989: Chapter 12.

58. DeMonte F, Peerless SJ, Rankin RN. Carotid angioplasty with evidence of distal embolization. *J Neurosurg.* 1989;70:138–141.

59. Belloni G, Bonaldi G, Moschini L, et al. Percutaneous angioplasty of atherosclerotic carotid arteries (abstract). *AJNR.* 1989;10:898.

60. Dietrich EB, Garrett HB, Ameriso J, et al. Occlusive disease of the common carotid and subclavian arteries treated by carotid subclavian bypass. *Am J Surg.* 1967;114:800–808.

61. Crawford ES, DeBakey ME, Morris GC Jr, et al. Surgical treatment of occlusion of the innominate, common, carotid and subclavian arteries. *Surgery.* 1969;65:17–31.

62. Beebe HG, Start K, Johnson ML, et al. Choice of operation for subclavian-vertebral arterial disease. *Am J Surg.* 1980;139:616–623.

63. Morris GC, Lechter A, DeBakey ME. Surgical treatment of fibromuscular disease of the carotid arteries. *Arch Surg.* 1968;96:636–643.

64. DeBakey ME, Crawford ES, Cooley DA, et al. Cerebral arterial insufficiency. One to 11 years result following arterial reconstructive operation. *Am J Surg.* 1965;161:921–945.

65. West H, Burton R, Roon AJ, et al. Comparative risk of operation and expectant management for carotid artery disease. *Stroke.* 1979;10:117–121.

66. Brown OW, Kerstein WD. The surgical management of transient ischemic attacks. *Angiology.* 1984;34:12–21.

67. Riles TS, Imparato AM, Mintzer R, et al. Comparison of results of bilateral and unilateral carotid endarterectomy five years after surgery. *Surgery.* 1982;91:258–262.

68. Loftus CM, Quest DO. Current status of carotid endarterectomy for atheromatous disease. *Neurosurgery.* 1983;12:718–723.

69. Baker RN, Carroll-Ramseyer J, Schauartz WS. Prognosis in patients with transient ischemic attacks. *Neurology.* 1968;18:1157–1165.

70. Cartlidge NEF, Whisnant JP, Elveback IR. Carotid and vertebral basilar transient cerebral ischemic attacks. *Mayo Clin Proc.* 1977;52:117–120.

71. De los Reyes RA, Ausman JI, Diaz FG, et al. The surgical management of vertebrobasilar insufficiency. *Acta Neurochi.* 1983;68:203–216.

72. Higashida RT, Hieshima GB, Halbach VV. Intravascular techniques for angioplasty and thrombosis. In: Weinstein PR, Fadden AI, eds. *Current Neurosurgical Practice: Protection of the Brain from Ischemia.* Baltimore, MD: Williams and Wilkins; 1989: Chapter 29.

73. Powell JS, Clozel JP, Muller RKM, et al. Inhibitors of angiotensin converting enzyme to prevent myointimal proliferation after vascular injury. *Science.* 1989;245:186–188.

74. Tsai FY, Myers T, Parker J, et al. Experimental results of corticosteroid to prevent restenosis after angioplasty. Presented at the Annual Meeting of the Association of University Radiologists; April 17–21, 1988; Tulane University, New Orleans, LA.

75. MacDonald RG, Panush RS, Pepine CJ. Rationale for use of glucocorticoids in modification of restenosis after percutaneous transluminal angioplasty. *Am J Cardiology.* 1987;60:56B–60B.

76. Allcock JM, Drake CG. Ruptured intracranial aneurysms—the role of arterial spasm. *J Neurosurg.* 1965;22:21–29.

77. Alksne JF, Greenhoot JM. Experimental catecholamine-induced chronic cerebral vasospasm. Myonecrosis in vessel wall. *J Neurosurg.* 1974;4:440–445.

78. Chapleau CE, White RP, Robertson JT. Cerebral vasodilation and prostacyclin. The effects of aspirin and meclotenamate in vitro. *J Neurosurg.* 1980;53:188–192.

79. Chyatte D, Rush N, Sundt TM Jr. Prevention of chronic experimental cerebral vasospasm with ibuprofen and high dose methylprednisolone. *J Neurosurg.* 1983;59:925–932.

80. Conway LW, McDonald LW. Structural changes of the intradural arteries following subarachnoid hemorrhage. *Neurosurg.* 1972;37:715–723.

81. Debouley G. Distribution of spasm in the intracranial arteries after subarachnoid hemorrhage. *Acta Radiol.* 1963;1:257–266.

82. Echlin F. Experimental vasospasm, acute and chronic, due to blood in the subarachnoid space. *J Neurosurg.* 1971;35:646–656.

83. Ecker A, Riemenschneider PA. Arteriographic demonstration of spasm of the intracranial arteries, with specific reference to saccular arterial aneurysms. *J Neurosurg.* 1951;8:660–667.

84. Ellis EF, Nies AS, Dates JA. Cerebral arterial smooth muscle contraction by thromboxane A2. *Stroke.* 1977;8:480–486.

85. Endos S, Suzuki J. Experimental cerebral vasospasm after subarachnoid hemorrhage. The participation of adrenergic nerves of cerebral vessel walls. *Stroke.* 1979;10:703–711.

86. Fein JM, Flor WJ, Cohan JL, et al. Sequential changes of vascular ultrastructure in experimental cerebral vasospasm. Myonecrosis of subarachnoid arteries. *J Neurosurg.* 1974;41:49–58.

87. Fisher CM, Kistler JP, Davis JM. Relation of cerebral vasospasm to subarachnoid hemorrhage visualized by computerized tomographic scanning. *Neurosurgery.* 1980;6:1–9.

88. Flamm ES, Yasargil ME, Ransohoff J. Alteration of experimental cerebral vasospasm by adrenergic blockage. *J Neurosurg.* 1972;37:294–301.

89. Graf CJ, Nibbelink DW. Cooperative study of intracranial aneurysms and subarachnoid hemorrhage: report on a randomized treatment and study. *Stroke.* 1974;5:557–601.

90. Hunt WE, Hess RM. Surgical risk as related to time of intervention in the repair of intracranial aneurysms. *J Neurosurg.* 1968;28:14–20.

91. Mizukami M, Kawase T, Usami T, et al. Prevention of vasospasm by early operation with removal of subarachnoid blood. *Neurosurgery.* 1982;10:301–307.

92. Owada K, Hori S, Suzuki J. Results of cervical sympathectomy for cerebral vasospasm following aneurysmal rupture. In: Suzuki J, ed. Cerebral aneurysms. Sendai: Neuron Pub; 1979: pp 435–551.

93. Owada K. Hori S. Cervical sympathectomy for cerebral ischemic lesions; a follow-up study. *Tohoku Med J (Sendai).* 1977;90:183–204.

94. Ropper AH, Zervas NT. Outcome one year after subarachnoid hemorrhage from cerebral aneurysm. *J Neurosurg.* 1984;60:909–915.

95. Sahs A, Perret GE, Locksley HB, et al. Intracranial aneurysms and subarachnoid hemorrhage. Philadelphia: J.B. Lippincott Co; 1969.

96. Sano K, Saito I. Timing and indication for surgery of ruptured intracranial aneurysms with regard to cerebral vasospasm. *Acta Neurochir.* 1978;41:49–63.

97. Saito I, Sano K. Vasospasm after aneurysm rupture: incidence, onset and course. In: Wilkins RH, ed. *Cerebral Arterial Spasm.* Baltimore: Williams and Wilkins; 1980:294–301.

98. Sundt TM Jr. Chemical management of cerebral vasospasm. In: Whisnant JP, Sandok BA, eds. *Cerebral Vascular Disease. Proceedings of the 9th Princeton Conference, 1974.* New York: Grune & Stratton; 1975:77–81.

99. Tanabe Y, Sakata K, Yamida H, et al. Cerebral vasospasm and ultrastructural changes in cerebral arterial wall. *J Neurosurg.* 1978;49:229–238.

100. Tani E, Maeda Y, Fukumori T. Effect of selective inhibitor of thromboxane AZ synthetase on cerebral vasospasm after early surgery. *J Neurosurg.* 1984;61:24–29.

101. Tanishima T. Cerebral vasospasm: contractile ability of hemoglobin in isolated canine basilar arteries. *J Neurosurg.* 1980;53:787–793.

102. Wilkins RH. Attempted prevention or treatment of intracranial arterial spasm: a survey. In: Wilkins RH, ed. *Cerebral Arterial Spasm.* Baltimore, MD: Williams and Wilkins; 1970: pp 542–555.

103. Zubkov YN, Nikiforov BM, Shustin VA. Balloon catheter technique for dilatation of constricted cerebral arteries after aneurysmal SAH. *Acta Neurochi.* 1984;70:665–679.

104. Hieshima GB, Higashida RT, Wapenski J, et al. Balloon embolization of a large distal basilar artery aneurysm. *J Neurosurg.* 1986;65:413–416.

105. Eskridge JM, Hartling RP. Angioplasty of vasospasm (abstract). *AJNR.* 1989;10:877.

106. Higashida RT, Halbach VV, Dormandy B, et al. A new microballoon device for transluminal angioplasty of intracranial arterial vasospasm: indications, techniques, technical considerations. *AJNR.* 1990;11:233–238.

107. Higashida RT, Halbach VV, Cahan LD, et al. Transluminal angioplasty for treatment of intracranial arterial vasospasm. *J of Neurosurg.* 1989;71:648–653.

108. Tsai FY, Alfieri K, Wadley D, et al. Transluminal angioplasty of vasospastic cerebral arteries with unclipped aneurysm, the potential risk and its management. Submitted to *AJNR.*

18
Preventing Cerebral Complications of Cardiac Surgery

Marc I. Chimowitz and Anthony J. Furlan

Considering the number of potential threats during heart surgery, the brain has proved to be remarkably resistant to serious injury. Nonetheless, stroke and encephalopathy remain major causes of morbidity following open heart surgery (OHS) (Table 18.1). This chapter focuses on the incidence, etiology, and prevention of these complications. The data presented largely apply to coronary artery bypass graft (CABG) surgery since our knowledge of the cerebral complications of OHS is derived mostly from studies of this operation. However, in a study from our institution, the risk of stroke or encephalopathy during CABG surgery did not differ significantly from other forms of cardiac surgery not involving transplantation.[1]

Stroke

Incidence

Stroke (cerebral infarction) was a common complication of open heart surgery in the 1960s.[2,3] Since then, improved surgical techniques and cardioplegic agents, along with the introduction of membrane oxygenators and in-line filtration, which decrease the release of microaggregates into the circulation, have substantially lowered the stroke risk. Nonetheless, several studies since the 1970s have shown a persistent stroke rate associated with OHS ranging from 1% to 5%.[4-9] Since over 300 000 CABG operations are done annually in the United States, these studies indicate that from 3000 to 15 000 patients will suffer a stroke in the perioperative period.

Etiology

Several studies have attempted to identify risk factors for stroke during CABG surgery. In a prospective study of 421 patients undergoing CABG surgery at the Cleveland Clinic, 22 (5%) developed focal brain or ocular infarction, and 2% suffered major neurologic disability.[8] Of a large number of preoperative, intraoperative, and postoperative variables evaluated (Table 18.2), only a history of prior stroke approached a statistical correlation with increased stroke risk during CABG surgery. However, probable mechanisms of stroke were identified in 16 of 22 patients (Table 18.3).

Other studies have suggested various risk factors for increased stroke risk during CABG surgery, notably carotid occlusive disease, prior stroke, perioperative arrythmias, and pump time.

Carotid Artery Disease and Peri-CABG Stroke

Extracranial carotid artery disease is often suggested as an important cause of stroke during CABG surgery. This theory proposes that severe carotid occlusive disease combined with intraoperative hypotension results in cerebral ischemia. However, most perioperative strokes occur in the absence of carotid occlusive disease or have their onset in the postoperative period.[10] Furthermore, a recent intraoperative transcranial Doppler study failed to demonstrate ipsilateral blood flow velocity changes during CABG surgery in patients with high-grade internal carotid artery stenosis.[11] Nevertheless, it is common practice in some hospitals to perform a prophylactic staged or combined

TABLE 18.1. Summary of recent data on CNS complications of open heart surgery.

Authors	Year[a]	Study design	Type of OHS	No. of patients	% with CNA deficit		Method of ascertainment
					Focal infarct	Encepha-lopathy	
1. Hill et al.[3]	1968	Pathologic analysis autopsy cases	Mixture	133	b (fat emboli in 62% brains, nonfat emboli in 31% brains)	b	Pathological analysis of brains
2. Heller et al.[61]	1969	Prospective	Mixture	100	b (24% had post-operative delirium)	9%	Psychiatric inter-view, psychologi-cal testing
3. Javid et al.[62]	1969	Prospective	Mixture	100	13+%	35%	Clinical exam, psy-chological testing
4. Tufo et al.[30]	1969	Prospective	Mixture	100	13+%	43%	Clinical exam, psy-chological testing
5. Branthwaite[4]	1970	Retrospective + prospective	Mixture	417	9.4%	10.1%	Chart review, clini-cal exam
6. Hansotia et al.[63]	1972	Prospective	Mixture	177	b (51% with persis-tently abnormal EEG at discharge. Includes 11 patients who died)	b	Serial EEG
7. Cannon et al.[64]	1972	Retrospective	Mixture	400	1%[c]	b	Chart review
8. Hutchinson et al.[65]	1972	Retrospective	CABG alone	376	0.3%[c]	b	Chart review
9. Branthwaite[55]	1973	Prospective	Mixture	140	b (7.1% had clinical neurological damage)	b	Intraoperative use of cerebral function monitor
10. Branthwaite[29]	1973	Retrospective	Mixture	538	3%	4.8%	Chart review
11. Hodgman et al.[66]	1974	Retrospective	Mixture	100	b (20% had minor psy-chiatric problems)[c]	b	Chart review
12. Kolkka et al.[67]	1977	Prospective	Mixture	204	2.9%	17.2%	Clinical exam
13. Lee et al.[68]	1978	Retrospective	Mixture	943	0.7%	b	Chart review
14. Gonzalez-Scarano et al.[5]	1978	Retrospective case control	CABG alone	1427	1%	0.4%	Chart review
15. Loop et al.[6]	1978	Retrospective	CABG alone	8741	c 1.3%-2%	b	Chart review, com-puterized cardio-vascular informa-tion registry
16. Muraoka et al.[69]	1979	Prospective	Congenital heart	57	0% (10.5% had persis-tent CT scan changes)	0%	Chart review
17. Turnipseed et al.[15]	1979	Prospective	CABG alone	170	4.7%	b	Clinical exam
18. Breuer et al.[8]	1980	Prospective	CABG alone	421	5.2% (total) 2% (severe)	11.6%	Clinical exam
19. Coffey et al.[7]	1981	Retrospective	CABG alone	1669	0.8%	3.4%	Chart review
20. Reed et al.[9]	1984	Retrospective	CABG	5915	1.03%		Chart review

[a]Latest year patients in study underwent surgery reflecting technology of that time (i.e., not year study published).

[b]No clinical examination data are available.

[c]These retrospective studies are highly devoted to analyses of nonneurological issues and complications and mention CNS dysfunction. (Modified from Breuer et al., 1983.[8] Used by permission.)

TABLE 18.2. Potential risk factors not significant for stroke or prolonged encephalopathy in CABG surgery.

1. Preoperative variables
   age, sex, race, weight, height, hx prior stroke, TIA, migraine, smoking hx, hx noncoronary arteriography, calf claudication, other vascular syndrome, admission BP, cholesterol level, triglycerides, abn lipoproteins, glucose intolerance, carotid bruit, use of meds: ASA, Persantine, Coumadin, anti-CHF, anti-BP, anti-dysrhythmia, anti-angina, hx AMI, cardiac arrhythmia, NYHA functional class, CHF, old MI, LVH by EKG, degree of coronary artery disease by angio, prior cardiac/vascular surgery, preop spirometry (predicted, found), abnormal chest X-ray, abnormal arterial blood gases, abnormal neurologic exam preop
2. Operative variables:
   surgical team, day of week, time of day, first or second time myocardial revascularization, anesthetic agent used, type oxygenator (bubble vs. membrane), duration total bypass, aortic clamp time, various extracorporeal circulation pump parameters, use of hypothermia, lowest hematocrit during bypass, use of Haemonetics autologous blood recovery, intraop blood gases, hypertension, intraoperative use of drugs pre-, during, or post-bypass
3. Postoperative variables:
   hypertension, ventilatory parameters, plasma-free hemoglobin level, total units blood transfused, use of Sorensen autotransfusion device, reoperation within 48 hours, duration of intubation, postop use of Morphine, Pantopon, Valium, Pavulon, postop cardiac enzymes, postop BB-CPK

From Breuer et al., 1983.[8] Reprinted by permission.

TABLE 18.3. Myocardial revascularization: possible etiology of focal CNS deficits.[a]

Cause	No. of patients
Cardiac arrhythmia intra/perioperatively	6
Internal carotid artery atherosclerosis	5
Air embolism from left ventricle	2
Carotid artery trauma during internal jugular vein cannulation	1
Aortic atherosclerosis at site of clamping	1
Prolonged intraoperative blood pressure decrease	1

[a]Cause identified in 16 of 22 patients (73%).
From Furlan and Breuer, 1984.[1] Reprinted by permission.

carotid endarterectomy in asymptomatic patients discovered to have carotid stenosis (usually through the detection of a bruit) prior to CABG surgery.

Most studies have failed to demonstrate a correlation between peri-CABG stroke and asymptomatic carotid bruits,[8,10,12] although a recent retrospective study[9] demonstrated a small but significantly increased risk. The results of bruit studies should be interpreted cautiously and are of limited use because bruits are neither specific nor sensitive for the presence or degree of carotid occlusive disease[13,14] and often do not correlate with the location of the stroke.

Studies using carotid noninvasive tests to screen asymptomatic patients prior to CABG surgery have provided conflicting data regarding stroke risk in patients with carotid stenosis. Most studies have not shown an increased risk of stroke,[15-17] although others have.[18,19]

In a retrospective angiographic study, Furlan and Craciun[20] identified 155 stenotic ($\geq$50%) or occluded carotid arteries in 144 patients undergoing CABG surgery. Ipsilateral stroke occurred in 1 out of 90 (1.1%) with 50 to 90% stenosis, 1 out of 16 (6.2%) with >90% stenosis, and 1 out of 49 (2%) with occlusion. In a prospective study, Brener et al.[21] identified 193 stenotic or occluded carotid arteries in 153 patients using noninvasive screening in 4047 patients undergoing CABG surgery. Angiography confirmed the diagnosis in 95/153 patients. Ipsilateral TIA or stroke occurred in 8 out of 47 (17%) with occlusion, 2 out of 89 (2.2%) with $\geq$ 50% stenosis not repaired during CABG surgery, and 2 out of 57 (3.5%) with $\geq$50% stenosis repaired during CABG surgery.

In a recent study at the Cleveland Clinic, Hertzer et al.[22] randomized 129 patients with angiographically proven asymptomatic carotid stenosis (>70%) into two treatment subsets: one group of 71 patients underwent combined carotid endarterectomy and CABG; the other group of 58 patients underwent CABG followed by delayed carotid endarterectomy. There were two perioperative strokes (2.8%) in the group undergoing the combined procedure and four (6.9%) in the group undergoing CABG alone. The difference in stroke rate between these two groups was not statistically significant.

There is virtually no data on peri-CABG stroke risk in patients with *symptomatic* high-grade unilateral carotid stenosis or multiple-vessel occlusive disease, since most of these patients undergo staged or combined carotid endarterectomy. Hertzer

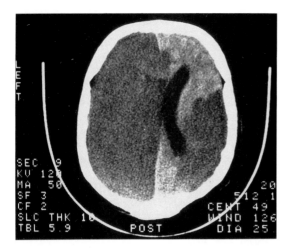

FIGURE 18.1. CT scan showing massive left hemisphere and smaller right hemisphere infarcts with herniation. At autopsy, the left internal carotid artery was occluded by atherosclerotic plaque and a superimposed fresh thrombus, and the left middle cerebral artery was occluded by an embolus.

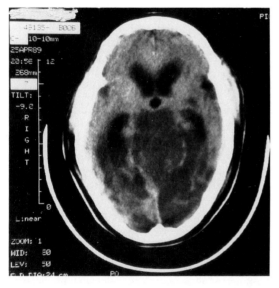

FIGURE 18.2. Seventy-eight-year-old man who failed to awaken after combined L. carotid endarterectomy and CABG surgery. Preoperative angiography of cervical vessels showed severe L. internal carotid artery stenosis, occlusion of R. vertebral artery, and severe narrowing of L. vertebral artery. CT scan shows extensive areas of infarction involving the brain stem, medial temporal lobes, and both occipital lobes. Additional findings at autopsy included 75% stenosis of the basilar artery and laminar necrosis of the L. frontal cortex. Mean arterial blood pressure during the 3 ½ hours of cardiopulmonary bypass ranged from 63 to 89 mm Hg.

et al.[22] recently reported a group of 23 patients with symptomatic or bilateral carotid stenosis ($\geq 70\%$) who underwent "unprotected" CABG, because their unstable coronary disease required urgent revascularization. Only two (8.7%) of these 23 patients developed a stroke perioperatively.

The results of these studies should be interpreted cautiously since each has at least one of the following serious design flaws: insufficient numbers of patients, retrospective analyses, lack of randomization, lack of information regarding degree of carotid disease and relation of stroke to side of stenosis, different definitions of what constitutes a stroke, incomplete information regarding investigation of other potential stroke mechanisms. However, it is possible to make some conclusions on the basis of these and other studies:

1. There is no evidence that asymptomatic patients with $>90\%$ stenosis of one carotid artery are at increased risk of stroke during CABG surgery.
2. The great majority of patients with asymptomatic unilateral $\geq 90\%$ stenosis or carotid occlusion do not sustain a stroke during CABG surgery. However, a small subset of these patients is likely to be at increased risk of stroke (Fig. 18.1), but the means to identify such patients pre- or intraoperatively have thus far eluded us.
3. There is no evidence that either staged or combined endarterectomy lowers stroke risk in these asymptomatic patients.
4. There is insufficient data on stroke risk in patients undergoing CABG with symptomatic high-grade carotid stenosis, bilateral carotid occlusive disease, and vertebrobasilar disease. We have personal knowledge of patients with bilateral carotid occlusion who have successfully undergone CABG, but, rarely, we have also seen patients who suffer a major stroke in the face of multivessel disease (Fig. 18.2).

Prior Stroke and Risk of Subsequent Open Heart Surgery

The data on this subject are limited. Previous studies have provided discrepant estimates of stroke risk in patients with prior stroke undergoing OHS, varying from no or marginally increased risk[5,8] to six times the risk of control patients.[9] However, these studies lack sufficient statistical power to permit definite conclusions.

In a recently completed retrospective study at our institution of 127 patients with a history of stroke who underwent OHS, 17 (13.4%) had a new stroke or worsening of prior deficits.[23] This rate is significantly higher (p < .005) than the expected rate of 5.2% predicted by our previous prospective study,[8] although the severe stroke rate was only 3.2%. Of note, almost all patients had no or minimal neurological deficit at the time of OHS. The stroke rate was higher (16.7%) in those patients whose previous strokes were recent (< 3 months prior to OHS) compared to those with remote strokes (12.3%), although this did not attain statistical significance. Sixty percent of the complications in the recent stroke group involved worsening of prior deficits, whereas 75% of the complications in the remote stroke group involved new deficits, suggesting different mechanisms of strokes in the two groups. Extracranial carotid disease was not a factor. In the remote group, perioperative cardiogenic embolus was considered the most likely mechanism since new areas of brain were affected and 50% had atrial fibrillation or flutter prior to their strokes. Patients with recent stroke exhibited periinfarction hemodynamic vulnerability, which led to infarct extension when mean arterial pressure fell during OHS.

Postoperative Arrhythmia and Stroke

Transient cardiac arrhythmias occur in 5% to 40% of patients after OHS.[24,25] Supraventricular arrhythmias are particularly common, prompting some authors to suggest prophylactic treatment with Inderal or Digoxin after OHS.[26] Data on the incidence of stroke associated with atrial fibrillation post-OHS are scanty. Taylor[27] and Reed et al.[9] reported a three- to fivefold increase in stroke risk post-CABG surgery in these patients. However, in a prospective study of 200 patients undergoing CABG surgery at the Cleveland Clinic Foundation, the stroke rate among patients with postoperative atrial fibrillation was 3.6%, compared to 3.5% in patients without cardiac dysrhythmias.[28] Ventricular arrhythmias have not been associated with an increased stroke risk post-CABG surgery.[27,28]

Pump Time and Stroke Risk

Pump time in excess of 2 hours has been associated with an increased frequency of stroke during CABG.[9,29,30] However, Breuer et al.[8] reported that the stroke rate in 36 patients undergoing prolonged bypass (> 2 hours) was not increased. Patients undergoing prolonged bypass tend to have compromised preoperative cardiorespiratory function and unstable hemodynamics intraoperatively, and it is likely that the reported increased stroke risk in patients undergoing prolonged bypass relates to these factors, rather than to the actual pump time.

Encephalopathy

Incidence

The incidence of clinically detectable diffuse encephalopathy following OHS varies from 3% to 12%.[7,8,31] Subtle, but significant, cognitive deficits detected by neuropsychological testing may occur in up to 30% of patients undergoing CABG surgery.[32,33]

Etiology

Post-CABG encephalopathy is often multifactorial and can be related to medications, hypoxia, fever, sepsis, metabolic derangements, hemodynamic instability, and intensive care psychosis. In the study by Breuer et al.,[8] no pre- or intraoperative risk factors emerged for the development of prolonged encephalopathy, but two postoperative variables did correlate with confusion: use of intra-aortic balloon pump and use of pressor drugs, both markers for patients with severe hypotension. These results and those of others[34,35] suggest that decreased cerebral blood flow, especially in patients with arteriolar cerebral vascular disease and defective autoregulation, may be an important cause of encephalopathy in some patients undergoing CABG surgery. Alternatively, multiple microemboli (i.e., < 20 μm) of air, fat, platelet/fibrin clumps generated during cardiopulmonary bypass have been proposed as a mechanism for diffuse encephalopathy.[27,36]

Coma After CABG Surgery

Nonmetabolic coma is a rare complication of OHS, occurring in < 1% of patients. Over a 4-year period, during which more than 12 000 procedures

TABLE 18.4. Causes of prolonged coma after open heart surgery.

Cause	No. of patients
Uncertain	19
Global ischemic/hypoxia	7
Hemisphere infarct with herniation	5
Multifocal infarcts	3
Total	34

From Furlan and Breuer, 1984. Reprinted by permission.

were performed at the Cleveland Clinic, our Stroke Service evaluated 34 patients who failed to awaken after OHS. The causes of coma in these patients are shown in Table 18.4. Although global ischemia/hypoxia was proved to be the cause in only seven patients, it was likely responsible for a large number of the uncertain group as well. It is important to note that massive hemisphere infarction (Fig. 18.1) or multifocal infarcts accounted for almost 25% of the total number of patients with coma. Whatever the cause of nonmetabolic coma after OHS, the prognosis is extremely poor; 85% of our patients died, 4 evolved into a persistent vegetative state, and only 1 patient had a useful neurologic recovery.

Preventing Brain Damage During CABG Surgery

Our experience and that of others indicate that there are few preoperative, intraoperative, or postoperative variables that can reliably predict the risk of stroke or encephalopathy during CABG surgery. However, there are certain prophylactic measures that should be taken to lower the risk of neurologic complications. Preoperatively, the only variable that has emerged as a clear-cut risk factor for stroke is prior stroke. Therefore, we suggest delaying CABG surgery for 3 months in patients with recent stroke, unless the patient has unstable angina, bacterial endocarditis, myxoma, or other urgent cardiac conditions. In such situations, the benefits of removing the embolic source or improving cardiac hemodynamics outweigh the risk of stroke extension during surgery.[37]

Although asymptomatic carotid occlusive disease has not been shown to increase the risk of stroke during CABG surgery, it remains probable that a small subset of these patients is at increased risk of stroke during the hemodynamic stress of CABG surgery. Currently, there is no reliable way to identify such patients preoperatively, although preliminary efforts to measure cerebral perfusion reserve in patients with carotid disease show promise. Studies using positron emission tomography (PET)[38-40] have shown that some patients with highly stenotic or occluded carotid arteries have high ipsilateral cerebral blood volume (CBV), consistent with vasodilation of resistance vessels in response to diminished cerebral perfusion pressure (CPP). Initially, vasodilation maintains cerebral blood flow (CBF) in response to diminished CPP, but once vasodilation becomes maximized, CBF falls proportionately to diminished CPP (i.e., loss of autoregulation). With low regional cerebral blood flow, regional oxygen metabolism is maintained by a compensatory rise in oxygen extraction. Other investigators, using two-dimensional Xenon-133, Xenon-133 single photon emission computerized tomography (SPECT), and SPECT with I-123 and Technetium-99-M labeled tracers, have also shown perfusion defects in some patients with asymptomatic carotid occlusive disease in the resting state.[41-44]

Unfortunately, none of these techniques has shown a predictable relationship between severity of extracranial occlusive disease and ipsilateral change in CBF or metabolism in the resting state. This has prompted some investigators to measure cerebral perfusion patterns after the application of a variety of hemodynamic stresses (cerebral vasodilators, eg., CO_2 or Acetazolamide; or physiological stimulation of sensorimotor cortex), on the theoretical grounds that the stress will unmask inadequacies in the compensatory mechanisms that maintain normal cerebral blood flow at rest (collateral circulation and arteriolar vasodilation). Overall, the results of these studies support the hypothesis that application of a hemodynamic stress will provoke or enhance perfusion defects in patients with hemodynamically significant extracranial carotid disease.[45-49] However, none of these studies determined if patients with perfusion defects detected by these tests are at greater risk of stroke during cardiopulmonary bypass. If futher studies confirm that patients with impaired perfusion reserve are at increased risk of stroke during CABG surgery, a more rational approach to prophylactic carotid endarterectomy and other preventative therapies may follow.

Intraoperatively and postoperatively, several prophylactic measures should be taken. First, meticulous medical management of these patients (control of metabolic parameters, maintaining adequate gas exchange, restricting polypharmacy, and prompt management of infection) will limit cerebral complications of OHS. Second, potential embolic situations, such as brittle aorta, ventricular thrombus, dysrhythmias, and air in the heart or bypass line should be watched for and dealt with appropriately. Echocardiography can detect ventricular intracavity air by means of the distinctive sonographic appearance of microbubbles, which would enable manual attempts to eradicate them. However, a recent study using intraoperative transesophageal echocardiography in patients undergoing CABG surgery showed that although microbubbles are often detected during surgery, they are not predictive of postoperative neurological complications.[50] There is some evidence that prostacyclin infusion during cardiopulmonary bypass lowers the incidence of encephalopathy during OHS by preventing adhesion of platelets to the extracorporeal tubing and subsequent microembolization.[51,52]

Third, marked drops in blood pressure should obviously be avoided. Although most patients on cardiopulmonary bypass do well with a mean pressure of 50 mm Hg, it would seem prudent to maintain a mean arterial pressure of at least 60 mm Hg in potentially high-risk patients (hypertensive, elderly, prior stroke, known occlusive disease) since the lower limit of mean arterial pressure at which CBF auto-regulation is abolished is higher in many of these patients.

Although EEG monitoring may allow early detection of focal or global brain ischemia intraoperatively,[53,54] it is impractical to monitor all surgical patients with EEG. However, preoperative testing of cerebral perfusion reserve and the development of an autoregulation profile might allow identification of a subgroup of high-risk patients who could then be selectively monitored with EEG or even intraoperative CBF measurement.[55,56] This would allow intraoperative detection of impaired CBF, which could be managed by elevating mean arterial pressure, hypothermic measures,[56] and pharmacological therapy to protect the brain from focal or global ischemia. Currently, there are no clinically established protocols for protecting the brain from ischemia; however, several drugs, including calcium antagonists[57,58] and N-methyl-D-aspartate receptor antagonists,[59,60] have been shown to reduce infarct size in animal models of focal and global ischemia and may become part of the clinician's armamentarium to ameliorate the effects of cerebral ischemia in the near future.

References

1. Furlan AJ, Breuer AC. Central nervous system complications of open heart surgery. *Stroke.* 1984;15: 912–915.
2. Gilman S. Cerebral disorders after open heart operations. *N Engl J Med.* 1965;272:489–498.
3. Hill JD, Aguilar MJ, Baranco A, et al. Neuropathological manifestations of cardiac surgery. *Ann Thorac Surg.* 1969;7:409–419.
4. Branthwaite MA. Neurological damage related to open-heart surgery: a clinical study. *Thorax.* 1972; 27:748–753.
5. Gonzalez-Scarano F, Hurtig HI. Neurologic complications of coronary artery bypass grafting: case control study. *Neurology.* 1981;31:1032–1035.
6. Loop FD, Cosgrove DM, Lytle BW, et al. An 11-year evolution of coronary arterial surgery (1967–1978). *Ann Surg.* 1979;190:444–455.
7. Coffey CE, Massey EW, Roberts KB, et al. Natural history of cerebral complications of coronary artery bypass graft surgery. *Neurology.* 1983;33:1416–1421.
8. Breuer AC, Furlan AJ, Hanson MR, et al. Central nervous system complications of coronary artery bypass graft surgery: prospective analysis of 421 patients. *Stroke.* 1983;14:682–687.
9. Reed GL III, Singer DE, Picard EH, et al. Stroke following coronary artery bypass surgery: a case control estimate of the risk from carotid bruits. *N Engl J Med.* 1988;319:1246–1250.
10. Hart RG, Easton JD. Management of cervical bruits and carotid stenosis in preoperative patients. *Stroke.* 1983;14:290–297.
11. von Reutern G-M, Hetzel A, Birnbaum D, et al. Transcranial Doppler ultrasonography during cardiopulmonary bypass in patients with severe carotid stenosis or occlusion. *Stroke.* 1988;19:674–680.
12. Ropper AH, Wechsler LR, Wilson LS. Carotid bruit and the risk of stroke in elective surgery. *N Engl J Med.* 1982;307:1388–1390.
13. Ivey TD, Strandness DE Jr, Williams DB, et al. Management of patients with carotid bruit undergoing cardiopulmonary bypass. *J Thor Cardiovasc Surg.* 1984;87:183–189.

14. Barnes RW, Rittgers SE, Putney WW. Real-time Doppler spectrum analysis. *Arch Surg.* 1982;117: 52–57.

15. Turnipseed WD, Berkoff HA, Belzer FO. Postoperative stroke in cardiac and peripheral vascular disease. *Ann Surg.* 1980;192:365–368.

16. Barnes RW, Marszalek PB. Asymptomatic carotid disease in the cardiovascular surgical patient: is prophylactic endarterectomy necessary? *Stroke.* 1981;12:497–500.

17. Breslau PJ, Fell G, Ivey TD, et al. Carotid arterial disease in patients undergoing coronary artery bypass operations. *J Thorac Cardiovasc Surg.* 1981; 82:765–767.

18. Kartchner MM, McRae LP. Guidelines for noninvasive evaluation of asymptomatic carotid bruits. *Clin Neurosurg.* 1981;28:418–428.

19. Brener BJ, Brief DK, Alpert J, et al. A four-year experience with preoperative noninvasive carotid evaluation of two thousand twenty-six patients undergoing cardiac surgery. *J Vasc Surg.* 1984;1:326–338.

20. Furlan AJ, Craciun AR. Risk of stroke during coronary artery bypass graft surgery in patients with internal carotid artery disease documented by angiography. *Stroke.* 1985;16:797–799.

21. Brener BJ, Brief DK, Alpert J, et al. The risk of stroke in patients with asymptomatic carotid stenosis undergoing cardiac surgery: a follow-up study. *J Vasc Surg.* 1987;5:269–279.

22. Hertzer NR, Loop FD, Beven EG, et al. Surgical staging for simultaneous coronary and carotid disease: a study including prospective randomization. *J Vasc Surg.* 1989;9:455–463.

23. Rorick M, Furlan AJ. Risk of cardiac surgery in patients with prior stroke. *Neurology.* 1990;40:835–837.

24. Michelson E, Morganroth J, MacVaugh H. Postoperative arrhythmias after coronary artery and cardiac valvular surgery detected by long-term electrocardiographic monitoring. *Am Heart J.* 1979;97:442–448.

25. Ghosh P, Pakrashi BC. Cardiac dysrhythmias after thoracotomy. *Br Heart J.* 1972;34:374–376.

26. Raffman J, Fieldman A. Digoxin and Propranolol in the prophylaxis of supraventricular tachydysrhythmias after coronary artery bypass surgery. *Ann Thor Surg.* 1981;31:496–501.

27. Taylor KM. Brain damage during open-heart surgery. *Thorax.* 1982;37:873–876.

28. O'Neill BJ III, Furlan AJ, Hobbs RD. Risk of stroke in patients with transient postoperative atrial fibrillation/flutter. *Stroke.* 1983;14:133.

29. Branthwaite MA. Prevention of neurological damage during open-heart surgery. *Thorax.* 1975; 30:258–261.

30. Tufo HM, Ostfeld AM, Shekelle R. Central nervous system dysfunction following open-heart surgery. *JAMA.* 1970;212:1333–1340.

31. Shaw PJ, Bates D, Cartlidge NEF, et al. Early neurological complications of coronary artery bypass surgery. *Br Med J.* 1985;291:1384–1387.

32. Sotaniemi KA, Mononen H, Hokkanen TE. Long-term cerebral outcome after open-heart surgery. A five-year neuropsychological follow-up study. *Stroke.* 1986;17:410–416.

33. Calabrese JR, Skwerer RG, Gulledge AD, et al. Incidence of postoperative delirium following myocardial revascularization: a prospective study. *Cleve Clin J Med.* 1987;54:29–32.

34. Henriksen L. Evidence suggestive of diffuse brain damage following cardiac operations. *Lancet.* 1984; 1:316.

35. Stockard JJ, Bickford RG, Schauble JF. Pressure dependent cerebral ischemia during cardiopulmonary bypass. *Neurology.* 1973;23:521–529.

36. Brennan RW, Patterson RH, Kessler J. Cerebral blood flow and metabolism during cardiopulmonary bypass: evidence of microembolic encephalopathy. *Neurology.* 1971;21:665–672.

37. Zisbrod Z, Rose DM, Jacobwitz IJ, et al. Results of open heart surgery in patients with recent cardiogenic embolic stroke and central nervous system dysfunction. *Circulation.* 1987;76 (suppl V):V109–V112.

38. Gibbs JM, Wise RJS, Leenders KL, et al. Evaluation of cerebral perfusion reserve in patients with carotid artery occlusion. *Lancet.* 1984;1:310–314.

39. Powers WJ, Press GA, Grubb RL Jr, et al. The effect of hemodynamically significant carotid artery disease on the hemodynamic status of the cerebral circulation. *Ann Int Med.* 1987;106:27–35.

40. Levine RL, Lagreze HL, Berkoff HA, et al. Noninvasive testing of cerebral perfusion reserve prior to coronary artery bypass graft surgery. *Angiology.* 1988;39:421–428.

41. Robertson WM, Welch KMA, Tilley BC, et al. Cerebral blood flow asymmetry in the detection of extracranial cerebrovascular disease. *Stroke.* 1988; 19:813–819.

42. Bonte FJ, Stokely EM, Devous MD. Single photon emission computed tomography of regional brain blood flow in cerebral vascular disease and stroke. *Non-invasive Medical Imaging.* 1984;1:9–16.

43. Bayko OB, Park HM, Edwards MK. I-123 HIPDM SPECT imaging and cerebral angiography for EC-IC bypass evaluation. *Radiographics.* 1987;5: 563–577.

44. Podreka I, Suess E, Goldenberg G. Initial experience with Technetium-99m HM-PAO Brain Spect. *J Nucl Med.* 1987;28:1657–1666.

45. Powers WJ, Fox PT, Raichle ME. The effect of carotid artery disease on the cerebrovascular response to physiologic stimulation. *Neurology.* 1988;38:1475–1478.

46. Vorstrup S, Brun B, Lassen N. Evaluation of the cerebral vasodilatory capacity by the Acetazolamide test before EC-IC bypass surgery in patients with occlusion of the internal carotid artery. *Stroke.* 1986;17:1291–1298.

47. Bullock R, Mendelow AD, Bone I, et al. Cerebral blood flow and CO-2 responsiveness as an indicator of collateral reserve capacity in patients with carotid artery disease. *Br J Surg.* 1985;72:348–351.

48. Bishop CCR, Powell S, Insall M, et al. Effect of internal carotid artery occlusion on middle cerebral blood flow at rest and in response to hypercapnia. *Lancet.* 1986;1:710–712.

49. Ringelstein EB, Sievers C, Ecker S, et al. Non-invasive assessment of CO-2 induced cerebral vasomotor response in normal individuals and patients with internal carotid artery occlusions. *Stroke.* 1988;19:963–969.

50. Topol EJ, Humphrey LF, Borkon AM, et al. Value of intraoperative left ventricular microbubbles detected by transesophageal two-dimensional echocardiography in predicting neurologic outcome after cardiac operation. *Am J Cardiol.* 1985;56:773–775.

51. Longmore D. The effects of prostacyclin on reducing cerebral damage following open heart surgery. In: Becker R, Katz J, Polonius M-J, Speidel H, eds. *Psychopathological and Neurological Dysfunction following Open-Heart Surgery.* New York, NY: Springer-Verlag; 1982:pp 320–342.

52. Pokar H, Bleese N, Fischer-Dusterhoff H, et al. Prevention of postoperative psychic and neurological disturbances after open-heart surgery using prostacyclin: a clinical study. In: Becker R, Katz J, Polonius M-J, Speidel H, eds. *Psychopathological and Neurological Dysfunction following Open-Heart Surgery.* New York, NY: Springer-Verlag; 1982: pp 312–319.

53. Salerno TA, Lince DP, White DN, et al. Monitoring of electroencephalogram during open-heart surgery: a prospective analysis of 118 cases. *J Thor Cardiovasc Surg.* 1978;76:97–100.

54. Kritikov PE, Branthwaite MA. Significance of changes in cerebral electrical activity at onset of cardiopulmonary bypass. *Thorax.* 1977;32:534–538.

55. Branthwaite MA. Cerebral blood flow and metabolism during open-heart surgery. *Thorax.* 1974;29:633–638.

56. Henriksen L, Hjelms E, Rygg IH. Cerebral blood flow measured in patients during open-heart surgery using intra-arterially injected Xenon-133: the effect of rewarming on cerebral blood flow. *J Cereb Blood Flow Metab.* 1981;1(suppl):432–433.

57. Deshpande JK, Wieloch T. Flunarizine, a calcium-entry blocker, ameliorates ischemic brain damage in the rat. *Anesthesiology.* 1986;64:215–224.

58. Salgado AV, Jones SC, Furlan AJ, et al. Bimodal treatment with nimodipine and low molecular weight dextran for focal cerebral ischemia in the rat. *Ann Neurol.* 1989;26:621–627.

59. Simon RP, Swan JH, Griffiths T, et al. Blockade of N-methyl-D-aspartate receptors may protect against ischemic damage in the brain. *Science.* 1984;226:850–852.

60. Steinberg GK, Saleh J, Kunis D, et al. Protective effect of N-methyl-D-aspartate antagonists after focal cerebral ischemic in rabbits. *Stroke.* 1989;20:1247–1252.

61. Heller SS, Frank KA, Malm JR, et al. Psychiatric complications of open-heart surgery. *N Engl J Med.* 1970;283:1015–1020.

62. Javid H, Tufo HM, Nafaji H, et al. Neurological abnormalities following open-heart surgery. *J Thorac Cardiovasc Surg.* 1969;58:502–509.

63. Hansotia PL, Myers WO, Ray JF III, et al. Prognostic value of electroencephalography in cardiac surgery. *Ann Thoracic Surg.* 1975;19:127–134.

64. Cannon DS, Miller DC, Shumway NE, et al. The long-term follow-up of patients undergoing saphenous vein bypass surgery. *Circulation.* 1974;49:77–85.

65. Hutchinson JE III, Green GE, Mekhjian HA, et al. Coronary bypass grafting in 376 consecutive patients, with three operative deaths. *J Thorac Cardiovasc Surg.* 1974;67:7–16.

66. Hodgman JR, Cosgrove DM. Post-hospital course and complications following coronary bypass surgery. *Cleve Clin Q.* 1976;43:125–129.

67. Kolkka R, Hilberman M. Neurologic dysfunction following cardiac operation with low-flow, low-pressure cardiopulmonary bypass. *J Thorac Cardiovasc Surg.* 1980;79:432–437.

68. Lee MC, Geiger J, Nicoloff D, et al. Cerebrovascular complications associated with coronary artery bypass (CAB) procedure. *Stroke.* 1979;10:13.

69. Muraoka R, Yokota M, Aoshima M, et al. Subclinical changes in brain morphology following cardiac operations as reflected by computed tomographic scans of the brain. *J Thorac Cardiovasc Surg.* 1981;81:364–369.

19
Prevention of Stroke from Cerebral Vascular Malformations*

Ricardo Garcia-Monaco, Pierre Lasjaunias, and Alex Berenstein

Cerebral vascular malformations (CVMs) produce both hemorrhagic and ischemic stroke. Cerebral hemorrhage is the most frequent type of stroke, and almost 50% of arteriovenous malformations (AVMs) present with parenchymatous hematoma.

Ischemic stroke is less frequent but is also seen in large AVMs or arteriovenous fistulas. It is commoner in children and is due to venous thrombosis within the vascular lesion, arterial "steal," or associated Moya-Moya or coagulation disturbances.

Epidemiology and Classification

The prevalence of cerebral AVMs in a given population is difficult to estimate, but about 0.14 to 0.8% of the population may present with a cerebral AVM in a year.[1,2,3] The incidence in autopsy series according to the various types is shown in Table 19.1. (Cerebral aneurysms and their relationship to stroke are not dealt with in this chapter.)

There are many classifications of brain vascular lesions based on surgical[4,5] or anatomopathological features.[6] A simple classification of cerebral vascular malformations is shown in Table 19.2. Arteriovenous lesions can also be classified by their pathological and biological behavior[7] (Table 19.3), and we feel that this classification is more useful for clinical and therapeutic management.

An arteriovenous shunt is an abnormal capillary bed with a shortened arteriovenous transit time.

There are two broad categories of arteriovenous shunts: arteriovenous fistulas and AVMs. In arteriovenous fistulas the shunt between the artery and vein is direct without evidence of a nidus, whereas AVMs are composed of a network of abnormal vascular channels (nidus) between the arterial feeder(s) and the draining vein(s). They are termed micro-AVMs when the nidus is <1 cm (Fig. 19.1).

Most AVMs are single, but multiple AVMs also occur, more commonly in children (20% in our series) than in adults (9% in our series). Multiple arteriovenous fistulas are also seen in patients with Rendu Osler Weber disease. Systematic lesions are either familial or nonfamilial with a predictable pathological anatomy, (e.g., Wyburn Mason syndrome or AVM compromising the optic tract).

Arterial variations are seen on angiography in 24% of cerebral AVMs,[8] more frequently than in patients examined for occlusive disease or in autopsy series. Persistence of embryonic channels (trigeminal, hypoglossal, etc.) and variations in the circle of Willis occur especially when the area of shunting is located in the watershed zone. When the lesion develops within the dominant area of supply, only the distal branching pattern of the anastomotic arteries undergo anatomical variations. The arterial territories of these variants must be known for one to decide on their potential surgical or embolization risks. These anatomical anomalies represent vulnerable areas that favor the development of flow-related aneurysms, a further factor in hemorrhage.

The incidence of cerebral vascular malformations in autopsies performed after cerebral hemorrhage is seen in Table 19.1. However, the number

*Reprinted in part from Berenstein A, Lasjaunias P. *Surgical Neuroangiography*. Vol 4. New York: Springer-Verlag; 1991.

TABLE 19.1. Incidence of cerebral AVMs in autopsy series.

	General autopsy	Autopsy for cerebral hemorrhage	
CVM	6%	7%	
Arteriovenous malformations	0.15%	3%	(× 20)
Cavernomas	0.05%	0.5%	(× 10)
Venous angiomas	0.25%	0.8%	(× 3)
Telangiectasias	0.15%	2.7%	(× 18)

Modified from Ref. 7. Used by permission.

of telangiectasias in relation to other vascular malformations in autopsy series if they have not bled is not known. Arteriovenous malformations and telangiectasias are seen 18 to 20 times more frequently in autopsies in patients with cerebral hemorrhage. These two lesions are almost equally present in the general population (0.15%) as in autopsies associated with cerebral hemorrhage (3%). However there is a discrepancy between autopsy findings (Table 19.4) and clinical series results (Table 19.5); the clinical incidence of supratentorial CVMs is higher than in autopsy series (9 to 20%). The opposite is true in infratentorial CVMs. Telangiectasias are significantly more frequent in the posterior fossa (60 to 70%), mainly in the brain stem (Table 19.6), and are usually silent until they bleed. Thus, infratentorial hemorrhages are more lethal than supratentorial bleeding, which probably explains the discrepancy between clinical and autopsy series.

The size of the cerebral AVM and the sex of the patient are not associated with an increased risk of hemorrhage, as shown in long-term clinical prospective studies.[9] However, temporal AVMs have a higher tendency to bleed than those in other areas.[8,9] The incidence of hemorrhagic stroke increases with age, and patients are at increased risk after the age of 60.[9]

TABLE 19.2. Types of cerebral vascular malformations.

Arterial (aneurysms)
Arteriovenous (arteriovenous malformations and fistulas)
Capillary (telangiectasias)
Venous (cavernous malformations)

Modified from Ref. 7.

TABLE 19.3. Classification of cerebral arteriovenous malformations.

Arteriovenous (AV) shunts
  Single
    Micro AV shunts (mAVM or mAVF)
    Macro AV shunts (compartmented nidus or AVF)
  Multiple Nonfamilial
    Systematized (Wyburn Mason)
    Nonsystematized (multiple separate niduses or "separated" compartment within 1 nidus)
  Familial
    Systematized (Rendu Osler)
    Nonsystematized (multiple separate niduses with or without AVF)

Associated vascular variants
  Arterial or venous

Secondary vascular changes
  Angiogenesis, kinking, and dolicho vessels
  Arterial aneurysms, venous ectasias, and pouches
  Venous and arterial stenoses or thrombosis
  External carotid supply—dural arteriovenous shunting
  Arterial and venous collateral circulation

Secondary morphological changes
  Hydrocephalus, cerebral atrophy, cavities
  Perivascular ischemia (MRI), calcification
  Bone hypertrophy

Modified from Ref. 7. Used by permission.

Mechanisms of Stroke in Cerebral Arteriovenous Malformations

Stroke from cerebral AVMs represents a significant change in the compliance of the vascular system. Epidemiological and clinical data indicate that usually these patients live normal lives, but they become symptomatic usually in adulthood or late childhood. Clearly, the AVMs are in equilibrium with the cerebrovascular system until trigger factors produce cerebral hemorrhage, brain ischemia, seizures or other symptoms. These trigger factors are still not understood, but examination of AVMs may demonstrate vulnerable areas which are responsible.

Stroke and Cerebral Hemorrhage from Cerebral AVMs

Cerebral hemorrhage is the most frequent cause of stroke in these patients, but every hemorrhage does not produce a stroke, and asymptomatic

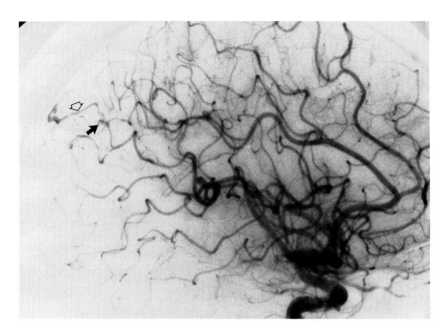

FIGURE 19.1. Internal carotid angiogram shows a parietal micro AVM. Notice the nidus (arrow) and normal-sized draining vein (open arrow). (Reprinted with permission from Ref. 14.)

bleeding is common. Bleeding can occur from rupture of the nidus, from arterial rupture, or from venous rupture, either close to or remote from the lesions (Table 19.7). Observations made during surgery of previous subclinical hemorrhages around the nidus[3,10] indicate that one third of AVMs show evidence of previous hemorrhage.[3] Bleeding from AVMs produces both hematomas and intraventricular hemorrhages. Sudden headaches, sometime with seizures, may occur with local hemorrhages.[11] These minor bleeding events increase the incidence of hemorrhage but decrease the apparent morbidity and mortality from cerebral hemorrhage.

Two different pathophysiological mechanisms produce cerebral hemorrhage; (1) the arterial or antegrade pressure-related rupture, and (2) venous

or retrograde pressure-related rupture. Both are related and can provoke rupture at the weak point of the lesion separately or together. Hemorrhage secondary to ischemic infarction may also occur.

Nidus Rupture

The "weak" area of the lesion causing cerebral hemorrhage may be at the nidus. There are different types of nidus; for instance, AVMs with small or micronidus may have a greater tendency to bleed, based upon the clinical observation that most of these patients present with hemorrhage. Actually, the size of the nidus is not related to the risk of cerebral hemorrhage.[9] In clinical practice, small or microlesions mostly present with cerebral hemorrhage since they cannot interfere

TABLE 19.4. Overall distribution of CVM regardless of type. Autopsy series.

Cerebral hemisphere, corpus callosum	64.8–70%
Intraparenchymatous, deep-seated	8.5– 9%
Brain stem	13 –16.1%
Cerebellum	11.8–17%

Modified from Ref. 7. Used by permission.

TABLE 19.5. Overall distribution of CVM regardless of type. Clinical series.

Cerebral hemisphere, corpus callosum	76.6–90%
Intraparenchymatous, deep-seated	2 – 8%
Brain stem	2.6– 7%
Cerebellum	5 – 9.6%

Modified from Ref. 7. Used by permission.

TABLE 19.6. Topographic repartition of CVM. Autopsy series.

	Supratentorial	Infratentorial
Arteriovenous malformations	70–76%	24–30%
Cavernomas	61–74%	26–39%
"Venous angiomas" (DVAs)	57–60%	40–43%
Telangiectasias	30–37%	63– 70%

Modified from Ref. 7. Used by permission.

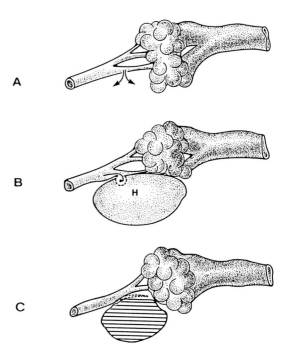

sufficiently to produce seizures, or neurological deficits.

Vessel ectasia within the nidus represent a vulnerable area of the AVM, leading to rupture and bleeding. They are difficult to visualize at angiography, unless outlined in hyperselective studies.

In intralesional ectasias, false arterial and false venous aneurysms close to the nidus may occur. Arterial false aneurysms (Fig. 19.2) are usually seen during the acute stage of an intracranial hemorrhage of arterial origin and are usually in close contact with the nidus. The aneurysms are small, but may enlarge and produce early secondary rupture. This is one of the few indications for emergency treatment. Sometimes false aneurysms resolve uneventfully with occlusion of the ruptured artery (Fig. 19.3).

FIGURE 19.2. Schematic representation of false arterial aneurysm. A: Arterial rupture (arrows) proximal to the nidus leading to hemorrhage. B: Hematoma (H) compression and clotting "help" to stop the bleeding. Communication between artery and hematoma forms the false aneurysm (dotted lines). C: Complete clotting of hematoma "seals" the arterial fissure leading to disappearance of the false arterial aneurysm (see also Fig. 19.3).

TABLE 19.7. Mechanisms of hemorrhage in a BAVM.

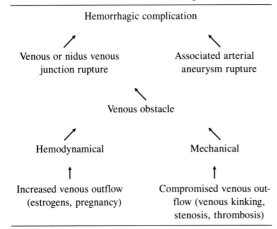

Modified from Ref. 7. Used by permission.

The false venous aneurysm (Fig. 19.4) is a vascular ectasia located distal to the nidus. It may represent a previously fissured vein close to the hematoma that underwent partial recanalization and annexation to the venous outlet (open ectasia), or a thrombosed draining vein leaving a proximal stump opacified through the nidus at the acute stage following a hemorrhage (closed ectasia) (Fig. 19.5). This may be an indication for emergency treatment. The venous origin of a false aneurysm is difficult to demonstrate, but most of these intralesional pouches have a recent history of hemorrhage. They are seen more frequently in deeply located lesions, such as in a sulcus infratemporally or within the brain, at the site of a hematoma.

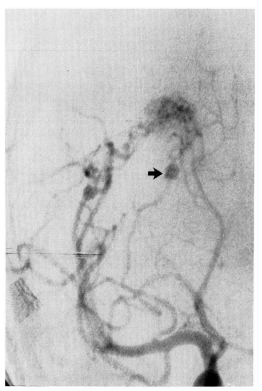

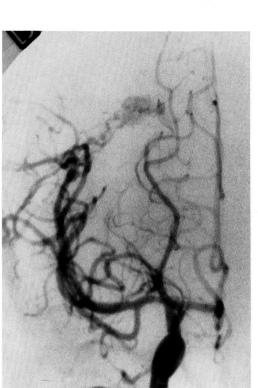

FIGURE 19.3. Patient with a parenchymatous intraventricular hemorrhage. A: Internal carotid angiogram shows a caudate AVM. A false arterial aneurysm (arrow) is visualized in close contact to the hematoma. B: Control angiogram performed 3 weeks later shows spontaneous disappearance of the false arterial aneurysm. ◄

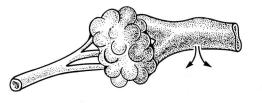

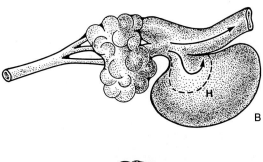

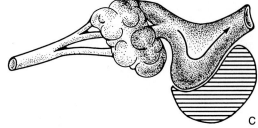

FIGURE 19.4. Schematic representation of a false venous aneurysm (open ectasia). A: Venous rupture (arrows) close to the venous nidus junction. B: Communication between ruptured vein and hematoma (H). C: After complete clotting of the hematoma, annexation of the false aneurysm to the venous outlet.

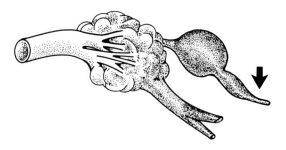

FIGURE 19.5. Schematic representation of a false venous aneurysm (closed ectasia). Thrombosed drainage vein (arrow) with a proximal ectatic stump communicated to the nidus. (Reprinted with permission from Ref. 27.)

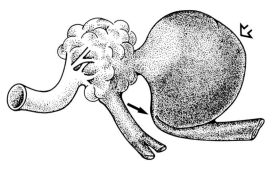

FIGURE 19.6. Schematic representation of a venous stenosis (arrow) leading to proximal venous ectasia (open arrow). (Reprinted with permission from Ref. 27.)

Venous Rupture

Veins represent a weak area within the lesion, and hemorrhages distant from the nidus usually relate to venous bleeding. According to Yasargil, most hemorrhages result from rupture of veins or the vein-nidus junction.[12] Examination of the angioarchitecture of the AVMs in patients who bleed shows venous stenosis (Fig. 19.6) in 50%.[8] This is more common in the hemorrhage group than in the overall population of AVMs. Venous stenosis alters hemodynamic conditions both in the AVM and in the neighboring brain parenchyma. Venous pressure in ruptured AVMs is higher than in nonruptured AVMs, as measured during open surgery. Thrombosis and kinking seen in the venous system draining the lesion provoke a retrograde increase of venous pressure. Direct venous compression by

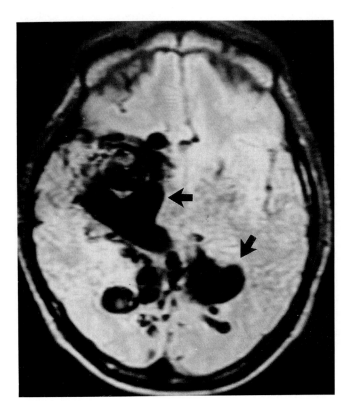

FIGURE 19.7. MRI of a patient with a deep-seated temporal AVM shows multiple venous ectasias (arrows). (Reprinted with permission from Ref. 8).

FIGURE 19.8. Carotid angiography shows a cingulocallosal AVM mainly fed by an enlarged anterior cerebral artery. Note arterial aneurysms (arrows) and stenosis (open arrow) in the pedicle supplying the AVM.

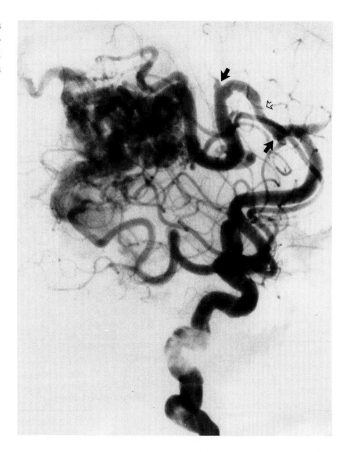

the sphenoid ridge or tentorial edge is also frequent and may account for the high incidence of hemorrhagic episodes in lesions in the incisural or the medial temporal lobe.

Venous obstruction may lead to partial venous ectasia (Fig. 19.7), representing the progressive response of the venous wall to both compromised outlet and turbulence. Obstruction is due to kinking, lengthening, mechanical compression within a sulcus, the tent, or the choroidal fissure. As long as the vein can enlarge, or more proximal venous outlets are recruited, no hemorrhage will occur. In our series, stenotic veins were more frequent in the population that bled, unlike ectasias.[8]

In large AVMs, cerebral hemorrhage is not frequent. These lesions usually present earlier with symptoms such as seizures, headaches, and neurological deficits. Most large AVMs do not have significant venous obstruction, since the veins enlarge and new venous outlets are recruited.

Venous obstruction may be the cause of hemorrhage in micro-AVMs. This is due to the normal arrangement of cortical veins.[13] Small bridging arteries anchor the cortical veins on the parenchyma and narrow them in the depth of the sulci, causing increased pressure upstream and secondary rupture.[14]

Arterial Rupture

Arterial rupture causes AVM hemorrhage, especially when associated with an arterial aneurysm. In patients with AVMs who have bled, arterial aneurysms are significantly more frequent than in the overall population of AVMs. About 41% to 50% cerebral AVM-arterial aneurysms present with hemorrhage, and 78% of these events probably result from aneurysmal rupture.[15,16]

The incidence of associated aneurysms (Fig. 19.8) and hemorrhage increases with age. In a given individual, the significance of the 2% to 3%

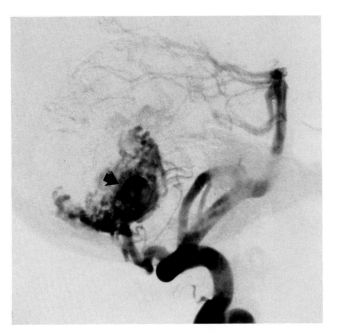

A

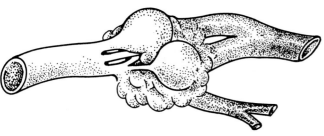

B

FIGURE 19.9. A: Vertebral angiogram shows a huge intralesional aneurysm (arrow) in an inferior vermian AVM supplied mainly by the PICA B: Schematic representation of intralesional arterial aneurysm. (Reprinted with permission from Refs. 21 and 27.)

risk of hemorrhage per year may not apply to the AVM itself. The chance of developing an arterial aneurysm and bleeding from it is fourfold between 10 and 50 years of age.[17]

The incidence of arterial aneurysms and cerebral arteriovenous malformations varies from 2.7%[18] to 16.7%.[16] These numbers are low compared to reports including complete high-quality diagnostic angiography. The difficulty in understanding the relationship between cerebral AVMs and arterial aneurysms is due in part to the underestimation of their association. The 23% found in our series[17] may reflect our use of high-quality pancerebral angiography and represent the true incidence in the overall population of cerebral AVMs.

Arterial aneurysms are an additional risk factor relevant to treatment. There are two types of arterial aneurysms associated with cerebral AVMs:

1. Flow-related aneurysms developing from the pedicle supplying the cerebral AVM
2. Dysplastic aneurysms.

There are two types of flow-related aneurysms. One group develops near the base of the brain (proximal arterial aneurysm), and the other is seen close to the nidus (distal arterial aneurysm) (Fig. 19.9). From 37% to 82% of the arterial aneurysms are considered flow-related,[15,17] including infundibula >3 mm in size.[15,16,19]

In AVMs most aneurysms are in the "feeding" arteries irrespective of the circulation, and the presence of an AVM predisposes to the formation of aneurysms. There is experimental and clinical evidence that aneurysms may occur after chronic increase of arterial flow.[7,17] The pathogenesis of AVMs and arterial aneurysms is not the same.

Arterial aneurysms worsen the prognosis of the AVM. In the cooperative aneurysm study, mortality was 50% with conservative treatment and 37% with surgical treatment.[20] Data of treatment by the endovascular approach to AVMs associated with arterial aneurysms are scanty, but following occlusion of the AVM, proximal arterial aneurysms have shown regression.[17]

Experience in Our Unit

In the past 6 years, we have had no complications with the embolization of pedicles of AVMs associated with arterial aneurysms. This has resulted in the diminution or disappearance of some of these aneurysms.

Arterial aneurysms of the anterior communicating artery associated with convexity AVMs pose a problem. However, an augmented diastolic fraction on Doppler in the internal carotid artery opposite to the shunt will confirm its role in the blood supply to the AVM. After treatment of the shunt (surgical or endovascular), regression of arterial aneurysms occurs.[12,17] In our series 44% of the associated aneurysms were multiple and 24% were dysplastic, or remote from the shunt.[17] In these patients there was no personal or familial history of vascular disease. Similarly there were no cases of multiple aneurysms in the group of multiple AVMs (9% of our series of AVMs in the adult population).

Arterial aneurysms are found predominantly in corticoventricular (66%) and cortical locations (30%). In deep-seated lesions, arterial aneurysms are rare (4%). Review of our cases shows the same incidence of arterial aneurysms in supra and infratentorial AVMs.[21] We believe that the presence of flow-related aneurysms indicates which nourishing arterial pedicles should be given priority in the sequential planning of endovascular therapy of cerebral AVMs (Fig. 19.10). Since at least 50% of patients (75% in our series) occurring

under these circumstances bleed[15,16] it is possible that some hemorrhages occurring in the course of a cerebral AVM are due to an arterial aneurysm not previously recognized. Dysplastic aneurysms develop on arterial branches independent of the AVM[15,20] and are not considered flow related.

Stroke and Cerebral Ischemia from Cerebral AVMs

Cerebral ischemia due to AVMs leads to neurological deficits and seizures because of hemodynamic factors within the AVM or remote from it. There are two broad groups: arterial and venous ischemia.

Arterial Ischemia

"Steal"

In our experience, symptomatic "steal" phenomenon has never been clearly demonstrated. The concept is that blood flows toward the low-resistance area in an arteriovenous malformation, producing a hemodynamic "steal" of cerebral parenchyma. Results of cerebral blood-flow studies with Xenon-131 are equivocal even with cerebral stimulation (visual or speech). For instance, visual activity "steals" blood from the AVM toward the occipital cortex.[22] "Steal" at angiography consists of nonvisualization of vessels in normal brain, but careful examination always visualizes the "missing" branches through leptomeningeal anastomosis. Most of the "stolen territories" are not symptomatic, even if flow within the AVM is enough to "steal" the contrast material from the ipsilateral hemisphere.

Arterial Stenosis

Arterial occlusion of the feeders also causes cerebral ischemia, part of a "high-flow angiopathy,"[23] but quantitative relationships between the degree of the stenosis and the shunt are difficult to establish. However, if there is a concentric narrowing by intraluminal protrusion of the endothelial cells, mesenchymal cell proliferation, and thinning of the wall, intraluminal stenosis occurs.

Occasionally arterial stenoses are extrinsic (due to dural or venous compression) and may be reversed if the external constraint is removed.

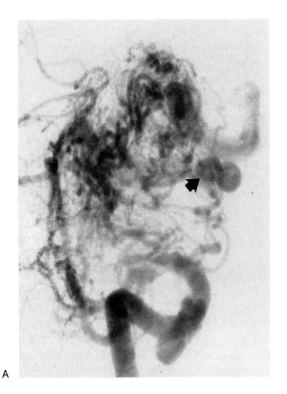

A

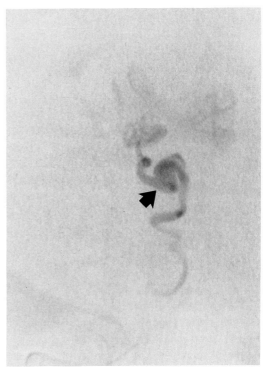

B

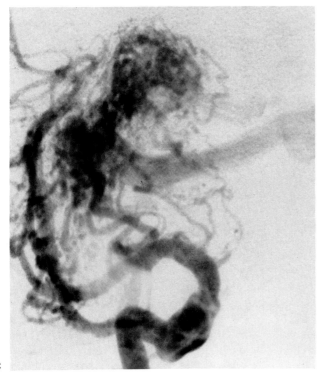

C

FIGURE 19.10. A: Left internal angiogram shows a deep-seated AVM with a proximal AA (arrow) in a lenticulostriate artery. B: Selective injection of this pedicle allows better visualization of the AA (arrow). C: Following embolization the aneurysm is no longer visible (reprinted with permission from Ref. 17).

FIGURE 19.11. A: Right carotid angiography in AP view shows a left sylvian AVM and inferior displacement of the watershed area (arrow) as response to a congenital constraint. B: Schematic representation of displacement of the watershed area as observed in A. C: Normal watershed zone between the anterior cerebral artery territory and the sylvian territory. D: Acquired development of collateral circulation in the watershed area.

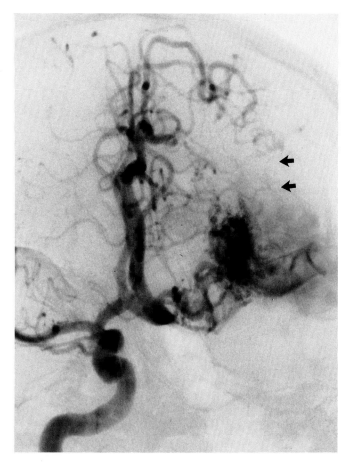

A

Extrinsic narrowing is usually seen in high-flow lesions with mass effect. The displacement of the watershed zones (Fig. 19.11) and their changes after embolization seen during follow-up angiography indicate their role and importance in collateral compensation. The various types of watershed zone changes demonstrate the possible evolution of the lesion over the years. Congenital versus acquired watershed transfer can be assessed by careful examination, and postischemic angiogenetic features can also be identified.

Moya-Moya

Arterial stenosis with sprouting angiogenesis may produce a "Moya-Moya" pattern. It is rare (0.3 to 3%), seen in young patients (Fig. 19.12), and is not reversible. It may represent a vascular proliferation or a local response to arterial narrowing or a combination. Mawad et al.[24] reviewed 13 cases of Moya-Moya phenomenon associated with cerebral AVM and postulated that it represented the development of an acquired dysplasia.

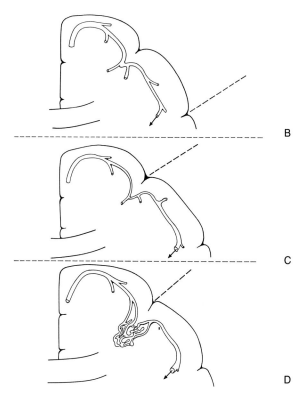

B

C

D

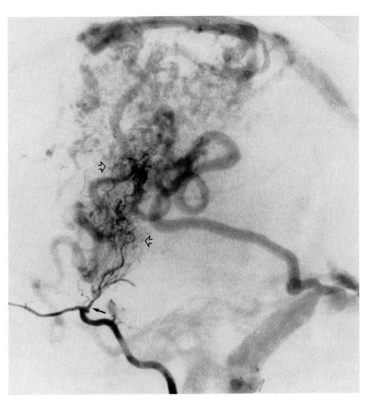

FIGURE 19.12. Lateral internal carotid angiogram shows a marked stenosis of the supraclinoid internal carotid artery (arrow), resulting in a Moya-Moya pattern (open arrow) of the lenticulostriate vessels that supply the deep compartment of a supratentorial AVM. (Reprinted with permission from Ref. 8.)

Although it is reported that Moya-Moya may protect the AVM from bleeding,[24] in Suzuki's series[25] (without an associated cerebral AVM) there was a 4% incidence of hemorrhage in the juvenile form and a 43% incidence in the adult form.

Venous Ischemia

The role of venous ischemia in cerebral arteriovenous lesions is usually not considered as a major one. Laine et al.[26] reviewed the key role of venous patterns in the presenting symptoms of AVMs and dural AVMs demonstrated the absence of arterial "steal" or any contribution by the pial arteries to the supply of dural AVMs indicating a major role of veins in this type of anomaly.[27] Spetzler, commenting on Nornes and Gripa,[28]

emphasized the importance of locally increased venous pressure as a secondary factor decreasing tissue perfusion. The congestion of the system that occurs hemodynamically or by stenosis or thrombosis will produce cerebral venous ischemia. The same occurs in dural AVMs draining into the cerebral veins; white matter does not tolerate venous congestion for long.

Decreased tissue perfusion secondary to venous ischemia may produce ischemic cerebral symptoms, such as motor or sensory deficits, neuropsychological alteration, or seizures. Venous stenosis raises proximal venous pressure and interferes with tissue perfusion if collateral circulation cannot overcome the obstruction to outflow (Fig. 19.13). Thrombosis in the venous drainage of a cerebral AVM is common and may be due to coagulation disorders, such as platelet aggregation[29] or

FIGURE 19.13. Arterial (A) and venous (B) phase of a carotid angiogram shows a superficial temporal AVM. Junctional venous stenosis (arrow) and anatomical disposition (absence of cavernous sinus) lead to rerouting of the venous outflow and developing of collateral venous circulation.

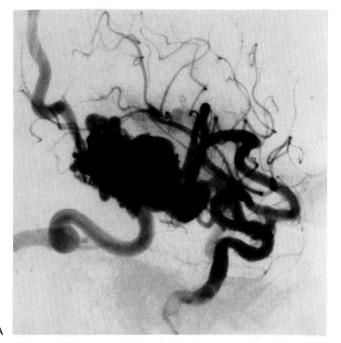

A

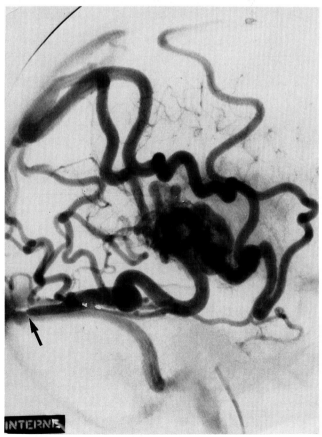

B

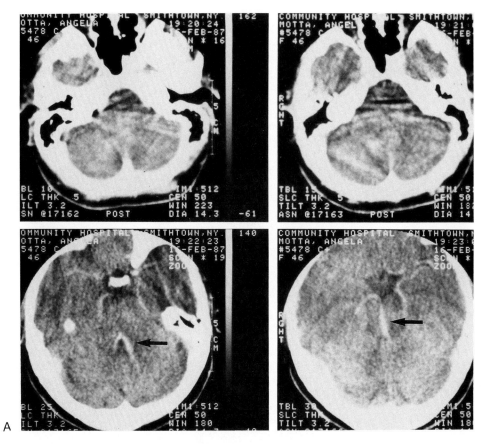

FIGURE 19.14A. Patient with a pontine hematoma. CT shows a posterior fossa DVA (arrows).

protein C deficiency. Calcifications in the AVM are usually seen in the venous walls of medullary, transcerebral, or subpial veins in relation to hypoxia at the venous watershed zones. These lesions are more commonly seen in children.

Stroke from Cerebral Venous Malformations and Venous Anomalies

One of the most controversial venous lesions is the cavernous type, referred to as venous angiomas or cavernous hemangiomas, and located intra- or extradurally. "True and false venous malformations" should be distinguished. Venous angiomas and cavernous hemangiomas are not real vascular malformations; the former represents an anatomic variant, while the latter is a benign vascular tumor. However, they are often erroneously considered to be venous malformations in the literature.

They are discussed in this chapter under the title of "False Venous Malformations," and they may cause stroke. We would also stress their differences from true venous malformations, such as cavernomas or Sturge Weber disease.

False Venous Malformation

Venous Angiomas

These are better termed *developmental venous anomalies*, since they represent an extreme anatomic variant of normal cerebral veins.[31] The two extreme types (superficial and deep) illustrate the

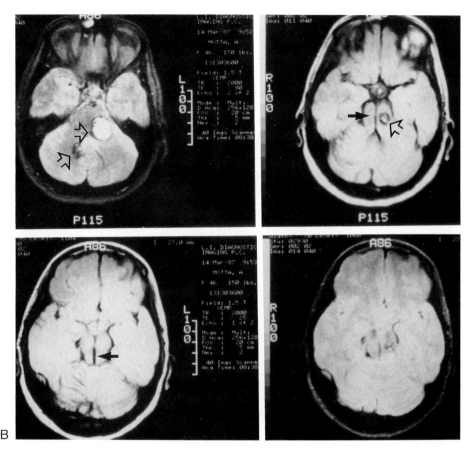

B

FIGURE 19.14B. MRI in the same patient shows the DVA (arrow) and associated multiple cavernomas (open arrows) not seen in the CT. The topography of the hematoma has no direct relationship with that of the DVA but with a cavernoma. (Reprinted with permission from Ref. 30.)

hemodynamic balance of the transcortical venous drainage in the periependymal zones. Therefore, the term *venous angioma* is inappropriate, since it is not a tumor or malformation but an anatomic variant. They drain normal cerebral tissue within a functionally normal arterial territory and are opacified at angiography in the same time sequence as the normal veins. The angiographic appearance consists of small medullary veins that converge toward a transcerebral collector, which in turn drains into a normal superficial or deep vein.

Venous angiomas illustrate the transhemispheric anastomotic pathways that develop due to hemodynamic demands.[30] They are stable, well-tolerated, and do not create any structural damage in developing brain. Venous thrombosis may occur, causing brain ischemia, a hemorrhagic infarction, or cere-bral hemorrhage. Magnetic resonance imaging (MRI) often demonstrates the cavernoma (vide infra) responsible for the bleeding (Fig. 19.14). Surgical treatment should be avoided in view of the potential adverse effects secondary to occlusion of the venous drainage of a normal territory.

Cavernous Hemangiomas

These are typical tumors, with proliferation characteristics of hemangiomas. They are extracerebral, and occur at the intracranial or intraspinal dural or extradural space.[32] Angiography usually shows a faint, homogenous capillary blush often leading to a preoperative diagnosis of meningioma. Cavernous hemangiomas are prominent in females, presenting with a progressive mass effect and eventually growing during menstruation or pregnancy. They seldom bleed and are absent from hemorrhagic autopsy series. Thus they differ significantly from the malformations. They represent true tumors and are nosologically close to the lingual or orbital ones.

True Venous Cerebral Malformations

These are abnormal venous channels of the cavernous type, with slow blood circulation, and are also termed *cavernomas* or *cavernous malformations*. Their incidence is 0.05%, and they occur anywhere in the cerebral or spinal cord tissue. They present clinically in adulthood or childhood, or even in the neonatal period. Cavernous malformations are not visualized by angiography ("angiographically occult") except for rare, partial venous filling seen at the time of a hemorrhagic episode. Their association with venous angiomas or the confusion with cavernous hemangiomas accounts for most of the reports of apparent positive angiography. However, they are well seen by MRI[33] and in some cases also by computerized tomography (CT). Only 4.5% of the cavernomas are symptomatic; thus they cannot be considered as dangerous as arteriovenous malformations or telangiectasias. Fundamentally nonproliferative, they grow by confluence of the vascular spaces and can achieve cystic forms following lysis and convergence of intralesional hematomas. Cavernous malformations (with telangiectasias and micro-AVMs) are a frequent cause of pontine hematoma; so an MRI scan should be performed in such cases despite negative angiography. Surgical removal of these lesions depends on their depth, the vicinity of cerebrally eloquent areas, and the presence of a residual cavity of hematoma.

Sturge Weber disease, another type of true venous malformation, does not present as a stroke and therefore is beyond the scope of this chapter.

Cryptic and Angiographically Occult Vascular Malformations

The term *cryptic vascular malformation* applies to those lesions presenting with cerebral hemorrhage in which a vascular malformation is suspected but is not demonstrated by diagnostic, surgical, or even anatomopathological methods.

Angiographically occult vascular malformation refers to vascular malformations not visualized at angiography. However, many "angiographically occult" lesions result from low-quality examinations. Selective catheterization, magnification and subtraction techniques reduce the number of "occult" lesions. In clinical practice, any angiographically occult malformation represents either a cavernoma or a small or micro-AVM, partially or totally thrombosed or compressed. Cavernomas are usually visible on CT and especially on MRI.[33] Therefore, a cerebral hematoma, with negative angiography, should be followed by MRI. Thrombosis of AVMs after hemorrhage may occur, especially in small lesions. Complete thrombosis renders them invisible at angiography.

The same concept of "occult lesions" at angiography can be applied to MRI, and MRI occult lesions (i.e., normal scans) may occur with positive angiography. This is seen in certain types of dural AVMs or micro-AVMs, which, because of their small size and superficial location, are not visualized by MRI. Therefore, a combination of diagnostic examinations (MRI, CT, and angiography) reduces the incidence of unexplained hemorrhagic stroke.

Treatment of Cerebral Arteriovenous Malformations

Recent developments in microsurgical techniques, endovascular therapy, and introduction of multibeam radiotherapy have considerably improved the treatment of AVMs. Anatomical obliteration is the ideal goal, achieved either by a single technique or by a combined approach, such as embolization followed by surgery or radiotherapy. If the same result can be achieved by any one of a number of different techniques with a similar risk, we believe that the less "aggressive" treatment should be used. Providing this condition is verified, endovascular therapy or radiotherapy is preferable to open craniotomy.

Although complete anatomic obliteration is the ideal treatment, partial endovascular therapy can be used. However it must have a specific target, such as venous congestion or associated aneurysms with an AVM, particularly if it causes uncontrollable seizures or a progressive deficit. Therefore, although technically feasible, feeders should not be embolized if they are not felt to play such a role.

Partial treatment does not mean transient treatment, and embolization should be performed with permanent embolic agents such as NBCA and not with particles, coils, or other agents that allow eventual recanalization of the feeders and the nidus of the AVM. In the management of AVMs, therapeutic decisions do not depend exclusively on the disease but also on the available therapeutic skills such as embolization, neurosurgery, or radiotherapy. Strategies and choices will differ from one center to another, and their results can be judged only on the data obtainable on adequate follow-up.

References

1. Garretson H. Intracranial arteriovenous malformations. In: Wilkins RH, Rengachary SS, eds. *Neurosurgery*. New York: McGraw-Hill;1985: pp 1448–1458.
2. Jellinger K. Vascular malformations of the central nervous system: a morphological overview. *Neurosurg Rev*. 1986;9:177–216.
3. Stein BM, Wolpert SM. Arteriovenous malformations of the brain I: current concepts and treatment. *Arch Neurol*. 1980;37:69–75.
4. Drake CG. Cerebral arteriovenous malformations. *Clin Neurosurg*. 1979;26:145–208.
5. Spetzler RF, Martin NA. A proposed grading system for arteriovenous malformations *J Neurosurg*. 1986; 65:476–483.
6. MacCormick WF. The pathology of vascular (arteriovenous) malformations. *J Neurosurg*. 1966;24:807.
7. Berenstein A, Lasjaunias P. *Surgical Neuroangiography*. Vol. 4. New York, NY: Springer Verlag; 1990.
8. Willinsky R, Lasjaunias P, Terbrugge K, et al. Brain arteriovenous malformations: analysis of angioarchitecture in relationship to hemorrhage. *J Neuroradiol*. 1988;15:225–237.
9. Crawford PM, West CW, Chadwick DW, et al. Arteriovenous malformations of the brain: natural history of unoperated patients. *J Neurol Neurosurg and Psychiatry*. 1986;49:1–10.
10. Pertuiset B, Sichez J, Philippon H, et al. Mortalité et morbidité après éxérèse chirurgicale totale de 162 malformations artérioveineuses intracraniennes. *Rev Neurol*. 1979;135:319–327.
11. Yamada S. Arteriovenous malformations in the functional area: surgical treatment and regional cerebral blood flow. *Neurol Res*. 1982;4:283–322.
12. Yasargil M. *Microneurosurgery*. Vol. IIIa. Stuttgart: George Thieme Verlag; 1987.
13. Duvernoy H, Delon S, Vannson J. Cortical blood vessels of the human brain. *Brain Res Bull*. 1981; 7:519–579.
14. Willinsky R, Lasjaunias P, Comoy J, et al. Cerebral micro-arteriovenous malformations. Review of 13 cases. *Acta Neurochir*. 1988;91:37–41.
15. Batjer H, Suss R, Samson E. Intracranial arteriovenous malformations associated with aneurysms. *Neurosurgery*. 1986;18:29–35.
16. Miyasaka K, Wolpert S, Prager R. The association of cerebral aneurysm, infundibula, and intracranial arteriovenous malformations. *Stroke*. 1982;13:186–203.
17. Lasjaunias P, Piske R, Terbrugge K, et al. Cerebral arteriovenous malformations and associated arterial aneurysms *Acta Neurochir*. 1988;91:29–36.
18. Paterson J, McKissock W. A clinical survey of intracranial angiomas with special reference to their mode of progression and surgical treatment. A report of 110 cases. *Brain*. 1986;70:233–266.
19. Hayashi S, Arimoto T, Itakura T. The association of intracranial aneurysms and arteriovenous malformation of the brain: case report. *J Neurosurg*. 1981; 55:971–975.
20. Perret G, Nishioka H. Report of the cooperative study of intracranial aneurysms and subarachnoid hemorrhage: VI. Arteriovenous malformations: an analysis of 545 cases of craniocerebral malformations and fistulae reported to the cooperative study. J Neurosurg, 1966;25:467–490.
21. Garcia Monaco R, Goulao A, Alvarez H, et al. Posterior fossa arteriovenous malformations: angioarchitecture in relationship to hemorrhage. *Neuroradiology*. 1990;31:471–475.
22. Deutsch, G. Blood flow changes in arteriovenous malformations during behavioral activation. *Annals of Neurology*. 1983;13:38–43.
23. Pille-Spellman J, Backer K, Liszczal T. High flow angiopathy: cerebral blood vessels changes in experimental chronic arteriovenous fistulae. *AJNR*. 1986;7:811–816.
24. Mawad M, Hilal S, Michelsen W, et al. Occlusive vascular disease associated with cerebral arteriovenous malformations. *Radiology*. 1989;153:401–408.
25. Suzuki J. Moya Moya disease. New York: Springer Verlag; 1986.
26. Laine E, Jamin M, Clarisse J, et al. Les malformations artérioveineuses cérébrales profondes. *Neurochirurgie*. 1981;27:147–160.
27. Lasjaunias P, Manelfe C, Chiu M. Angiographic architecture of intracranial vascular malformations and fistulas—pretherapeutic aspects. *Neurosurg Rev*. 1986;9:253–263.

28. Nornes H, Gripa N. Hemodynamic aspect of cerebral arteriovenous malformations. *J Neurosurg.* 1980;53:456–464.

29. Sutherland G, King M, Drake C, et al. Platelet aggregation within cerebral arteriovenous malformations. *J Neurosurg.* 1988;68:198–204.

30. Lasjaunias P, Terbrugge K, Rodesch G, et al. Vraies et fausses lésions veineuses cérébrales. Pseudo-angiomes veineux et hémangiomes caverneux. *Neurochirurgie.* 1989;35:132–139.

31. Lasjaunias P, Burrows P, Planet C. Developmental venous anomalies (DVA): the so called venous angiomas. *Neurosurg Rev.* 1986;9:239–244.

32. Simard J, Garcia Bengochea F, Ballinger W, et al. Cavernous angioma. A review of 126 collected and 12 new clinical cases. *Neurosurgery.* 1986;18:162–172.

33. Gomori J, Grossman R, Goldberg H, et al. Occult cerebral vascular malformations: high field MR imaging. *Radiology.* 1986;158:707–713.

20
Prevention of Aneurysmal Subarachnoid Hemorrhage

J.M. Findlay and B.K.A. Weir

Approximately 1 to 20% of the general adult population harbor a saccular cerebral aneurysm, which is an acquired lesion resulting from prolonged hemodynamic stress at unsupported bifurcations and angles in major cerebral arteries traversing the subarachnoid space. A more liberal application of computerized tomography (CT) in the investigation of unusual headaches could facilitate recognition of minor hemorrhages that frequently precede major, devastating aneurysm ruptures. Rebleeding is a major cause of death and disability in survivors of aneurysm rupture, and the rate of rebleeding is highest on the first 2 days following the initial hemorrhage. If treated with bed rest alone, approximately 20% of patients will rebleed within 14 days, 30% in 30 days, 40% in 180 days, and thereafter patients will continue to rebleed at the rate of about 3% per year. Although it has become apparent that the timing of surgery to clip ruptured aneurysms and protect the patient from rehemorrhage is not the most important determinant of overall patient outcome, the results of the International Cooperative Study on the Timing of Aneurysm Surgery and a more recent randomized trial examining the timing of aneurysm surgery indicate that best results are obtained when surgery is carried out in the first several days after hemorrhage.

While antifibrinolytic treatment has been shown to reduce the risk of rebleeding, this beneficial effect is offset by a concomitant increase in the risk of delayed ischemia; thus use of antifibrinolytic agents is restricted to patients at low risk for vasospasm in whom there exist contraindications to early surgery. When recognized, all unruptured aneurysms should be considered for repair by experienced aneurysm surgeons. Each case must be considered individually on the basis of the aneurysm's location, size, and shape, combined with the patient's age, medical condition, and wishes. Our understanding of the natural history of such aneurysms remains imperfect. Screening investigations for asymptomatic aneurysms cannot be recommended to any patient groups with a firm set of guidelines at this time. The development of high-resolution CT or magnetic resonance imaging (MRI) capable of demonstrating even small aneurysms will lead to a wider investigation of family members of aneurysm patients and, consequently, a better understanding of their relative risk of bearing one of these dangerous lesions.

Prevention of Rebleeding from Ruptured Aneurysms

Diagnosis of Subarachnoid Hemorrhage

Bleeding into the subarachnoid space can occur in a wide variety of pathological conditions, but the most common cause of spontaneous subarachnoid hemorrhage (SAH) is the rupture of intracranial saccular aneurysms. Aneurysms account for approximately 60% of SAHs associated with an angiographically or autopsy-defined etiology.[1] Subarachnoid hemorrhage is the most frequent presentation of cerebral aneurysms.[2] The variable severity of the hemorrhage provides a diversity of clinical patterns ranging from slight headache to deep coma and imminent death.

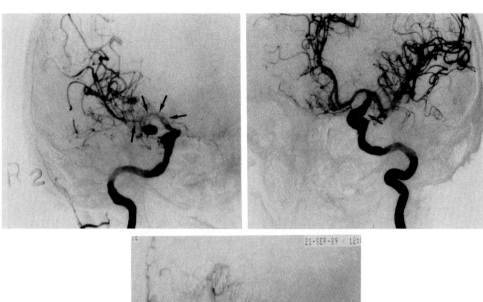

FIGURE 20.1. Case 1 A 53-year-old woman suffered a sudden severe headache and visited her family physician a total of three times before referral to hospital. A computed tomographic scan of the head demonstrated resolving blood in the right sylvian fissure. A cerebral angiogram demonstrated a large right middle cerebral artery aneurysm (upper left) with severe vasospasm in the adjacent right middle cerebral and internal carotid arteries (arrows). The major arteries on the left side of the circle of Willis (upper right) were free of arterial narrowing, and an infundibular widening of the left posterior communicating artery was noted (arrows). Twelve days after the initial subarachnoid hemorrhage, and following successful repair of the aneurysm, a right cerebral angiogram demonstrated adequate clipping of the aneurysm sac and partial resolution of vasospasm (lower center).

In as many as one half of patients, premonitory symptoms or "warning signs" occur in the weeks prior to a major rupture.[3-6] These symptoms may be due to expansion of the aneurysm sac, a minor leakage of blood, or other, ill-defined mechanisms.[4] Although sometimes as unremarkable as local head, eye, or facial pain and as nonspecific as dizziness,[4,5] even complaints of sudden, severe headaches, meningism, photophobia, and diplopia are frequently misdiagnosed by physicians[6,7,8] (Fig. 20.1). Charles Drake has written:

It is dismaying to realize that many patients go unrecognized, at least until a massive brain-destroying hemorrhage has occurred. Only a small fraction of the patients are seen after the initial bleed when the greatest therapeutic reward could occur. The challenge for the future, then, will be the early recognition of the initial bleeding, the warning bleeding. It will require public education about the problem in a continuing fashion, as well as continuing emphasis on it for students and physicians. The potential for prevention of death or dreadful disability is large for thousands in the prime of life each year.

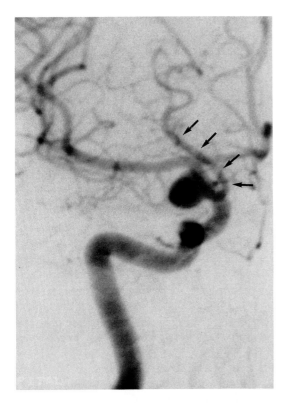

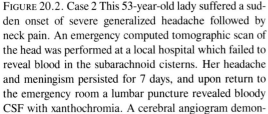

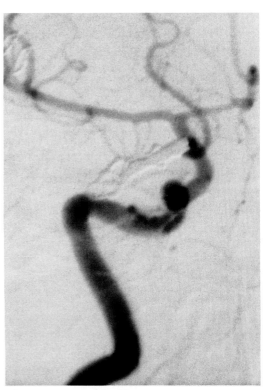

FIGURE 20.2. Case 2 This 53-year-old lady suffered a sudden onset of severe generalized headache followed by neck pain. An emergency computed tomographic scan of the head was performed at a local hospital which failed to reveal blood in the subarachnoid cisterns. Her headache and meningism persisted for 7 days, and upon return to the emergency room a lumbar puncture revealed bloody CSF with xanthochromia. A cerebral angiogram demon-strated a large internal carotid aneurysm arising at the origin of a fetal-type posterior communicating artery (upper, left, arrows indicate the posterior communicating artery, which is the sole blood supply to the right occipital cortex). Immediate surgery was performed to obliterate the aneurysm, and postoperative angiography revealed clipping of the aneurysm with preservation of the posterior communicating artery (upper, right).

An unavoidable percentage of patients will continue to present with a lethal or highly morbid initial aneurysm rupture, and a further group with minor, sentinel bleeds will be missed because of the very nonspecific nature of their symptoms. Every effort, however, must be made to identify those patients with recognizable minor SAHs in whom prompt treatment yields the most satisfying results.[6]

When SAH is suspected, the next appropriate step is to submit the patient for CT, which confirms the presence of intracranial bleeding and provides prognostic information. The CT demonstration of intraventricular hemorrhage, intracerebral hemorrhage, or diffuse collections of subarachnoid blood is predictive of increased mortality,[10] whereas a normal CT study is correlated with a favorable outcome. Diffuse or focal, thick collections of subarachnoid blood predict vasospasm.[11] Computerized tomography may also identify patients with alternative etiologies for SAH, such as an arteriovenous malformation, and in patients with multiple aneurysms focal collections of clot indicate the particular sac that has bled. Currently, the only indication for lumbar puncture following SAH is to establish the diagnosis in the occasional patient (about 5 to 10% of patients with SAH) whose CT study does not show blood or any evidence of raised intracranial pressure (ICP) but who have a strongly suggestive history (Figure 20.2). In addition to the danger of inducing brain herniation in patients with elevated ICP, lumbar puncture carries the risk of lowering ICP, which tamponades the aneurysm, thereby precipitating rebleeding.[12]

At this time MRI has not surpassed the diagnostic usefulness of CT for SAH. Computed tomography is quicker, more accessible, and cheaper. It has been suggested that MRI will become more sensitive in detecting oxyhemoglobin metabolized into methemoglobin in the cerebrospinal fluid (CSF) over time, assisting in the diagnosis of patients who present late after SAH.[13,14] Magnetic resonance imaging has also proved to be a useful adjunct in identifying which of multiple aneurysms has bled.[15]

Risk of Rebleeding

Until recently, it has been believed that the highest risk of rebleeding from a ruptured aneurysm occurred in the second part of the first week and in the beginning of the second week after the initial SAH.[16,17] However, in a 1983 report from the Cooperative Aneurysm Study by Kassell and Torner,[18] including 2265 patients, the rate of rebleeding was maximal within the first 24 hours after SAH (4.1%). The rebleed rate dropped sharply until the end of 48 hours, when it was approximately 1.5% per day, and then declined thereafter for a cumulative rebleeding rate at 14 days of 26.5% (rates quoted for those patients not receiving antifibrinolytic therapy). This study and several previous smaller studies were summarized by Jane et al.[19] with similar conclusions. Hillman et al. reporting on a population of 933 800 within Sweden, where they believe almost every patient stricken with SAH and surviving long enough for transport are seen in their institution, found that in one 34-month period 9.6% of SAH patients suffered from "ultra-early" rebleeding within 24 hours of SAH.[20]

A recent report from the Danish Aneurysm Study, which examined 1076 patients over a 5-year period,[21] found a rather low risk of rebleeding within the first 24 hours (0.8%). In this study the maximum risk of rebleeding occurred between days 4 and 9 after SAH, and the cumulative rate of rebleeding was 16.8% within the first 2 weeks after initial SAH. In this series patients who suffered at least one rebleed had a mortality rate of 80%, compared to 41% for patients without a rebleed, and

patients with poor neurological grades had significantly more rebleeding episodes. Similarly, in separate reports from the Cooperative Aneurysm Study, it was found that rebleeding episodes were fatal in 78% of patients[22] and that poor neurological status was significantly related to both mortality and the likelihood of recurrent hemorrhage.[23] Patients admitted who were poorly responsive or unresponsive were 6 times more likely to die and 2.6 times more likely to suffer a rebleed than those who were admitted alert.

In a recent series of 510 patients seen in several different British hospitals, the incidence of recurrent hemorrhage during the period awaiting surgery was 13.7%, although the fact that <50% of patients were admitted to a neurosurgical unit before the fourth day postictus suggested that this figure was an underestimate.[24] Following rebleeding there was an immediate mortality of 34% in good-grade patients and 52% in poor-grade patients. In the long term, only 4.4% of good-grade and 8% of poor-grade patients made a good recovery following a second bleed, as compared to 70.6% and 52.8%, respectively, for those who did not rehemorrhage.

Thus it can be seen that rebleeding exacts a tremendous toll on survivors of SAH. Along with the direct effect of the initial hemorrhage and delayed cerebral ischemia due to vasospasm, rebleeding is a major source of mortality and morbidity in the natural history of aneurysmal SAH[25] (Figure 20.3). While the greatest propensity for hemorrhage to recur is in the first several weeks after the initial ictus, at least 50% will rebleed during the first 6 months, and thereafter the risk drops off to at least 3% a year.[19]

Timing of Aneurysm Surgery

From the foregoing it should be evident that the basic indication of surgery and aneurysm clipping as soon as possible and at least within the first several days after SAH is to prevent catastrophic rehemorrhage.[26] There are several other potential advantages of such "early surgery." An attempt can be made to remove subarachnoid clot in contact with the major cerebral arteries, thereby reducing the risk of vasospasm.[27,28] More importantly, the early obliteration of the aneurysm sac allows aggressive hypervolemic, hypertensive treatment to prevent cerebral ischemia in the event of vasospasm.[29]

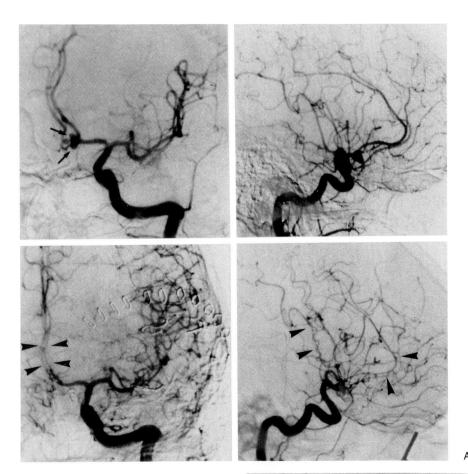

FIGURE 20.3. Case 3 A 52-year-old woman suffered several bleeding episodes from an intracranial aneurysm over the course of 1 week. A cerebral angiogram demonstrated the source of the hemorrhage to be a bilobed anterior communicating artery aneurysm filling from the left side (upper left, left AP, oblique projection; upper right, lateral projection). Three days following surgery for repair of the aneurysm and 10 days following the primary subarachnoid hemorrhage, the patient became obtunded with severe bilateral lower extremity weakness. Cerebral angiography demonstrated severe vasospasm of both anterior cerebral arteries and distal branches of the left middle cerebral artery (lower left and right, arrowheads). She was treated with hypertensive, hypervolemic therapy as well as the calcium antagonist nimodipine. She improved gradually and computed tomography scanning failed to reveal evidence of cerebral infarction due to vasospasm. Three months later an incidentally discovered right middle cerebral artery bifurcation aneurysm (B) was electively repaired without complication.

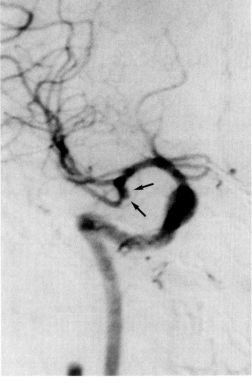

Early surgery avoids to some extent the complications of inactivity forced upon patients awaiting delayed operation and may result in a shorter hospitalization.

Early surgery, however, bears potential disadvantages.[30] It seemed likely that in the early stage after SAH, surgeons would be faced with a swollen brain that, together with clot-laden subarachnoid cisterns, would make exposure of the aneurysm difficult and the risk of intraoperative rupture and neural damage greater than after waiting for more than a week. It was feared that early surgery might exacerbate the problem of vasospasm and delayed ischemia, although Hunt's work suggested that the incidence and severity of spasm was not statistically related to the presence or absence of operative intervention.[31] There was concern that early surgery might, by preventing fatal rehemorrhages, preserve the life of patients destined to remain in poor neurological condition, thereby decreasing mortality at the expense of increased morbidity. Neurosurgeons naturally wished to have the lowest postoperative morbidity and mortality, and this concerned them more than the overall management results—a more valid assessment of surgical treatment strategies.[32]

The optimal timing of aneurysm surgery became the subject of much neurosurgical debate in the 1980s. A number of reports appeared in the literature examining this problem, and many of these uncontrolled, anecdotal series suggested outcome at least as favorable with early operation as with delayed operation.[33-38] In response to this controversy, Kassell and colleagues conducted the International Cooperative Study on Timing of Aneurysm Surgery.[39,40]

Between 1980 and 1983, 3521 patients with ruptured aneurysm were admitted to 113 hospitals in 14 countries. These patients were 41% of the total admitted with SAH, but exclusions were made for the following reasons: admitted more than 3 days post-SAH, 46%; no aneurysm, 30%; multiple bleeds, 11%; urgent evacuation of hematoma, 5%; other reasons, 8%. Forty-nine percent were admitted day 0, and 31% day 1 post-SAH. The surgeon responsible decided when to operate, and patients were then stratified according to the planned surgical interval. Some who believed in the efficacy of early intervention recorded a days 0 to 3 choice; others chose a later time. Early surgery was

planned for 45% (1595) of patients and delayed surgery (days 7-14) for 30% (1055). The two groups were comparable with respect to prognostic factors such as age, sex, hypertension, and neurological state. Neurological complications were as follows: rebleeding, early 6%, late 13%; focal ischemic deficit, early 27%, late 32%; hydrocephalus, early 13%, late 12%; seizures, early 4%, late 5%. The striking difference, as anticipated, was that early clipping of aneurysms conferred protection against rebleeding. Fully 21% of the late planned surgical group never actually came to surgery because of rebleeding or deterioration. The unadjusted mortality for patients in all consciousness levels was less for the early surgery groups (18% versus 26%). Similarly, an unadjusted favorable outcome at 6 months was more likely for the early surgery group (64% versus 57%). Adjustments for prognostic factors did not change the apparent favorable influence of early surgery. The differences between groups, however, did not achieve statistical significance. The causes of death and disability were vasospasm, early 14%, late 15%; rebleeding, early 4%, late 9%; direct effect of bleed, early 8%, late 8%; surgical complication, early 4%, late 4%; other, early 11%, late 9%. The analysis of the first 4 days showed that results for alert patients operated on day 0 were better than for those from day 1, which in turn were better for results in the 2- to 9-day period. It was concluded that surgery performed on day 0 to 3 gave results that were at least as good as, if not better than, those obtained when surgery was planned for day 11 and beyond. The benefits of early surgery appear to relate to reduction in rebleeding.

It became apparent in the Timing study that modern neuroanesthesia, optimal brain relaxation, and careful microsurgical technique overcomes the potential technical problems imposed upon the surgeon operating within the acute stage of SAH. Another observation of the Timing of Aneurysm Surgery study was that timing per se is not the most important determinant of outcome. It appears that there is no significant difference between early and late aneurysm surgery in terms of overall outcome. A recent analysis of 244 patients admitted to the Mayo Clinic led to the same conclusion, and it was felt that in this series most management morbidity and mortality could be traced to the effects of the initial hemorrhage.[41] These authors suggested that early surgical intervention was advantageous in "good-grade" patients in order to capitalize on a reduced rebleeding risk, and delayed surgery in "poor-grade" patients until their condition has stabilized or improved unless intracranial hypertension (due to an intracranial hematoma, for example) is contributing to the patient's poor neurological condition.

The first prospective, randomized study on the timing of operation for ruptured supratentorial aneurysms was published in 1989.[42] Two hundred sixteen patients who were admitted in Hunt and Hess grades I to III within 72 hours of their last SAH were randomly assigned to 1 of 3 operation groups: 0 to 3 days after SAH (acute surgery), 4 to 7 days after SAH (intermediate surgery), and later than 7 days after SAH (late surgery). Although no volume expansion or hypertension was employed in the patients, 159 of them were randomly assigned to placebo or nimodipine in an independent and coexistent trial. The different groups were well balanced with respect to key prognostic factors that could affect patient outcome. The neurological grade deteriorated preoperatively significantly more often in the late surgery group than in the acute surgery group because of rebleeding or delayed ischemia. As in the Timing of Aneurysm study, operation within 3 days after SAH was associated with a trend toward better overall results at the end of 3 months, although the difference was not significant. The percentage of patients who were classified as independent, dependent, and dead, respectively, for the different groups were: early surgery 92%, 3%, 6%; intermediate surgery 79%, 16%, 6%; and late surgery 80%, 7%, 13%. There were no deaths caused by rebleeding in the early surgery group, but 2 occurred in the intermediate surgery group and 4 in the late surgery group. The management mortality in both the early and intermediate surgery group was 6%, and in the late surgery group it was 13%. Although this difference did not reach statistical significance, the trend toward better results in the early surgery group was clear, and the authors concluded by recommending operation at the acute stage, combined with intravenous nimodipine, since this treatment significantly reduced the incidence of delayed deficit due to cerebral ischemia.

These results support the contention[34,43] that the expeditious conduct of surgery on ruptured aneurysms by experienced aneurysm surgeons is preferred unless (1) the patient is neurologically devastated, in which case no surgery is usually indicated, or (2) the aneurysm clipping promises to be especially difficult (i.e., a large, complex basilar tip aneurysm). In such cases it is usually safer to wait until the effects of the hemorrhage have subsided and maximal brain relaxation can be obtained. Antifibrinolytic agents may be of value during this time period (see below).

Antifibrinolytic Treatment

Antifibrinolytic therapy has been shown to reduce the rate of rehemorrhage after aneurysm rupture, but the beneficial effect on outcome is negated by a concomitant increase in the incidence of vasospasm and delayed cerebral ischemia. Kassell et al.[44] assessed 672 patients in the International Cooperative Study on the Timing of Aneurysm Surgery. Those receiving antifibrinolytic therapy had a significantly lower rebleeding rate but higher rates of ischemic deficits and hydrocephalus. The net result demonstrated no difference in mortality in the first month following the initial bleeding. The patients were studied between 1980 and 1982. Sixty-eight neurosurgical centers participated. More than 75% of patients in both groups were admitted within 1 day of the hemorrhage. Although the antifibrinolytic and the nonantifibrinolytic groups were not selected randomly, they were remarkably similar with respect to prognostic factors for death and rebleeding. The mortality rate at 14 days for the antifibrinolytic group was 13.2%, and at 30 days it was 22.3%. For the nonantifibrinolytic group, the mortality rates were 13% and 20%, respectively. In the untreated group, the estimated cause of death at one month was rebleeding in 45% and vasospasm in 24%. Paradoxically, the situation was almost identically reversed in those who were treated with antifibrinolytic agents (24% and 42%). The 14-day rebleeding rate was 11.7% for those treated with antifibrinolytics, which was almost identical to the rate for the earlier cooperative study.

In 1984, Vermeulen et al.[45] reported on the results of a multicenter, randomized, double-blind, placebo-controlled trial of the antifibrinolytic agent tranexamic acid in 479 patients with SAH. There was no significant difference in outcome in the treated and control groups 3 months after the hemorrhage. When the analysis was restricted to the 285 patients with angiographically demonstrated aneurysm, there was still no significant difference between the groups. The absence of the overall beneficial effect was not due to the lack of antifibrinolytic activity, because the rate of rebleeding was reduced from 24% in the control group to 9% in the tranexamic acid–treated group. This was a highly significant difference. Sadly, as had been intimated from earlier studies, there was a concurrent increase in the incidence of ischemic complications: it increased from 15% in the control group to 24% in the treated group. The conclusion was that until some method could be found to minimize ischemic complications, tranexamic acid was of no benefit in patients with SAH. The 3-month outcomes for 130 tranexamic acid treated cases of aneurysm were as follows: dead, 28%; dependent, 12%; and independent, 59%. Comparable figures for the 155 placebo-treated cases of aneurysm were 32%, 12%, and 56%.

One explanation for this increased risk of delayed cerebral ischemia with the usage of antifibrinolytic agents is that inhibition of already limited CSF fibrinolytic activity further delays clearance of vasogenic hemolyzing erythrocytes from the basal cisterns. Because of this risk, and because of the more widespread adoption of early aneurysm clipping to prevent rebleeding, antifibrinolytic agents no longer have a major role in the management of aneurysmal SAH. Rare candidates for this therapy still exist, however. Such a patient might be one in whom the risk of vasospasm is judged to be minimal, and when overwhelming contraindications to early or any surgery are present.

Regrowth of Aneurysms from Residual Neck Following Successful Clipping

Drawing from his own experience with intracranial aneurysms, Drake has emphasized the problem of rerupture of incompletely obliterated aneurysms,[46,47] and recently his group has reported hemorrhage of aneurysms that regrew from 1 to 2-mm aneurysm neck remnants years after what

was believed to be technically adequate aneurysm clipping.[48] It is important to place the aneurysm clip flush with the origin of the neck of the aneurysm, and a strong argument can be made in favor of routine postoperative angiography. If a large portion of the aneurysm remains, then reoperation should be performed. It was the policy of the Karolinska Institute between 1970 and 1980 to perform routine postoperative angiography, which demonstrated residual aneurysmal sac in 27 cases out of 715. Repeat studies were done on average 6 years later. One had increased in size and bled twice, 5 were spontaneously obliterated, 2 diminished, 13 were unchanged, and in 7 cases no late follow-up angiography was performed.[49] In our opinion, a significant residual neck poses a definite but probably slight risk of subsequent rerupture, and therefore repeat operation would be considered. Yasargil reported rebleeding from clipped anterior communicating aneurysms in 7 out of 375 cases; 4 of them died.[50] Particularly in younger patients, the presence of a residual neck might lead to a follow-up angiogram or MRI 3 to 5 years postclipping in selected cases. The physician, however, has a real obligation not to generate needless and crippling anxiety in patients who have already undergone the horror of aneurysmal rupture.

Proximal Vessel Occlusion

The oldest surgical treatment for ruptured aneurysms, occlusion of the proximal vessel, will only assuredly prevent rebleeding if it is combined with a procedure to occlude the parent vessel distally, the so-called "trapping procedure."[51,52] Inherent in this approach is the risk of cerebral ischemia. Parent artery occlusion is employed only when direct aneurysm neck clipping is impossible by virtue of aneurysm size or location, and intravascular detachable balloons appear to be the superior technique.[53] When a test occlusion results in cerebral ischemia, then an extracranial to intracranial bypass procedure should be considered.[54] In addition to the risks of recurrent hemorrhage from the treated aneurysm and ischemia, carotid ligation also bears the risk of putting added hemodynamic stress on other points of the intracranial circulation and promoting the growth of a second aneurysm, which may rupture.[55]

Prevention of Bleeding from Unruptured Aneurysms

The Cooperative Aneurysm Study found that among 3321 patients presenting with aneurysmal SAH and undergoing cerebral angiography, the incidence of multiple aneurysms was 20%; 3.5% had three lesions and 1.4% had four or more lesions.[56] A second aneurysm occurred on the ipsilateral side in 21% of their patients, on the contralateral side in 47%, and the combination of midline (i.e., anterior communicating artery) and lateral aneurysm occurred in 29%; both aneurysms occurred in the midline in only 3%, and the combination of an anterior and posterior circulation aneurysm was seen in only 3% to 5% of cases. Multiple aneurysms involving the middle cerebral or internal carotid arteries tend to develop symmetrically or ipsilaterally on the main vessel.

In patients with multiple aneurysms, it is important to determine which lesion has ruptured so that surgical treatment can be directed at it first. Attention may be drawn to a particular aneurysm by the presence of neurological signs, such as a third nerve palsy associated with a posterior communicating aneurysm. Computed tomography may be particularly helpful in determining the site of aneurysm rupture by identifying areas of more pronounced SAH or adjacent intraparenchymal hematomas.[57] Recently MRI has also been shown to be useful in detecting the bleeding site.[15] Helpful angiographic criteria that correlate with the ruptured sac include larger aneurysm size, a multiloculated or irregular shape to the aneurysm, the presence of adjacent arterial narrowing, prolonged opacification of the aneurysm sac, and the location of the aneurysm on the anterior communicating artery.[58]

At the time of craniotomy for the ruptured aneurysm, all other aneurysms that can be safely accessed through the operative exposure should be clipped. Yasargil has suggested clipping the ruptured aneurysm first in all cases if feasible.[50] A decision must then be made about the treatment of any other ruptured aneurysms left remaining. A similar problem is the asymptomatic aneurysm identified incidentally in patients being investigated for symptoms other than those related to a possible aneurysm. The precise incidence of

TABLE 20.1. Prevention of Aneurysmal Bleeding.

Clip (or otherwise obliterate) ruptured aneurysms
  Recognize the minor bleed
  Early aneurysm surgery
  Avoid lumbar puncture or intracranial drains preoperatively if possible

Clip unruptured aneurysms
  Elective clipping of "multiple" aneurysms after recovery from initial clipping
  Elective clipping of "incidental" aneurysms
  Screening of groups at risk
    Relatives of "familial" cases
    Polycystic kidney disease, coarctation of the aorta, fibromuscular dysplasia
    Cases with previous carotid ligation for aneurysm
    Cases with residual aneurysmal neck noted on postoperative angiography
    Cases with previous remote "wrapping" or "coating"

unruptured cerebral aneurysms in a general population is not known. Stehbens performed a literature survey of 14 autopsy series, dated between 1890 and 1966, and found that the incidence of intracranial saccular aneurysms was between 0.2% and 9%; the average of these percentages was 2.4%.[59] The angiographic frequency of cerebral aneurysms in a general population was recently found to be 1%.[60] It has been estimated that, in general, the rate of hemorrhage for all types of unruptured aneurysms is 1% a year.[19] The cumulative probability of having a rupture over a given number of years can be calculated from the formula $P = 1 - n^y$, where P = probability, n = yearly chance of *not* having the event, and y = number of years. For example, the probability that a 30-year-old patient will bleed from an unruptured, asymptomatic aneurysm during his/her lifetime (assuming he/she lives to 76) is 37%; the risk for a 50-year-old is 23%.

Heiskanen reviewed 61 patients having at least two aneurysms in which only the ruptured one was clipped. By 10 years four fatal and three nonfatal ruptures had occurred in the previously unruptured lesions. Three additional cases had recurrent hemorrhage > 10 years later.[61] We strongly favor the elective clipping of such aneurysms 3 months or so after the patient has recovered from the initial bleed. The operative mortality and morbidity are well under the expected natural history.

It has long been recognized that the threat of an unruptured aneurysm varies somewhat with aneurysm size. The Cooperative Aneurysm Study suggested that lesions ≥7 mm in diameter may be regarded as threatening.[62] The Mayo Clinic reviewed 130 patients who harbored a total of 161 unruptured aneurysms and found that none of the 102 aneurysms < 10 mm in diameter ruptured, and that 15 of the 51 aneurysms of ≥ 10 mm in diameter did eventually rupture, 14 of which were fatal.[63] It is difficult to reconcile these data in view of the fact that most aneurysms that have ruptured are < 10 mm.[64] The authors suggested this may be due to deflation shrinkage in aneurysm size after hemorrhage.

Bearing in mind that combined mortality and severe morbidity for SAH approaches 60%,[21] we feel that in the absence of definitive prospective natural history data, surgical repair should be considered for all aneurysms identified on cerebral angiography. Each case should be considered on the basis of the aneurysm's location, size, and shape, combined with the patient's age (and therefore the number of years at risk for bleeding), medical condition, and the patient's wishes. Less surgically accessible, larger aneurysms adversely influence operative safety,[65] and this latter fact must be borne in mind if one chooses to electively repair only large, (i.e., >10 mm in diameter) unruptured aneurysms. In the senior author's practice, incidental aneurysms as small as 3 mm have been electively repaired. When conservative therapy is chosen for a small aneurysm, follow-up cerebral angiography or MRI 1 or 2 years later may be appropriate to ensure that the aneurysm has not grown, in which case it should be repaired. Hypertension should be corrected when present. Finally, repair of asymptomatic, unruptured aneurysms should be undertaken by surgeons whose personal mortality and morbidity rates do not exceed 5% in such cases.

If large enough, aneurysms can become symptomatic through compression and irritation of meninges or nearby neural structures,[66] and they rarely present as sources of emboli causing cerebral ischemic symptoms.[67,68] Such symptomatic but unruptured aneurysms are occasionally "giant" in size (>25 mm in diameter). Although direct repair of all such aneurysms is desirable, the patient with an enlarging aneurysm causing sudden pain and a cranial nerve palsy is at far greater immediate risk for rupture than a patient presenting with mass effects from a giant aneurysm. Surgical planning should be done accordingly.

An infundibulum is a funnel-shaped widening of the origin of a cerebral vessel, and it is seen most commonly at the posterior communicating artery. An incidence of 7% infundibular changes was observed in 1020 angiograms.[69] Such junctional dilatations have been associated with both SAH[70] and evolution into actual saccular aneurysms, which can hemorrhage.[71,72] Itakura, after reviewing the literature on this subject, concluded that the following characteristics were shared by cases of "de novo" aneurysm development from infundibula: (1) most cases are young women; (2) most have multiple aneurysms; (3) the junctional dilatation is on the proximal portion of the posterior communicating artery; and (4) the junctional dilatation changes into a true aneurysm in 6 to 9 years.[71] Such developments appear to be very uncommon, however, and the authors generally regard true infundibula to be innocuous except in the setting of SAH when blood appears localized to the region of the infundibulum on CT and no other source of bleeding can be seen on repeated cerebral angiography. Perhaps in the future high-resolution CT or magnetic resonance angiography (MRA) capable of imaging the major cerebral vessels in detail will facilitate the monitoring of infundibula and permit a better understanding of their natural history.

Screening for Unruptured Aneurysms

Even if all minor hemorrhages were detected and the underlying aneurysm repaired prior to major rupture, there would still be an unavoidable percentage of patients that will die or be neurologically devastated as a direct effect of their first one or more SAHs that occur prior to medical intervention. Our present level of understanding makes it difficult to anticipate the prevention of aneurysm formation. Consequently, the screening of supposed high-risk populations for asymptomatic aneurysms so that they can be prophylactically repaired has been considered.

There exists a number of hereditary and congenital diseases that are associated with a higher incidence of cerebral aneurysms than the general population. Cerebral aneurysms have been reported in both autosomal dominant (Marfan's syndrome, polycystic kidney disease, fibromuscular dysplasia, tuberous sclerosis) and autosomal recessive (pseudoxanthoma elasticum, Ehler-Danlos syndrome disorders.[73] Cerebral aneurysms have also been reported in the congenital conditions of coarctation of the aorta[73] and vascular abnormalities of the head and neck[74] that are without a recognized hereditary tendency. In the cases of polycystic kidney disease and aortic coarctation, concomitant severe hypertension complicating these conditions is etiologically related to the development of cerebral aneurysms.[75] Both groups of patients are reasonably screened with cerebral angiography in order to detect and correct threatening lesions[73] The remaining diseases are thought to predispose to development of aneurysms at sites of hemodynamic stress by virtue of connective tissue fragility in the cerebral vessel wall. With the possible exception of fibromuscular dysplasia, these conditions are sufficiently rare that screening for aneurysms does not represent a practical approach.

Separate from aneurysms associated with the aforementioned disease states are those that occur in identical twins[76] and in members of the same family.[77] The possibility of genetic determination of cerebral aneurysms has been considered in this subset of aneurysm patients. It has been suggested that these patients may be deficient in type III collagen, rendering their arteries more susceptible to aneurysm formation,[78,79] but a recent study has cast doubt on this possibility.[79]

Stehbens believes[81] that aside from rare hereditary connective tissue disorders, there is no evidence of a congenital, developmental, or inherited weakness of the vessel wall underlying the development of aneurysms. His review of the evidence indicated that aneurysms are entirely acquired, degenerative lesions: the effect of hemodynamic stress. It has been well documented that occlusion of a feeding vessel enhances the possibility of aneurysm formation at large arterial forks subjected to augmented hemodynamic stress.[55] An implication of the "degeneration theory" is that hypertension is an aggravating factor in the etiology of aneurysms, although this relationship has not been found in all studies.[82]

The introduction of high-resolution CT or MRA or other imaging modality capable of showing aneurysms will lead to a wider investigation of relatives of patients suffering from rupture of an aneurysm, and a better understanding of their risk of bearing an unruptured aneurysm. At the present time cerebral angiography cannot be recommended for family members using any absolutely firm set of guidelines. The many reported cases of familial clusters of aneurysms make it likely that there does exist a subset of aneurysm patients in whom the development of aneurysms is somehow genetically determined. If a reasonably healthy adult patient with a significant life expectancy has two first-degree relatives with documented cerebral aneurysm, we currently recommend complete cerebral angiography. In the future it is to be hoped that high resolution CT[83] or MRA[84,85] will be a safer, cheaper, and more accessible screening modality to offer to these relatives, and any other patients considered at risk for the development of cerebral aneurysms.[86]

References

1. Torner JC. Epidemiology of subarachnoid hemorrhage. *Sem Neurol.* 1984;4:354–369.
2. Sahs AL, Nibbelink DW, Torner JC, eds. *Aneurysmal Subarachnoid Hemorrhage.* Baltimore, MD: Urban and Schwarzenberg; 1981.
3. Gillingham FJ. The management of ruptured intracranial aneurysms. *Scott Med J.* 1967;12:377–383.
4. Okawara S. Warning signs prior to rupture of an intracranial aneurysm. *J Neurosurg.* 1973;38:575–580.
5. Waga S, Ohtsubo K, Handa H. Warning signs in intracranial aneurysms. *Surg Neurol.* 1975;3:5–20.
6. Leblanc R. The minor leak preceding subarachnoid hemorrhage. *J Neurosurg.* 1987;66:35–39.
7. Kassell NF, Kongable GL, Torner JC, et al. Delay in referral of patients with ruptured aneurysms to neurosurgical attention. *Stroke.* 1985;16:587–590.
8. Verweij RD, Wijdicks FM, Van Gijn J. Warning Headache in Aneurysmal Subarachnoid Hemorrhage. *Arch Neurol.* 1988;45:1019–1021.
9. Drake CG. Management of cerebral aneurysm. *Stroke.* 1981;12:273–283.

10. Adams HP Jr, Kassell NF, Torner JC. Usefulness of computed tomography in predicting outcome after aneurysmal subarachnoid hemorrhage: a preliminary report of the Cooperative Aneurysm Study. *Neurology.* 1985;35:1263–1267.

11. Kistler JP, Crowell RM, Davis KR, et al. The relation of cerebral vasospasm to the extent and location of subarachnoid blood visualized by CT scan: a prospective study. *Neurology.* 1983;33:424–436.

12. Duffy GP. Lumbar puncture in spontaneous subarachnoid hemorrhage. *Br M J.* 1982;285:1163–1164.

13. Jenkins A, Hadley DM, Teasdale GM, et al. Magnetic resonance imaging of acute subarachnoid hemorrhage. *J Neurosurg.* 1988;68:731–736.

14. Di Chiro G, Brooks RA, Girton ME, et al. Sequential MR studies of intracerebral hematomas in monkeys. *AJNR.* 1986;7:193–199.

15. Stone JL, Crowell RM, Gandhi YN, et al. Multiple intracranial aneurysms: Magnetic resonance imaging for determination of the site of rupture. Report of a case. *Neurosurgery.* 1988;23:97–100.

16. Pakarinen S. Incidence, aetiology, and prognosis of primary subarachnoid hemorrhage. A study based on 589 cases diagnosed in a defined urban population during a defined period. *Acta Neurol Scand.* 1967;43(suppl 29):1–128.

17. Suzuki J, Hori S. Prediction of reattacks following rupture of intracranial aneurysms. *Neurol Med Chir.* 1975;15(part 1):35–39.

18. Kassell NF, Torner JC. Aneurysmal rebleeding: a preliminary report from the Cooperative Aneurysm Study. *Neurosurgery.* 1983;13:479–481.

19. Jane JA, Kassell NF, Torner JC, et al. The natural history of aneurysms in arteriovenous malformations. *J Neurosurg.* 1985;62:321–323.

20. Hillman J, von Essen C, Leszniewski W, et al. Significance of "ultra-early" rebleeding in subarachnoid hemorrhage. *J Neurosurg.* 1988;68:901–907.

21. Rosenorn J, Eskesen V, Schmidt K, et al. The risk of rebleeding from ruptured intracranial aneurysms. *J Neurosurg* 1987;67:329–332.

22. Nishioka H, Torner JC, Graf CJ, et al. Cooperative study of intracranial aneurysms in subarachnoid hemorrhage: a long term prognostic study: II. Ruptured intracranial aneurysms managed conservatively. *Arch Neurol.* 1984;41:1142–1146.

23. Torner JC, Kassell NF, Wallace RB, et al. Preoperative prognostic factors for rebleeding and survival in aneurysm patients receiving antifibrinolytic therapy: report of the Cooperative Aneurysm study. *Neurosurgery* 1981;9:506–513.

24. O'Neill P, West CR, Chadwick DW, et al. Recurrent aneurysmal subarachnoid hemorrhage: incidence, timing and effects. A re-appraisal in a surgical series. *Br J Neurosurg.* 1988;2:43–48.

25. Flamm ES. The timing of aneurysm surgery 1985. *Clin Neurosurg.* 1985;33:147–158.

26. Kassell NF, Drake CG. Timing of aneurysm surgery. *Neurosurgery.* 1982;10:514–519.

27. Mizukami M, Usami T, Tazawa T, et al. Prevention of vasospasm by removal of subarachnoid blood in early operation. *Neurol Med Chir.* 1981;21:1069–1077.

28. Taneda M. Effect of early operation for ruptured aneurysms on prevention of delayed ischemic symptoms. *J Neurosurg.* 1982;57:622–628.

29. Kassell NF, Peerless SG, Durward QJ, et al. Treatment of ischemic deficits from vasospasm with intravascular volume expansion and induced arterial hypertension. *Neurosurgery.* 1982;11:337–343.

30. Ljunggren B, Brandt L. Timing of aneurysm surgery. *Clin Neurosurg.* 1985;33:159–175.

31. Hunt WE. Timing of surgery for intracranial aneurysm. In: Wilkins RH, ed. *Cerebral Arterial Spasm.* Baltimore: Williams & Wilkins; 1980.

32. Lougheed WM. Selection, timing and technique of aneurysm surgery of the anterior circle of Willis. *Clin Neurosurg.* 1968;16:95–113.

33. Kassell NF, Boarini DJ, Adams HP Jr, et al. Overall management of ruptured aneurysm: Comparison of early and late operation. *Neurosurgery.* 1981;9:120–128.

34. Weir B, Aronyk K. Management mortality and the timing of surgery for supratentorial aneurysms. *J Neurosurg.* 1981;54:146–150.

35. Saito I, Sano K. Timing and indication of surgery for ruptured cerebral aneurysms. *Neurol Med Chir.* 1981;21:261–267.

36. Suzuki K, Kodama N, Yoshimoto T, et al. Ultra-early surgery of intracranial aneurysms. *Acta Neurochir (Wien)* 1982;63:185–191.

37. Ljunggren B, Brandt L, Sundbarg G, et al. Early management of aneurysmal subarachnoid hemorrhage. *Neurosurgery.* 1982;11:412–418.

38. Ljunggren B, Saveland H, Brandt L, et al. Early operation and overall outcome in aneurysmal subarachnoid hemorrhage. *J Neurosurg* 1985;62:547–551.

39. Kassell NF, Tornor JC, Haley EC, Jr., et al. The International Coopeative Study on the Timing of Aneurysm Surgery. Part 1: Overall management results. *J Neurosurg.* 1990;73:18–36.

40. Kassell NF, Torner JC, Jane JA, et al. The International Cooperative Study on the Timing of Aneurysm Surgery. Part 2: Surgical results. *J Neurosurg.* 1990;73:37–47.

41. Chyatte D, Fode NC, Sundt TM Jr. Early versus late intracranial aneurysm surgery in subarachnoid hemorrhage. *J Neurosurg.* 1988;69:326–331.

42. Ohman J, Heiskanen O. Timing of operation for ruptured supratentorial aneurysms: a prospective randomized study. *J Neurosurg.* 1989;70:55–60.

43. Disney L, Weir B, Petruk K. Effect on management mortality as a deliberated policy of early operation on supratentorial aneurysms. *Neurosurgery.* 1987; 20:695–701.

44. Kassell NF, Torner JC, Adams HP Jr. Antifibrinolytic therapy in the acute period following aneurysmal subarachnoid hemorrhage: preliminary observations from the Cooperative Aneurysm study. *J Neurosurg.* 1984;61:225–230.

45. Vermeulen M, Lindsay KW, Murray GD, et al. Antifibrinolytic treatment in subarachnoid hemorrhage. *N Engl J Med.* 1984;311:432–437.

46. Drake CG, Vanderlinden RG. The late consequences of incomplete surgical treatment of cerebral aneurysms. *J Neurosurg.* 1967;27:226–238.

47. Drake CG, Allcock JM. Postoperative angiography and the "slipped" clip. *J Neurosurg.* 1973;39:683–689.

48. Lin T, Fox AJ, Drake CG. Regrowth of aneurysm sacs from residual neck following aneurysm clipping. *J Neurosurg.* 1989;70:556–560.

49. Feuerberg I, Lindquist C, Lindqvist M, et al. Natural history of postoperative aneurysm rests. *J Neurosurg.* 1987;66:30–34.

50. Yasargil MG. *Microneurosurgery.* Vol. 2. Stuttgart: Georg Thieme Verlag; 1984.

51. Kak VK, Taylor AR, Gordon DS. Proximal carotid ligation for internal carotid aneurysms. A long-term follow-up study. *J Neurosurg.* 1973;39:503–513.

52. Miller JD, Jawa DK, Jennett B. Safety of carotid ligation and its role in the management of intracranial aneurysms. *J Neurol Neurosurg Psychiatry.* 1977;40:64–72.

53. Fox AJ, Vinuela F, Pelz DM, et al. Use of detachable balloons for proximal artery occlusion in the treatment of unclippable cerebral aneurysms. *J Neurosurg.* 1987;66:40–46.

54. Peerless SJ, Hampf CR. Extracranial to intracranial bypass in the treatment of aneurysms. *Clin Neurosurg.* 1984;32:114–154.

55. Diste GN, Beck D. De novo aneurysm formation following carotid ligation: case report and review of the literature. *Neurosurgery.* 1989;24:88–92.

56. Sahs AL, Perret GE, Locksley HB, et al. Intracranial aneurysms in subarachnoid hemorrhage. A cooperative study. Philadelphia: Lippincott; 1969.

57. Nehls DG, Flom RA, Carter LP, et al. Multiple intracranial aneurysms: determining the site of rupture. *J Neurosurg.* 1985;63:342–348.

58. Wood EH. Angiographic identification of the ruptured lesion in patients with multiple cerebral aneurysms. *J Neurosurg.* 1964;21:182–198.

59. Stehbens WE. The pathology of intracranial arterial aneurysms and their complications. In: Fox JL, ed. *Intracranial Aneurysms.* Vol. 1. New York, NY: Springer-Verlag; 1983: pp 272–357.

60. Atkinson JLD, Sundt TM Jr, Houser OW, et al. Angiographic frequency of anterior circulation intracranial aneurysms. *J Neurosurg.* 1989;70:551–555.

61. Heiskanen O. Risk of rebleeding from unruptured aneurysms in cases with multiple intracranial aneurysms. *J Neurosurg.* 1981;55:524–526.

62. Locksley HB. Report on the cooperative study of intracranial aneurysms and subarachnoid hemorrhage: Section V, part II. Natural history of subarachnoid hemorrhage, intracranial aneurysms and arteriovenous malformations. Based on 6368 cases in the Cooperative Study. *J Neurosurg.* 1966;25: 219–239.

63. Wiebers DO, Whisnant JP, Sundt TM Jr, et al. The significance of unruptured intracranial saccular aneurysms. *J Neurosurg.* 1987;66:23–29.

64. Weir B. Intracranial aneurysms and subarachnoid hemorrhage: An overview. In: Wilkins RH, Rengachary SS, eds. *Neurosurgery.* New York: McGraw-Hill; 1985.

65. Wirth FP, Laws ER Jr, Piepgras D, et al. Surgical treatment of incidental intracranial aneurysms. *Neurosurgery.* 1983;12:507–511.

66. Hyland HH, Barnett HJM. The pathogenesis of cranial nerve palsies associated with intracranial aneurysms. *Proc R Soc Med.* 1954;47:141–146.

67. Fisher M, Davidson RI, Marcos EM. Transient focal cerebral ischemia as a presenting manifestation of unruptured cerebral aneurysms. *Annals Neurol.* 1980;8:367–372.

68. Stewart RM, Sampson DL, Diehl J, et al. Unruptured cerebral aneurysms presenting as recurrent transient neurologic deficits. *Neurology.* 1980;30: 47–51.

69. Hassler O, Saltzman G-F. Angiographic and histologic changes in infundibular widening of the posterior communicating artery. *Acta Radiol.* 1963; 1:321–327.

70. Archer CR, Silbert S. Infundibula may be clinically significant. *Neuroradiology.* 1978;15:247–251.

71. Itakura T, Ozaki F, Nakai E, et al. Bilateral aneurysm formation developing from junctional dilatation (infundibulum) of the posterior communicating arteries: case report. *J Neurosurg.* 1983; 58:117–119.

72. Misra BK, Whittle IR, Steers AJ, et al. De novo saccular aneurysms. *Neurosurgery.* 1988;23:10–15.

73. Weir B. *Aneurysms Affecting the Nervous System.* Baltimore: Williams & Wilkins; 1987:54–74.

74. George B, Mourier KL, Galbert F, et al. Vascular abnormalities in the neck associated with intracranial aneurysms. *Neurosurgery.* 1989;24:499–508.

75. Stehbens WE. Hypertension and cerebral aneurysms. *Med J Aust.* 1962;2:8–10.

76. Weil STM, Olivi A, Greiner AL, et al. Multiple intracranial aneurysms in identical twins. *Acta Neurochir (Wien)* 1988;95:121–125.

77. Lozano AM, Leblanc R. Familial intracranial aneurysms. *J Neurosurg.* 1987;66:522–528.

78. Neil-Dwyer G, Barlett JR, Nicholls AC, et al. Collagen deficiency in ruptured cerebral aneurysm. A clinical and biochemical study. *J Neurosurg.* 1983;59:16–20.

79. Ostergaard JR, Oxlund H. Collagen type III deficiency in patients with rupture of intracranial saccular aneurysms. *J Neurosurg.* 1987;67:690–696.

80. Leblanc R, Lozano AM, Vanderest M, et al. Absence of collagen deficiency in familial cerebral aneurysms. *J Neurosurg.* 1989;70:837–840.

81. Stehbens WE. Etiology of intracranial berry aneurysms. *J Neurosurg.* 1989;70:823–831.

82. McCormick WF, Schmalstieg EJ. The relationship of arterial hypertension to intracranial aneurysms. *Arch Neurol.* 1977;34:285–287.

83. Schmid UD, Steiger HJ, Huber P. Accuracy of high resolution computed tomography in direct diagnosis of cerebral aneurysms. *Neuroradiology.* 1987;29:152–159.

84. Ross JS, Masaryk TJ, Modic MT, et al. Intracranial Aneurysms: Evaluation by MR Angiography. *AJNR* 1990;11:449–456.

85. Pernicone JR, Siebert JE, Potchen EJ, et al. Three-dimensional phase-contrast MR angiography in head and neck: preliminary report. *AJNR* 1990;11:457–466.

86. Weir BKA. The management of intracranial aneurysms—prospects for improvement. *Clin Neurosurg* 1986;34:154–160.

21
Prevention of Recurrent Stroke

N.M. Bornstein and A.D. Korczyn

When meditating over a disease, I never think of finding a remedy for it, but instead, a means of preventing it.

Louis Pasteur

Cerebrovascular disease (CVD) is the third leading cause of death in the developed world and represents a major cause of disability in the aged. In the United States, CVD ranks as the eighth cause of years of potential life lost before age 65.[1] The 1989 edition of a popular brochure "Stroke Facts" states: "In America someone dies of cardiovascular disease every 32 seconds. In 1986 nearly one out of two Americans died of heart and vascular disease; stroke claimed 147,000 lives in 1986. Stroke accounts for half of all patients hospitalized for acute neurological disease. Stroke related health care in 1989 is estimated by the American Heart Association at 13.5 billion dollars." Detailed, accurate knowledge of the natural history of stroke, its incidence, and management is required to predict outcome and evaluate treatment.

There is wide agreement in the literature on the factors associated with an increased risk of first stroke. These include hypertension, left ventricular hypertrophy (LVH), ischemic heart disease (IHD), congestive heart failure (CHF), atrial fibrillation (AF), diabetes mellitus (DM), hyperlipidemia, transient ischemic attacks (TIA), and cigarette smoking.[2] Identification and treatment of these factors (particularly hypertension) has played a major role in the currently observed decline in stroke mortality.[1,3-13] Causal factors (particularly those which are treatable, such as hypertension and smoking),[4] should be distinguished from biological indicators of enhanced susceptibility such as age, sex, and diabetic control.

Available evidence suggests that treatment of hypertension is the only significant contributor to the decline of stroke,[3,4] although it is our opinion that elimination of rheumatic heart disease is also an important factor. Improvements in the detection and control of hypertension may have contributed to the decline in the incidence of stroke in Rochester, Minnesota.[5] The difference between sexes in effective management of hypertension, noted earlier in women, could explain the difference between men and women in the trend of stroke decline. In addition to the control of hypertension, factors such as decreased severity of the disease and improved diagnostic and/or therapeutic modalities may also have contributed.[6-8]

The decline in stroke mortality is due to lower incidence as well as to a lower mortality rate.[7] Dyken[14] observed that survival after stroke has been improving in both the acute and long term. Previous studies identified numerous factors affecting survival after stroke, including stroke severity and conscious level at admission, age, history of previous strokes, presence of cardiac disease, diabetes, and hypertension.[9,15,16]

Although the decline in incidence and mortality of CVD has been reported in the United States, Japan, and Finland, it is not a universal phenomenon.[11] According to national statistics, CVD mortality in Israel[12] (and other countries) showed an increase from the 1960s to the end of the 1970s.[13] In Sweden, Terent[17] reported an increased incidence of stroke among women but could not explain it.

The Problem of Recurrence

Stroke is mostly the result of atherosclerosis and so is an acute event on a background of progressive disease. While TIAs are a warning sign of an impending stroke, little effort has been made to study the effect of stroke on recurrent strokes.

Recurrent stroke is a major cause of morbidity and mortality among stroke survivors. Most large series indicate stroke recurrence rates of 16% to 42% and mortality rates of 35% to 65% over 5 years.[16,18-30] The reported rates vary widely due to referral bias, difference in criteria for selection of patients, variation of follow-up periods, and the definition of stroke recurrence. When recurrence is defined as worsening of existing symptomatology, rates are higher than when evidence of a new event is required.

The probability of stroke recurring is highest during the first year,[16] and the recurrent stroke in most cases is identical in type to the initial stroke.[19,20,23,24] Reduced survival relates to several factors, particularly hypertensive heart disease and peripheral vascular disease.

Hypercoagulability following acute stroke may account partly for the immediate increased risk of stroke recurrence.[31] Also, according to the National Institute of Neurology and Communicative Disorders and Stroke (NINCDS) Stroke Data Bank figures, early recurrence was associated with a history of hypertension, diabetes, elevated blood sugar on admission, and severity of weakness.[32] Davis et al.[28] analyzed the effects of various medical conditions on the risk of an initial ischemic stroke in 1804 residents of Rochester, Minnesota, followed for 13 years. The risk factors identified in this study for initial stroke differ from those for recurrent strokes in the Lehigh Valley study.[29] The data from Rochester, Minnesota,[19] failed to show that the level of blood pressure before the first stroke or that the effective management of hypertension had any effect on stroke recurrence rates during a follow-up of 30 years. There were no significant differences in the recurrence rates at 1, 5, and 10 years of observation between men and women. On the other hand, in the Framingham study,[16] stroke recurrence was more frequent in men and was strongly influenced by cardiac comorbidity (IHD and CHF) prior to the initial stroke, as well as by the presence of hypertension.

In the Lehigh Valley study[25] a logistic regression model was employed to study the relative contribution of 7 risk factors to the likelihood of recurrent stroke. TIAs, myocardial infarction, and heart disease were more important risk factors than hypertension, diabetes, age, or sex. Cardiac comorbidity was an important risk factor for recurrent stroke in other studies.[19,23,26] Hypertension was not an important risk factor for stroke recurrence, but both Beevers et al.[27] and Sacco et al.[16] reported that control of blood pressure reduced the risk of stroke recurrence. These results have rather negative implications for management since the risk factors for recurrent stroke are associated rather than causal factors.

Hypertension, a known risk factor for first-ever strokes, is not apparently an important factor for recurrent strokes. However, stroke occurrence does not depend so much on the immediate blood pressure as on its duration; therefore, the effect of hypertensive control will be seen only years after achieving stabilization of desired blood pressure levels. By the time the first stroke occurs, widespread vascular damage is already present; thus even if proper control is now implemented, its effects may not be observed for years.

Medical Prevention of Recurrent Stroke

Modification of Risk Factors

The first step in preventing stroke recurrence must be the treatment of recognized risk factors, with special emphasis on their interaction. These are multiplicative, rather than cumulative, risks. For example, the risk of stroke in young women is more likely if they are smokers, hypertensive, *and* take the birth-control pill.

Leonberg and Elliott,[18] in a prospective study of 88 survivors of a first ischemic stroke, determined the effect on long-term prognosis of stroke from an energetic and sustained program of control of eight risk factors. After 5 years there was a reduced (16%) stroke recurrence rate. Transient ischemic attacks and myocardial infarction (MI) occurred more frequently in patients who had recurrent stroke.

Antiplatelet Agents

Randomized clinical trials (RCTs) of antiplatelet agents in patients with TIAs or minor strokes have been conducted since 1969.[33-35] Because of the relatively small sample size of many of the trials, meta-analysis of published RCTs of all antiplatelet agents was performed. Retrospective pooling of data from multiple small studies is less subject to random error and avoids the systematic bias produced when many trials are conducted but few are published.

Sze et al.[36] performed a meta-analysis of RCTs comparing aspirin and/or sulfinpyrazone or dipyridamole with placebo. Aspirin achieved a nonsignificant reduction in stroke of 15% compared to placebo. The Antiplatelet Trialists Collaboration Study[37] compared 25 completed RCTs of antiplatelet treatment for patients with TIA, occlusive stroke, unstable angina, or MI. Overall, the antiplatelet treatment reduced vascular mortality by 15% (SD 4%) and stroke or MI by 30% (SD 4%).

Debate continues as to whether the correct dose of aspirin should be high (1000 to 1300 mg daily), intermediate (300 mg daily), or low (80 mg daily). Most studies used between 1000 and 1300 mg of aspirin daily, and only one study, the UK-TIA aspirin trial,[35] compared the effect of 300 mg and 1200 mg daily. There was no difference in therapeutic effect, except that the lower dose was significantly less gastrotoxic.

In the current Dutch trial[38] of patients with TIA or nondisabling stroke, 30 mg versus 300 mg of aspirin and 50 mg of atenolol versus placebo are being compared. The study will take 3 years and may help decide the issue of low or intermediate dosage.

In the largest aspirin study yet published, the European Stroke Prevention Study (ESPS),[39] 2500 patients with TIAs or recent minor stroke were randomized to placebo or 325 mg aspirin plus 75 mg dipyridamole/day. There was a 33.5% reduction in death or stroke in the drug group by intention-to-treat analysis. The end-point reduction was equal in men and women.

This beneficial effect was greater than that found in any other secondary prevention studies, apart from Accidents Ischémiques Cérebraux Liés à l'Athérosclérose (AICLA),[34] since most previous studies showed only a 20% risk reduction of stroke.

This may simply reflect the increased statistical power of the large number of patients in the ESPS study.[39]

Ticlopidine, a new antiplatelet drug, has been described in detail elsewhere in this book. Unlike aspirin, it does not inhibit cyclooxygenase, and unlike dipyridamole, it does not inhibit phosphodiesterase. It blocks the platelet-release reaction, inhibits platelet aggregation induced by ADP, and platelet adhesion. In the Canadian-American Ticlopidine Study (CATS),[40] efficacy analysis demonstrated a 30% reduction (95% confidence interval, 7.5% to 48.3% reduction) in the relative risk of the "composite end point" of stroke/MI/vascular death. The risk reduction for fatal and nonfatal recurrent stroke was similar at 33.5%. With the use of an "intention-to-treat," analysis, the relative risk reduction for fatal and nonfatal stroke fell to 20.5%. Thus, ticlopidine definitely reduces the risk of serious vascular events, but by how much is not certain; it could be < 10% or as much as 50%.

Anticoagulation

Data from randomized studies in the 1960s indicated that anticoagulants do not prevent stroke and, in patients treated for several months, add to the morbidity and mortality. However, these early studies were methodologically weak, with lack of randomization, small number of patients, and inadequate follow-up. More important, they did not attempt to differentiate artery-to-artery embolism from cardiogenic embolism.

Cardiogenic embolism is a separate issue and accounts for about one in six ischemic strokes. Atrial fibrillation is found in 0.4% of the adult population and nonrheumatic AF is probably the most common source for brain embolism; 6% to 24% of all ischemic strokes are associated with AF.[41,42] Atrial fibrillation occurring in the absence of valvular disease affects more than one million Americans, and it is associated with >75 000 cases of stroke a year—almost half of all episodes of cardiogenic embolism.[43] Rheumatic mitral stenosis, prosthetic valves, mitral valve prolapse, calcified annulus, and calcific aortic stenosis are also sources of cardioembolic stroke.

The prognosis of AF is of current interest due to the increased awareness of the risk of thromboembolic complications from this condition.[44-48]

TABLE 21.1. Embolic complications in the Copenhagen AFASAK study.

Complication	Warfarin group (N = 335)		Aspirin group (N = 336)		Placebo group (N = 336)	
	ON	OFF	ON	OFF	ON	OFF
Transient ischemic attack	0	1	2	0	3	0
Minor stroke	0	1	1	0	2	1
Nondisabling stroke	0	2	7	0	3	1
Disabling stroke	4	1	4	1	7	1
Fatal stroke	1	0	3	0	4	0
Visceral	0	1	2	0	2	1
Extremities	0	0	1	0	0	0
Total	11		21		25	

Reprinted with permission from Letter to the Editor, New England Journal of Medicine 990:323.

Recurrent stroke is common (10% to 20% yearly) in patients with nonvalvular AF. Early recurrence of cerebral infarction within the first 2 weeks is best documented for cardiogenic embolism and originally was believed to be as high as 1% per day.[46-48] Consensus regarding the indications for acute anticoagulation after cardioembolic stroke however, has proved to be elusive. Lodder et al.[49] evaluated the long-term anticoagulation treatment in two series of patients with AF and ischemic stroke and found no significant difference in either survival or the rate of recurrent stroke between the two groups.

However, there are two current studies of anticoagulants and antiplatelet agents in nonrheumatic chronic atrial fibrillation that may significantly change medical practice. These are AFASAK,[50] a placebo-controlled, randomized trial of warfarin and aspirin to prevent thromboembolic complications, and SPAF[51] "Stroke prevention in atrial fibrillation," a similar study incorporating aspirin and warfarin.

In the Copenhagen AFASAK trial,[50] warfarin, aspirin and placebo were compared for their effects on stroke, TIA, and systemic embolism, over 2 years, in 1007 patients. All vascular end points were significantly reduced in the warfarin group compared to aspirin or placebo (Table 21.1).

The SPAF study, a multicenter trial in the United States, is still in progress. By November 1989, 1244 patients were enrolled. Results so far indicate that antithrombotic therapy with warfarin or aspirin is effective in the short term in reducing the risk of stroke or systemic embolism in patients with atrial fibrillation (Figures 21.1 and 21.2).

The Boston anticoagulant study (BAATAF), unlike the previous two, was an unblinded but randomized trial of warfarin in 420 patients. It showed an 86% reduction in stroke risk.[52]

These studies will almost certainly change our views of prevention of stroke, both initial and recurrent, and will encourage long-term anticoagulation in all patients with atrial fibrillation, as long as no contraindications exist.

Surgical Prevention

EC/IC Bypass

A large, multicenter clinical trial comparing extracranial-intracranial bypass with medical therapy for the prevention of stroke in symptomatic patients with carotid occlusion or surgically inaccessible stenosis was negative.[53] It has been criticized because large numbers of eligible patients underwent surgery outside the study protocol at participating centers and because patients with cerebral embolism (who are not likely to benefit from the operation), were not excluded. However, patients with occlusion or high-grade carotid stenosis, who would be expected to benefit from the increased cerebral perfusion provided by this procedure, did not benefit either. A significant number of the patients in either study group was also treated with aspirin; so the conclusion is that EC-IC bypass is not superior to medical therapy alone. A separate analysis of those who were not on aspirin (possibly because of intolerance) could have settled the issue.

As it stands, the operation is generally not performed for secondary prevention of cerebral ischemia. In view of the enormous expense and administrative difficulties in monitoring such a large, surgical trial, it is unlikely to be repeated.

Carotid Endarterectomy

Since the first report of this operation in 1954,[54] it has become increasingly popular, and about 107 000 carotid endarterectomies were performed

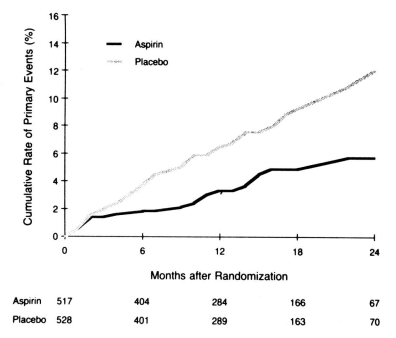

| Aspirin | 517 | 404 | 284 | 166 | 67 |
| Placebo | 528 | 401 | 289 | 163 | 70 |

FIGURE 21.1. Rates of stroke or systemic embolism in patients receiving aspirin or placebo (SPAF) study. (Reprinted with permission from *N Engl J Med*. 1990;322:863–868.)

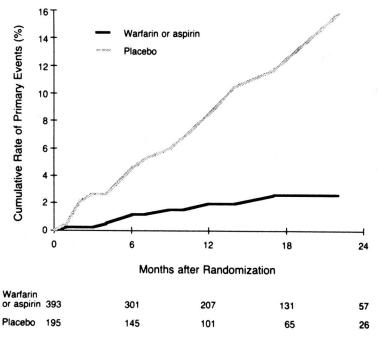

| Warfarin or aspirin | 393 | 301 | 207 | 131 | 57 |
| Placebo | 195 | 145 | 101 | 65 | 26 |

FIGURE 21.2. Rates of stroke or systemic embolism in patients receiving active therapy or placebo (SPAF) study. (Reprinted with permission from *N Engl J Med*. 1990;322:863–868.)

in the United States in 1985.[55] The most common indications for this operation are TIAs or minor stroke.

Neither of the two prospective randomized studies of carotid endarterectomy[56,57] demonstrated a beneficial effect on outcome compared to medical therapy; but neither study met modern standards of clinical trial methodology. The value of the operation has been vigorously discussed, resulting in numerous reviews and position statements.[58-63] The Committee on Health Care Issues of the American Neurological Association[61] concluded that "the procedure may be of value if the surgical complication rate is very low but that the net effect in the United States as a whole may be unfavorable." Several attempts are in progress to assess the efficacy of carotid endarterectomy in symptomatic patients. These are:

1. National Institutes of Health Multicenter Trial: North American Symptomatic Carotid Endarterectomy Trial. Randomization of patients began in February 1988; 3000 patients to be randomized and followed until February 1993.
2. Veterans Administration Cooperative Study: The Role of Carotid Endarterectomy in Preventing Stroke from Symptomatic Carotid Stenosis. Randomization of patients began in July 1988; 600 patients will be entered by June 1992 and followed until June 1995.
3. European Multicenter Carotid Endarterectomy Trial. Randomization began in 1984 (C.P. Warlow, senior principal investigator).

A minimum perioperative morbidity and mortality figure suggested by the Stroke Council of the American Heart Association was a 30-day mortality rate from all causes not >2% and morbidity and mortality for carotid endarterectomy <7%.

At present, there is widespread concern in North America that the numbers of patients referred for these trials is rapidly diminishing. This is a result of published critical reviews of carotid surgery[58,64] as well as adverse comments in the lay press.[65,66] It is earnestly hoped that this does not result in "throwing out the baby with the bath water."[67]

Conclusion

1. The greatest risk of stroke is stroke itself, the recurrent rate being about 10% annually. About

one in four hospital admissions for stroke are, in fact, recurrent stroke.[68] The risk of recurrent stroke after the initial event is fivefold that of a matched population.
2. Identification of risk factors for recurrent stroke is critical but, largely undetermined. They appear to be different from those for the original stroke.
3. The decline of stroke due to control of risk factors may already be optimal, since the annual mortality is no longer declining.[69]
4. Medical trials for new antiplatelet drugs and standard anticoagulants have shown significant reduction of stroke and other vascular outcomes. Surgical prevention studies, however, have so far proved to be disappointing.
5. Further clinical research on this important issue is needed, and prevention of recurrent stroke should be a major and immediate concern for health care planners.

References

1. Center of Disease Control. Premature mortality due to cerebrovascular disease—United States, 1983. *JAMA*. 1987;258:182.
2. Dyken ML, Wolf PA, Barnett HJM, et al. Risk factors in stroke, a statement for physicians by the subcommittee on risk factors and stroke of the stroke council. *Stroke*. 1984;15:1105–1111.
3. Whisnant JP. The role of the neurologist in the decline of stroke. *Ann Neurol*. 1983;14:1–7.
4. Whisnant JP. The decline of stroke. *Stroke*. 1984; 15:160–168.
5. Garraway WM, Whisnant JP. The changing pattern of hypertension and the declining incidence of stroke. *JAMA*. 1987;258:214–217.
6. Hachinski V. Decreased incidence and mortality of stroke. *Stroke*. 1984;15:376–378.
7. Howard G, Toole JF, Becker C, et al. Changes in survival following stroke in five North Carolina counties observed during different periods. *Stroke*. 1989;20:345–350.
8. Ahmed OI, Orchard TJ, Sharma R, et al. Declining mortality from stroke in Allegheny County, Pennsylvania. Trends in case fatality and severity of disease, 1971–1980. *Stroke*. 1988;19:181–184.
9. Baum HM, Robins M. National Survey of Stroke. Survival and prevalence. *Stroke*. 1981;12(suppl 1):59–68.
10. Cooper SE. Stroke mortality declines; still major health problem. *JAMA*. 1984;252:594.

11. Bonita R, Stewart A, Beaglehole R. International trends in stroke mortality: 1970–1985. *Stroke*. 1990; 21:989–992.

12. Epstein L, Zaaroor M. Mortality from ischemic heart disease and cerebrovascular disease in Israel 1969–1978. *Stroke*. 1982;13:570–573.

13. Pisa Z, Uemurat K. Trends in mortality from ischemic heart disease and other cardiovascular disease in 27 countries. *World Health State Q*. 1982;35:11–49.

14. Dyken ML. 'Natural' history of ischemic stroke. In: *Cerebral Vascular Disease*, eds MJG Harrison and ML Dyken, Butterworths, London, 1983, pp 139–170.

15. Chambers BR, Norris JW, Shurvell BL, et al. Prognosis of acute stroke. *Neurology*. 1987;37:221–225.

16. Sacco RL, Wolf PA, Kannel WB, et al. Survival and recurrence following stroke, the Framingham study. *Stroke*. 1982;13:290–295.

17. Terent A. Increasing incidence of stroke among Swedish women. *Stroke*. 1988;19:598–603.

18. Leonberg SC, Elliott FA. Prevention of recurrent stroke. *Stroke*. 1981;12:731–735.

19. Meissner I, Whisnant JP, Garraway WM. Hypertension management and stroke recurrence in community (Rochester, Minnesota, 1950–1979). *Stroke*. 1988;19:459–463.

20. Schmidt EV, Smirnov VE, Ryabova VS. Results of the seven-years prospective study of stroke patients. *Stroke*. 1988;19:942–949.

21. Matsumoto N, Whisnant JP, Kurland LT, et al. Natural history of stroke in Rochester, Minnesota, 1955 through 1969: an extension of a previous study, 1945 through 1954. *Stroke*. 1973;4:20–29.

22. Baker RN, Schwartz WS, Ramseyer JC. Prognosis among survivors of ischemic stroke. *Neurology*. 1968;18:933–941.

23. Viitanen M, Eriksson S, Asplund K. Risk of recurrent stroke, myocardial infarction and epilepsy during long-term follow-up after stroke. *Eur Neurol*. 1988;28:227–731.

24. Homer D, Whisnant JP, Schoenberg BS. Trends in the incidence rates of stroke in Rochester, Minnesota, since 1935. *Ann Neurol*. 1987;22:245–251.

25. Sobel E, Alter M, Davanipour Z, et al. Stroke in the Lehigh valley: combined risk factors for recurrent ischemic stroke. *Neurology*. 1989;39:669–672.

26. Hypertension-Stroke Cooperative Study Group. Effect of antihypertensive treatment on stroke recurrence. *JAMA*. 1974;229:409–418.

27. Beevers DG, Hamilton M, Fairmant MJ, et al. Antihypertensive treatment and the course of established cerebral vascular disease. *Lancet*. 1973;1:1407–1409.

28. Davis PH, Dambtosia JM, Schoenberg BS, et al. Risk factors for ischemic stroke: A prospective study in Rochester, Minnesota. *Ann Neurol*. 1987;22:319–327.

29. Alter M, Sobel E, McCoy RL, et al. Stroke in the Lehigh valley: Risk factors for recurrent stroke. *Neurology*. 1987;37:503–507.

30. Solzi P, Ring H, Najenson T, Luz Y. Hemiplegic after a first stroke: Late survival and risk factors. *Stroke*. 1983;14:703–709.

31. Landi G, Barbarotto R, Morabito A, et al. Prognostic significance of fibrinopeptide A in survivors of cerebral infarction. *Stroke*. 1990;21:424–427.

32. Sacco RL, Foulkes MA, Mohr JP, et al. Determinants of early recurrence of cerebral infarction, the Stroke Data Bank. *Stroke*. 1989;20:983–989.

33. The Canadian Cooperative Study Group. A randomized trial of aspirin and sulfinpyrazone in threatened stroke. *N Engl J Med*. 1978;299:53–59.

34. Bousser MG, Eschwege E, Hagenau M, et al. "AICLA" controlled trial of aspirin and dipyridamole in the secondary prevention of atherothrombotic cerebral ischaemia. *Stroke*. 1983;14:5–14.

35. UK-TIA Study Group. United Kingdom transient ischaemic attack (UK-TIA) aspirin trial: interim results. *Br Med J*. 1988;296:316–320.

36. Sze PC, Reitman D, Pincus MM, et al. Antiplatelet agents in the secondary prevention of stroke: meta-analysis of randomized controlled trials. *Stroke*. 1988;19:436–442.

37. Antiplatelet Trialists Collaboration. Secondary prevention of vascular disease by prolonged antiplatelet treatment. *Br Med J*. 1988;296:320–331.

38. The Dutch TIA Study Group. The Dutch TIA trial: protective effects of low-dose aspirin and atenolol in patients with transient ischemic attacks or nondisabling stroke. *Stroke*. 1988;19:512–517.

39. ESPS Group. European Stroke Prevention Study. *Stroke*. 1990;21:1122–1130.

40. Gent M, Blakely JA, Easton JD, et al. The Canadian American Ticlopidine Study (CATS) in thromboembolic stroke. *Lancet*. 1989;1:1215–1220.

41. Ostrander LD, Jr., Brandt RL, Kjelsberg MO, et al. Electrocardiographic findings among the adult population of a total natural community, Tecumseh, Michigan. *Circulation*. 1965;31:888–898.

42. Cardiogenic Brain Embolism. The second report of the cerebral embolism task force. *Arch Neurol*. 1989;46:727–743.

43. Halperin JL, Hart RG. Atrial fibrillation and stroke: new ideas, persisting dilemmas. *Stroke*. 1988;19: 937–941.

44. Wolf PA, Kannel WB, McGee DL, et al. Duration of atrial fibrillation and imminence of stroke: the Framingham study. *Stroke*. 1983;14:664–667.

45. Wolf PA, Abbott RD, Kannel WB. Atrial fibrillation: A major contribution to stroke in the elderly. *Arch Intern Med*. 1987;147:1561–1564.

46. Cerebral Embolism Task Force. Cardiogenic brain embolism. *Arch Neurol*. 1986;43:71–84.

47. Kelley RE, Berger JR, Alter M, et al. Cerebral ischemia and atrial fibrillation: prospective study. *Neurology*. 1984;34:1285–1291.

48. Kannel WB, Abbott RD, Savage DD, et al. Epidemiologic features of chronic atrial fibrillation, the Framingham study. *N Engl J Med*. 1982;306:1018–1022.

49. Lodder J, Dennis MS, Van Raak L, et al. Cooperative study on the value of long term anticoagulation in patients with stroke and non-rheumatic atrial fibrillation. *Br Med J*. 1988;296:1435–1438.

50. Petersen P, Boysen G, Godtfredsen J, et al. Placebo-controlled, randomized trial of warfarin and aspirin for prevention of thromboembolic complications in chronic atrial fibrillation. The Copenhagen AFA-SAK Study. *Lancet*. 1989;175–179.

51. Stroke Prevention in Atrial Fibrillation Study Group Investigators. Preliminary report of the stroke prevention in atrial fibrillation study. *N Engl J Med*. 1990;322:863–868.

52. The Boston Area Anticoagulation Trial for Atrial Fibrillation. The effects of low dose warfarin on the risk of stroke in patients with non-rheumatic atrial fibrillation. *N Engl J Med*. 1990;323:1505–1511.

53. The EC/IC Bypass Study Group. Failure of extracranial-intracranial arterial bypass to reduce the risk of ischemic stroke: Results of an international randomized trial. *N Engl J Med*. 1985;313:1191–1200.

54. Eastcott HHG, Pickering GW, Rob CG. Reconstruction of internal carotid artery in a patient with intermittent attacks of hemiplegia. *Lancet*. 1954;2:994–996.

55. Pokras R, Dyken ML. Dramatic changes in the performance of endarterectomy for diseases of the extracranial arteries of the head. *Stroke*. 1988;19:1289–1290.

56. Fields WS, Maslenikov V, Meyer JS, et al. Joint study of extracranial arterial occlusion. *JAMA*. 1970;211:1993–2003.

57. Shaw DA, Venables GS, Cartlidge NEF, et al. Carotid endarterectomy in patients with transient cerebral ischemia. *J Neurol Sci*. 1984;64:45–53.

58. Winslow CM, Solomon DH, Chassin MR, et al. The appropriateness of carotid endarterectomy. *N Engl J Med*. 1988;318:721–727.

59. Beebe HG, Clagett GP, DeWeese JA, et al. Assessing risk associated with carotid endarterectomy. A statement for health professionals by an Ad Hoc Committee on Carotid Surgery Standards of the Stroke Council, American Heart Association. *Stroke*. 1989;20:314–315.

60. American Academy of Neurology, Therapeutics and Technology Assessment Subcommittee. Interim assessment: carotid endarterectomy. *Neurology*. 1990;40:682–683.

61. Committee on Health Care Issues, American Neurological Association. Does carotid endarterectomy decrease stroke and death in patients with transient ischemic attacks? *Ann Neurol*. 1987;22:72–76.

62. Caplan LR. Carotid-artery disease. *N Engl J Med*. 1986;315:886–887.

63. Callow AD, Caplan LR, Correll JW, et al. Carotid endarterectomy: what is its current status? *Am J Med*. 1988;85:835–838.

64. Barnett HJM, Plum F, Walton JN. Carotid endarterectomy—an expression of concern. *Stroke*. 1984;15:941–943.

65. Califano JA Jr. Billions blown on health. *New York Times;*12 April 1989.

66. Lundtyke MA. Physician—inform thyself. *New York Times*;16 April 1989.

67. Thompson JE. Don't throw out the baby with the bath water. A perspective on carotid endarterectomy. *J Vasc Surg*. 1986;4:543–545.

68. Robins M, Baum HM. Incidence. National Survey of Stroke. *Stroke*. 1981;12 (suppl 1):1-45-55.

69. Cooper R, Hsieh SC. Slowdown in the decline of stroke mortality in the United States, 1978–1986. Stroke 1990;21:1274–1279.

Index

Acute myocardial infarction
 anticoagulants, 153
 cardioembolic stroke, 153
 ventricular aneurysm following, 154
Age factors, risk for stroke, 2, 88–89
AIDS, risk of stroke in young, 6
Alcohol use
 risk for stroke, 86
 risk of stroke in young, 6
Alpha blockers, 116
American Heart Association
 diet, 43
 Stroke Council, 83
Aneurysms
 proximal vessel occlusion, 254
 surgery
  complications of, 252
  regrowth following clipping, 254
  timing for surgery, 250–253
 unruptured
  prevention of bleeding, 255–256
  screening for, 256–257
 See also Subarachnoid hemorrhage
Angiographically occult lesions, 244
Angiography
 cardioembolic stroke and, 151
 carotid, 178–179
 limitations in use of, 55–56
 studies of progression/regression, 56
Angiotensin-converting-enzyme inhibitors, 116

Animal studies and atherogenesis, 23
 lipid theory of atherogenesis, 40
 nonprimate animal models, 51–52
 primate models, 52
Anticardiolipin antibodies
 risk for stroke, 91
 risk of stroke in young, 4–5
Anticoagulants, 2
 acute myocardial infarction, 153
 and bleeding risks, 155
 clinical studies
  cardioembolic stroke, 142–143, 145, 155–156
  cerebral venous thrombosis, 144, 145
  cervicocerebral arterial dissections, 143, 145
  completed stroke, 141–142
  management recommendations, 144–145
  progressing stroke, 141
  transient ischemic attacks, 140–141
 heparin, 139–140
 mechanisms of drug activity, 139
 nonvalvular atrial fibrillation, 153
 and prevention of stroke, 7
 prosthetic cardiac valves, 154
 recurrent stroke prevention, 263–264
 valvular heart disease, 154
 ventricular aneurysm, 154
 warfarin, 140
Antifibrinogenic treatment, 247
 subarachnoid hemorrhage, 253–254

Antihypertensive drugs
 effects of, 116–117
 effects on lipoproteins, 116
 hypertensive arteriolar strokes, 115
 hypertensive encephalopathy, 114
Antiplatelet agents
 mitral valve prolapse, 154
 recurrent stroke prevention, 263
 types of, 7–8
Apoproteins, 38
 apoprotein AI, 42
 apoprotein B100 , 41, 42
 plasma determination of, 41–42
Arrhythmia, postoperative and stroke, 223
Arterial dissection, warfarin, 145
Arterial enlargement, plaque restructuring and, 54–55
Arterial ischemia, cerebral vascular malformations, 237–240
Arterial neck bruits, 106–107
Arterial rupture, cerebral vascular malformations, 235–237
Arterial stenosis, cerebral vascular malformations, 237–239
Arteries
 changes in walls and atherogenesis, 66
 plaque and size
  distal segments, 54
  proximal segments, 54
Arteriography, and carotid endarterectomy, 172
Artery-to-artery embolization, 23

Aspirin and stroke prevention
  aspirin-ticlopidine therapy,
    132–135, 136–137
  dosage, 121–122, 263
  effect on atherogenesis, 124–125
  effect on stroke severity,
    122–124
  gender effects, 7
  post-surgical carotid endarterec-
    tomy, 180
  prevention of subclinical
    ischemia, 124
  primary prevention, 124
Asymptomatic bruits, patient
  management, 6
Asymptomatic carotid arterial
  lesions. *See* Bruits
Asymptomatic carotid stenosis
  angiography, 178–179
  asymptomatic, use of term, 177
  carotid endarterectomy
    prognosis after surgery,
      185–187
    risks related to, 184–185
  current surgical developments,
    189
  issues related to, 178
  prophylactic endarterectomy,
    187–189
  recurrent carotid stenosis, 187
  risk of stroke, 180–181
  risk of stroke without warning,
    182
  significant lesions, carotid bruits,
    178
  surgery, rationale for, 180
  TIAs and, 182–184
Asymptomatic contralateral
  stenosis, 189
Atherogenesis
  lipid theory of, 40–42
  models of
    human studies, 52–53
    nonprimate animal models,
      51–52
    primate models, 52
  pathology in, 50
  stages of
    complicated advanced lesions,
      51
    developed lesions, 50
    fibrous lesions, 50
    lipoid lesions, 50
Atheromas, histopathology of,
  38–40

Atherosclerosis
  animal models in study of, 23
  cellular aspects
    hypertension, 30
    lipoproteins, 28–29
    smoking, 30
  induction of
    atheroma induced by electrical
      stimulation, 66–75
    atheroma induced by intra-
      luminal balloon, 76
    drug inhibition of plaque, 66
    methods of inducing plaque,
      65
    production of plaque, 65–66
  nature of, 9
  pathogenesis of, 23–28
    early theories of, 23–24
    endothelial cells, 25
    growth factors, 26–27
    hemodynamic factors, 27–28
    monocytes/macrophages,
      24–25
    platelets, 26
    smooth muscle cells, 25–26
  pathology of, 19–23
  therapeutic approaches to
    calcium channel blockers, 32
    fatty acids, n-3 fatty acids,
      30–32
    heparin, 32
Atherothrombotic brain infarction
  atheromas, histopathology of,
    38–40
  atherosclerosis management
    correction of abnormal
      lipoprotein patterns, 43
    future strategies for stroke risk
      reduction, 38, 44
    management of hyperlipid-
      emias, 43–44
  clinical disorders related to,
    42–43
  lipid theory of atherogenesis,
    40–42
  past therapeutic measures, 37
  reduced HDL in, 39–40
  reduction of risk factors
    approach, 37
  risk factors for, 38
Atrial fibrillation
  anticoagulation and nonvalvular
    type, 153
  cardioembolic stroke, 152–153
  lone atrial fibrillation, 152

  nonvalvular atrial fibrillation,
    152
  risk of stroke, 85
  and thyrotoxicosis, 152–153
Average number of trials to the
  estimate (ANTE), 164

Balloon angioplasty, 11
  indications for, 207
  mechanism of, 205
  results of use, 207, 209
  technique in, 205–207
Benefit/risk assessment, of clinical
  trial, 166–167
Beta-blockers, 116
Biochemical factors, regression of
  atherosclerosis, 53
Blacks, risk for stroke, 89
Bleeding risks, and anticoagulants,
  155
Brain damage, after coronary
  artery bypass surgery,
  224–225
Bruits
  carotid bruits, 178
  cause of, 103
  clinical significance of, 103
  intracranial bruits, 105–106
  neck bruits, 106–111
    arterial neck bruits, 106–107
    frequency in carotid stenosis
      patients, 107–108
    frequency of carotid stenosis
      in, 109–110
    gender differences, 111
    venous neck bruits, 106
  noninvasive procedures and, 92
  ocular bruits, 103–104
  pathogenesis of, 103
  risk of stroke, 91–92
  variation over time, 103

Calcium antagonists, effectiveness
  of, 56
Calcium channel blockers, atherosclerosis, 32
Canadian American Ticlopidine
  Study, 8, 135–136
Cardiac disease
  risk for stroke, 3, 85
  risk of stroke in young, 4
Cardioembolic stroke
  angiographic features of, 151

cardiac evaluation of, 151
causes of, 151–155
  acute myocardial infarction,
    153
  atrial fibrillation, 152–153
  infective endocarditis, 155
  mitral valve prolapse, 154
  paradoxical embolism,
    154–155
  prosthetic cardiac valves, 154
  valvular heart disease, 154
  ventricular aneurysm, 154
characteristics of, 150
computerized tomography,
  150–151
diagnostic ambiguity, 150
heparin, 145
incidence/prevalence of, 149
pathophysiology, 149
prevention of first embolus,
  142–143
prevention of recurrence, 142
treatment of acute stroke, 155
Carotid bruits, 178
Carotid endarterectomy
  and arteriography, 172
  aspirin, post-surgical manage-
    ment, 200–201
  concerns related to, 171–172
  follow-up medical management,
    200–201
  lesions, types of, 195
  prognosis for asymptomatic
    carotid stenosis, 180
  prophylactic surgery, rationale
    for, 180
  recurrent stroke prevention, 264,
    266
  responses to disarray of
    procedure, 173–174
  results from cohorts in
    randomized studies,
    197–199
  results of analysis of studies,
    199–200
  rise/decline in use, 7, 172–173
  risks of, 172, 184–185
  stroke prevention data
    assessment of outcome,
      196–197
    methods of study, 195–196
Carotid stenosis
  bruits and, 107–110
  silent nature of, 107
Cavernous hemangiomas, cerebral

vascular malformation,
    243–244
Cavernous malformations, 244
Cerebral aneurysm
  prophylactic aneurysm clipping,
    11
  screening for, 11
Cerebral hemorrhage
  cerebral vascular malformations,
    230–231
  events in, 114
  prevention of, 114
Cerebral vascular malformations
  classifications of, 229, 230
  cryptic vascular malformation,
    244
  epidemiology, 229–230
  stroke and
    arterial ischemia, 237–240
    arterial rupture, 235–237
    arterial stenosis, 237, 239
    cavernous hemangiomas,
      243–244
    cerebral hemorrhage, 230–231
    false venous malformation,
      242–244
    Moya-Moya pattern, 239–240
    nidus rupture, 231–232
    steal phenomenon, 237
    true venous cerebral
      malformations, 244
    venous angiomas, 242–243
    venous ischemia, 240, 242
    venous rupture, 234–235
  treatment of, 244–245
Cerebral venous thrombosis
  anticoagulant therapy, 144
  heparin, 145
Cervicocerebral arterial
    dissections,
    anticoagulant therapy, 143
Cholesterol, 38
  actions of cholesterol-lowering
    agents, 44
  borderline levels, 44
  dangerous level, 9
  reduction and CHD, 43
  separation techniques, 41
  subfractionation, 39–41
  See also HDL; LDL
CLEAT syndrome, 5
Climate, risk of stroke, 93
Clinical trials
  categorical evaluations, 165, 167
  conventional paradigm, 161–162

how sure continuum, 165
  statistical risk, 167
predictive paradigm, 162–167
  average number of trials to the
    estimate, 164
  example of, 162–163
  fulfillment of prediction, 164
  predictive potential, 163
  predictive value, 163, 164
risks in
  benefit/risk assessment,
    166–167
  data risk, 165
  disease risk, 165
  treatment risk, 165–166
Color coded duplex sonography, 55
Coma, after coronary artery
    bypass surgery, 223–224
Completed stroke, heparin, 142
Complicated advanced lesions,
    characteristics of, 51
Computerized tomography
  cardioembolic stroke and,
    150–151
  detection of minor hemorrhages,
    247
  subarachnoid hemorrhage,
    249–250
Conventional paradigm. See
    Clinical trials
Coronary artery bypass surgery
  complications of
    brain damage, 224–225
    coma, 223–224
    encephalopathy, 223
    stroke, 219–223
Coronary heart disease
  dietary intervention, 40
  holistic approaches to, 37
  risk factors, 38
Cryptic vascular malformation,
    244
Cystathionine synthase, 88
Cytokines
  effects of, 24–25
  macrophage production of, 24

Data risk, of clinical trial, 165
Densitometric measurements,
    69–70
Developed lesions, characteristics
    of, 50
Developmental venous anomalies,
    242–243

Diabetes mellitus
    accelerated atherosclerosis and,
        43
    risk for stroke, 3, 90
Diet
    to decrease LDL/raise HDL,
        43–44
    reduction of CHD and, 40
    regression of atherosclerosis, 53
    risk for stroke, 87
Dipyridamole, 7, 263
Disease risk, of clinical trial, 165
Doppler sonography, 57, 58
Drug use
    risk for stroke, 86–87
    risk of stroke in young, 6

EC-IC bypass, recurrent stroke
        prevention, 264
Electrical stimulation, atheroma
        induced by, 66–75
Electrocardiograms, cardioembolic
        stroke, 151
Encephalopathy
    after coronary artery bypass
        surgery, 223
    etiology of, 223
    incidence of, 223
Endothelial cells
    atherosclerosis and, 25
    endothelial permeability, in
        carotid arteriosclerosis,
        67–70
    injury in hypertension, 115
Endothelial-derived relaxing factor,
        32
Epidermal growth factors, 26, 77
Erythrocytosis, risk for stroke, 3–4
Extracranial/intracranial bypass
        surgery, 37

False venous malformation,
        cerebral vascular
        malformations, 242–244
Familial hypercholesterolemia,
        molecular/cellular biology
        of, 40, 42
Fatty acids
    cellular and biochemical
        inhibitory effects, 31–32
    n-3 fatty acids, hypertension,
        30–32
    Omega-3 fatty acids, 9–10

Fatty streaks
    in atherosclerosis, 19, 20
    characteristics of, 50
Fibrinogen, risk for stroke, 3,
        90–91
Fibroblast growth factor, 26, 27
Fibrous plaque, characteristics of,
        50
Flunarizine, 75, 77
Foam cells, 9, 38
    components of, 20
    death of, 53
    formation of, 24
    theories on role of, 39
Fractional catabolic rate, 39, 42
Framingham study, 83, 84, 85, 87,
        90, 91, 117
Free radical production, 25

Gender
    effects of aspirin, 7
    neck bruits and, 111
    risk for stroke, 3, 89
Gene polymorphism, in stroke-
        prone, 42
Geographic area, risk of stroke, 92
Growth-factors
    atherosclerosis and, 26–27
    promoters/inhibitors of, 27
    types of, 26

Hard plaque, 50
HDL
    atherothrombotic brain
        infarction and, 39–40
    characteristics of, 41
    HDL3, 41, 42
    interventions for increasing,
        43–44
    macrophages and, 25
    major apoproteins of, 42
    reduced, in coronary heart
        disease, 39
    as subfraction of cholesterol, 41
Health screening, 11
Helsinki Heart Study, 38, 43
Hematocrit, high level, risk of
        stroke, 4, 90
Hemocysteinuria, risk of stroke in
        young, 5
Hemodynamic factors
    atherosclerosis and, 27–28
    regression of atherosclerosis and,

53–54
Heparin, 139–140
    atherosclerosis, 32
    cardioembolic stroke, 145
    cerebral venous thrombosis, 145
    completed stroke, 142
    dosage, 140
    fibroblast growth factor and, 27
    new heparinoids, development
        of, 140
    pharmacologic effect, 139–140
    progressing stroke, 141
    route of administration, 140
    stroke prevention, 145
    transient ischemic attack, 141
    warfarin used with, 140
Heredity, risk for stroke, 3, 89
High density lipoprotein
        cholesterol. See HDL
Homocysteinemia, 10
    risk for stroke, 88
Honolulu Heart Program, 85, 88,
        90
Hydralazine, 116
Hypercoagulable state, 140
Hyperlipidemia
    preventive management of,
        43–45
    risk for stroke, 4, 87
    risk of stroke in young, 5
Hypertension
    antihypertensive drugs, 114,
        116–117
    atherosclerosis and, 30
    cerebral hemorrhage and, 114
    hypertensive encephalopathy,
        113–114
    lacunar infarction and, 115
    nature of strokes due to, 113
    pathogenesis of atherosclerosis,
        115–116
        laminar flow, 115
        shear stress, 116
        turbulence, 115–116
    risk for stroke, 3, 84
Hypertensive crisis, 113
Hyperuricemia, physical inactivity,
        88

IDL, conversion of VLDL to, 41
Ileal bypass, effectiveness of, 56
Infection, risk for stroke, 88
Infective endocarditis,
        cardioembolic

stroke, 155
Intermediate density lipoprotein.
    See IDL, conversion of
    VLDL to
Internal elastic lamina, 66, 169
Intracranial arterial vasospasm,
    transluminal angioplasty,
    212–215
Intracranial bruits, 105
Intraluminal balloon, atheroma
    induced by, 76

Japanese, risk for stroke, 89–90
J-shaped curve, 115

Kaliuretic diuretics, 116

Lacunar infarction, 115
Laminar flow, hypertension and,
    115
Laser angioplasty, 11
LDL
    atherosclerosis and, 28–30
    characteristics of, 41
    elevated levels, effects of, 38–39
    interventions for reduction of, 43
    macrophages and, 24, 25
    major apoproteins of, 42
    oxidized LDL, 29
LDL/HDL ratio, 39, 40
Leukoaraiosis, 115
Lifestyle, importance of changing,
    43
Lipid Clinics Coronary Prevention
    Trial, 116
Lipid infiltration hypothesis, 29
Lipid lowering drugs
    effectiveness of, 56
    inhibition of experimental
    plaques, 66
Lipid Research Clinic – Coronary
    Primary Prevention Trial,
    38, 43
Lipid theory of atherogenesis
    animal studies, 40
    apoprotein determination, 41–42
    cholesterol subfractionation,
    40–41
    dynamic metabolism of
    lipoproteins in, 42
    human studies, 40
Lipoproteins

antihypertensive drugs, effects
    of, 116
atherosclerosis and, 28
dynamic metabolism of, 42
high/low levels, 44
lipoprotein (a), 41
molecular/cellular biology of, 42
turnover, 39
Low density lipoprotein. *See* LDL
Lupus anticoagulant, risk for
    stroke, 91

Macrophages, 50
    HDL3 receptors and, 39
    plaque progression and, 24–25
    regression of atherosclerosis and,
    53
    See also Foam cells
Mean Arterial Pressure, 114
Methionine loading, 88
Methyldopa, 116
Middle cerebral artery, 150
Migraine
    complicated migraine, 92
    risk of stroke, 92
    risk of stroke in young, 5
Mitral stenosis, 4
Mitral valve prolapse
    antiplatelet agents, 154
    cardioembolic stroke, 154
    incidence of, 154
    risk of stroke, 4, 85
Monocytes, plaque progression
    and, 24
Moya-Moya, cerebral vascular
    malformations, 239–240
Multiple factors in combination,
    risk of stroke, 93–94
Multiple Risk Factor Intervention
    Trial, 1, 43, 84
Myocardial infarction, cerebral
    embolism following, 143

Neck bruits
    arterial neck bruits, 106–107
    frequency in carotid stenosis
    patients, 107–108
    frequency of carotid stenosis in,
    109–110
    gender differences, 111
    venous neck bruits, 106
Neurosyphilis, risk of stroke in
    young, 6

Neutropenia, side effect of
    ticlopidine, 133
Nidus rupture, cerebral vascular
    malformations, 231–234
Nifedipine, 114
Nonvalvular atrial fibrillation,
    occurrence of stroke and,
    142–143

Obesity, physical inactivity, 88
Ocular bruits, 103
Omega-3 fatty acids, reduction of
    atherosclerosis, 9–10
Oral contraceptives
    physical inactivity, 88
    risk for stroke, 87–88
    risk of stroke in young, 5

Paradoxical emboli, 4
    cardioembolic stroke, 154–155
Percutaneous transluminal
    angioplasty
    balloon dilatation
        indications for use, 207
        mechanism of, 205
        technique in, 205–207
    development of, 205, 209–210
    effectiveness of, 211
    results of, 207, 209
Personality type, risk of stroke, 93
Pharmacotherapy
    anticoagulants, 139–145
    antihypertensive drugs, 114,
    116–117
    antiplatelet agents, 154, 263
    aspirin, 121–125
    concentration-dependent
        antiproliferative response,
        75
    effect on proliferative response,
        77
    effects on cultures of smooth
        muscle cells, 78
    lipid-lowering drugs, 56, 66
    platelet antiaggregation
        medication, 86
    ticlopidine, 127–137
Physical inactivity, risk for stroke,
    4
Plaque
    in atherosclerosis, 20–23
    complicated advanced lesions,
        characteristics of, 51

developed lesions, characteristics of, 50
experimental plaque, induction of
  atheroma induced by electrical stimulation, 66–75
  atheroma induced by intra-luminal balloon, 76
  drug inhibition of, 66
  methods of inducing plaque, 65
  production of, 65–66
fibrous plaque, characteristics of, 50
hard plaque, 50
progression of in one year, 39
  restructuring, 54–55
  arterial enlargement in, 54–55
shrinkage
  biochemical factors, 53
  cellular factors, 53
  hemodynamic factors, 53–54
soft plaque, 50
Platelet activating factors induced aggregation, 137
Platelet aggregation, ticlopidine therapy, 127–137
Platelet antiaggregating medication, 86
Platelet derived growth factor, 25, 26, 39, 50
Platelets, atherosclerosis and, 26
Potassium, level and risk for stroke, 4
Predictive paradigm. See Clinical trials
Predictive potential, of clinical trial, 163
Predictive value, of clinical trial, 163, 164
Primary prevention, aspirin, 124
Probucol, 29
Progressing stroke, heparin, 141
Prosthetic cardiac valves
  anticoagulants, 154
  cardioembolic stroke, 154
Proximal vessel occlusion, aneurysms, 254
Pump time, stroke and coronary artery bypass surgery, 223

Racial factors, risk for stroke, 3, 89–90
Recurrent carotid stenosis, 187

Recurrent stroke
  cardioembolic, prevention of, 142
  management of, 8
  medical prevention
    anticoagulation, 263–264
    antiplatelet agents, 263
    modification of risk factors, 262–263
  prevention of, 90
  probability of, 262
  surgical prevention
    carotid endarterectomy, 264, 266
    EC-IC bypass, 264
Regression of atherosclerosis, 9–11
  angiographic studies, 55–56
  arguments in favor of, 49
  human studies, 52–53
    hemodynamic factors, 53–54
  mechanisms of
    biochemical factors, 53
    cellular factors, 53
  plaque restructuring, 54–55
    arterial dilatation and, 54–55
  problems in evaluation of, 49
  treatment approaches
    calcium antagonists, 56
    ileal bypass, 56
    lipid-lowering drugs, 56
    repeat plasma exchange, 56
  ultrasound studies, 57–58
Repeat plasma exchange, effectiveness of, 56
Response to injury theory, 23, 66
Restriction fragment length polymorphisms, 44
Reverse cholesterol transport, 39, 40, 41
Risk factors
  abnormal lipids, 87
  age, 2, 88–89
  aggregation/interaction of, 6
  alcohol use, 86
  asymptomatic carotid arterial lesions (bruits), 91–92
  cardiac disease, 3, 85
  climate/seasons, 93
  diabetes mellitus, 3, 90
  diet, 87
  drug use, 86–87
  erthrocytosis, 3–4
  fibrinogen, 3, 90–91
  gender, 3, 89
  geographic location, 92

hematocrit increases, 90
heredity, 89
homocysteinemia, 88
hyperlipidemia, 4
hypertension, 3, 84–85
hyperuricemia, 88
infection, 88
lupus anticoagulant, 91
migraine, 92
modification and stroke prevention, 262
multiple factors in combination, 93–94
obesity, 88
oral contraceptives, 87–88
personality type, 93
physical inactivity, 4, 88
potassium, 4
previous stroke, 90
race, 89–90
search for new risks, 6
sickle cell disease, 91
smoking, 3, 86
socioeconomic factors, 93
transient ischemic attacks, 85–86
Risk factors in young
  AIDS, 6
  alcohol use, 6
  anticardiolipin antibodies, 4–5
  cardiac disease, 4
  drug use, 6
  homocysteinuria, 5
  hyperlipidemia, 5
  migraine, 5
  neurosyphilis, 6
  oral contraceptives, 5
  sickle cell disease, 5
  smoking, 6
  trauma, 5

Scavenger receptor, 24, 29, 39
Season, risk of stroke, 93
Sentinel headache, 11
Separation techniques, ultra-centrifugation, 41
Shear stress, in atherogenesis, 116
Sickle cell disease
  risk for stroke, 91
  risk of stroke in young, 5
Single photon emission compu-terized tomography, 224
Smoking
  atherosclerosis and, 30
  risk for stroke, 3, 86

Smooth muscle cells, 20, 65
  atherosclerosis and, 25–26
  proliferation of, 38
Socioeconomic factors, risk of
    stroke, 93
Soft plaque, 50
Statistical risk, of clinical trial, 167
Steal phenomena, cerebral vascular
    malformations, 237
Stroke
  after coronary artery bypass
      surgery
    carotid artery disease and, 219,
        221–222
      etiology of, 219
      incidence of, 219
      postoperative arrhythmia, 223
      prior stroke and risk, 222–223
      pump time and risk, 223
  decline in incidence of, 11, 38,
      261
  prevalence of, 83
Stroke Data Bank, 149, 262
Stroke prevention
  aspirin, 121–125
  in asymptomatic stage, 2–6
  future strategies for, 38, 44
  historical view, 1–2
  modification of risk factors
    anticoagulants, 7
    antiplatelet agents, 7–8
    carotid endarterectomy, 7
  in recurrent stage, 8
  in warning stage, 6–8
  See also individual topics
Subarachnoid hemorrhage
  antifibrinolytic treatment, 247,
      253–254
  computerized tomography in
      detection of, 249–250
  diagnosis of, 247–250
  proximal vessel occlusion, 254
  regrowth of aneurysms, 254
  risk of rebleeding, 250
  symptoms of, 248
  timing for surgery, 250–253
  unruptured aneurysms
    prevention of bleeding, 255–256
    screening for, 256–257
  warning signs, 24
Subendothelial space, electrical
    stimulation and plaque
    development, 70–75

Sublingual, use of term, 114
Sulfinpyrazone, 7, 263
Systemic lupus erythematosus, 4–5

Thrombi, acute ischemic attacks
    and, 23
Ticlopidine, 8, 263
  background information, 127
  clinical studies, 131–136
    Canadian-American ticlopidine
        study, 135–136
    criticism of large scale studies,
        136
    large scale studies, 132–136
    small clinical trials, 131–132
    ticlopidine aspirin stroke
        study, 132–135
  combined therapy, 136–137
  major side effect, 133
  mode/site of action, 129–131
  pharmacology, 127–129
Transforming growth factor, 26,
    27
Transient ischemic attacks, 1, 2
  aspirin as stroke prevention
      after, 121–125
  carotid occlusion and, 182–184
  heparin, 141
  as indication of heart disease,
      150
  intraplaque hemorrhage, 21–23
  nature of, 85
  neck bruits and, 109–110
  risk for stroke, 85–86
  stroke prevention measures,
      85–86
  warfarin, 140–141
Transluminal angioplasty
  effectiveness of, 214–215
  indications for, 213
  intracranial arterial vasospasm,
      212–215
  technique in, 213
  See also Percutaneous trans-
      luminal angioplasty
Trauma, risk of stroke in young,
    5
Treatment
  calcium antagonists, 56
  ileal bypass, 56
  lipid lowering drugs, 56
  repeat plasma exchange, 56

Treatment risk, of clinical trial,
    165–166
Triglycerides
  functions of, 41
  and VLDL, 41
True venous cerebral mal-
    formations, 244
Turbulence, hypertension and,
    115–116
Type A personality, risk of stroke, 93

UK-TIA Aspirin Trial, 7
Ultracentrifugation, 41
Ultrasound
  echotomography, 57, 58
  use in human studies, 57–58
United Kingdom TIA aspirin trial,
    121, 123

Valvular heart disease, cardioem-
    bolic stroke, 154
Venous angiomas, cerebral vascular
    malformations, 242–243
Venous ischemia, cerebral vascular
    malformations, 240–242
Venous neck bruits, 106
Venous rupture, cerebral vascular
    malformations, 234–235
Ventricular aneurysm
  anticoagulants, 154
  cardioembolic stroke, 154
Verapamil, 75
Very low density lipoprotein. See
    VLDL
VLDL
  characteristics of, 41
  conversion to IDL, 41
  as subfraction of plasma
      cholesterol, 41
  triglycerides and, 41

Warfarin
  arterial dissection, 145
  dosage, 140
  heparin used with, 140
  pharmacological effect, 140
  stroke prevention, 144–145
  transient ischemic attack,
      140–141
Women, risk of stroke, 87, 93